TREATMENT OF BIPOLAR DISORDER IN CHILDREN AND ADOLESCENTS

Treatment of Bipolar Disorder in Children and Adolescents

Edited by
BARBARA GELLER
MELISSA P. DELBELLO

THE GUILFORD PRESS
New York   London

© 2008 The Guilford Press
A Division of Guilford Publications, Inc.
72 Spring Street, New York, NY 10012
www.guilford.com

Printed in the United States of America

This book is printed on acid-free paper.

Last digit is print number: 9   8   7   6   5   4   3   2   1

The authors have checked with sources believed to be reliable in their efforts to provide information
that is complete and generally in accord with the standards of practice that are accepted at the time
of publication. However, in view of the possibility of human error or changes in medical sciences,
neither the authors, nor the editors and publisher, nor any other party who has been involved in the
preparation or publication of this work warrants that the information contained herein is in every
respect accurate or complete, and they are not responsible for any errors or omissions or the results
obtained from the use of such information. Readers are encouraged to confirm the information contained in this book with other sources.

Library of Congress Cataloging-in-Publication Data

Treatment of bipolar disorder in children and adolescents / edited by Barbara Geller,
Melissa P. DelBello.
     p. ; cm.
  Includes bibliographical references and index.
  ISBN: 978-1-59385-678-6 (hardcover : alk. paper)
  1. Manic depressive illness in children—Treatment. 2. Manic depressive illness in
adolescence—Treatment. I. Geller, Barbara. II. DelBello, Melissa P.
  [DNLM: 1. Bipolar Disorder—drug therapy. 2. Adolescent. 3. Bipolar Disorder—
complications. 4. Bipolar Disorder—psychology. 5. Child. WM 207 T784 2008]
  RJ506.D4T77 2008
  618.92'895—dc22

                                                                2008004582

About the Editors

Barbara Geller, MD, is Professor of Psychiatry at Washington University in St. Louis. An internationally recognized researcher for studies of child and adolescent bipolar disorders, Dr. Geller is principal investigator on multiple National Institute of Mental Health-funded projects. Dr. Geller earned her medical degree from Albert Einstein College of Medicine in New York, and completed her residency and fellowship at New York University–Bellevue Medical Center. She has served on numerous federal advisory committees, editorial boards, and advocacy group scientific advisory boards. Among her awards are the American Academy of Child and Adolescent Psychiatry Nathan Cummings Special Research Award and the National Alliance on Mental Illness Exemplary Psychiatrist Award. Widely published, Dr. Geller has written more than 125 articles on diagnostic characteristics, phenomenology, longitudinal course, family psychopathology, molecular genetics, and pharmacological treatment of pediatric manic–depressive disorders.

Melissa P. DelBello, MD, MS, is Associate Professor of Psychiatry and Pediatrics, Vice-Chair for Clinical Research, and Codirector of the Division of Bipolar Disorders Research at the University of Cincinnati College of Medicine. She is also Director, Research Education and Training, Child and Adolescent Psychiatry Division, at Cincinnati Children's Hospital Medical Center. Dr. DelBello earned her medical degree with honors from the University of Rochester School of Medicine in Rochester, New York. She completed her residency in psychiatry at the Payne Whitney Clinic, New York Hospital–Cornell Medical Center, and at the University of Cincinnati College of Medicine, and a fellowship in Child and Adolescent Psychiatry at Cincinnati Children's Hospital Medical Center. Dr. DelBello is the author or coauthor of over 100 journal articles or chapters, and her primary research interests include neuropharmacology and neurodevelopment of pediatric bipolar disorder.

Contributors

Shannon Rae Barnett, MD, is Assistant Professor of Psychiatry in the Division of Child and Adolescent Psychiatry at the Johns Hopkins University School of Medicine in Baltimore, Maryland. Dr. Barnett has worked on several multisite studies focusing on mood disorders in children and adolescents, including the Treatment of Early Age Mania, the Treatment for Adolescents with Depression Study, and the Treatment of Adolescent Suicide Attempters. In addition, Dr. Barnett is the Director of Adolescent Psychiatry Services at Johns Hopkins Bayview Medical Center, where she leads a treatment team with an emphasis on treating adolescents with mood disorders.

Samantha Blankenship, MSW, is the study monitor for the Treatment of Early Age Mania study at Washington University and has contributed to the work on the Pediatric Depression Study. She specializes in education and clinical research with young children and families, including intensive training in therapeutic interventions with preschool- and school-age children. Through her work at the Early Emotional Development Program at Washington University, Ms. Blankenship has coauthored multiple articles on preschool mood disorders.

Hallie R. Bregman, BA, is a research coordinator at the Child and Adolescent Neuropsychiatric Research Program at Cambridge Health Alliance, Cambridge, Massachusetts. She earned her bachelor's degree with honors in psychology from the University of Delaware, where she was awarded the Psychology Research Award in 2006.

Kiki D. Chang, MD, is Associate Professor of Psychiatry and Behavioral Sciences at the Stanford University School of Medicine, Division of Child Psychiatry. He is Director of the Pediatric Bipolar Disorders Clinic and Research Program, where he specializes in pediatric psychopharmacology and treatment of depression and bipolar disorder in children and adolescents. His research includes brain imaging, genetics, and medication and psychotherapy trials, with a special focus on early identification and prevention of bipolar disorder. Dr. Chang is the author of over 50 papers and book chapters regarding bipolar disorder.

Christoph U. Correll, MD, is Assistant Professor of Psychiatry and Behavioral Sciences, Albert Einstein College of Medicine, Bronx, New York. He has been working as a research psychiatrist at the Zucker Hillside Hospital, where he is the Medical Director of the Recognition and Prevention Program, a National Institute of Mental Health-funded research program for the early identification and treatment of youth at risk for psychosis. His research focuses on early-phase psychotic and bipolar disorders and the risk–benefit evaluation of psychotropic medications, particularly antipsychotics and mood stabilizers. He has received more than 20 research awards and has authored numerous articles in the area of the psychotic and bipolar prodrome, as well as adverse effects of antipsychotics in youth and adults.

Kristen H. Davidson, PhD, is in private practice in Rochester, New York, and is a clinical senior instructor in the Departments of Psychiatry and Pediatrics at the University of Rochester Medical Center. She has authored several articles and book chapters on the assessment and treatment of childhood mood disorders.

Melissa P. DelBello, MD, MS (*see* "About the Editors").

Robert L. Findling, MD, is the Director of the Division of Child and Adolescent Psychiatry at University Hospitals Case Medical Center and Professor of Psychiatry and Pediatrics at Case Western Reserve University. He is both a child and adolescent psychiatrist as well as a pediatrician. Dr Findling's research endeavors have focused on pediatric psychopharmacology and psychotic disorders in children. He has been honored with numerous awards and has received international recognition as a clinical investigator. Dr. Findling is the principal investigator of a National Institute of Child Health and Human Development contract examining lithium in the treatment of pediatric mania and also the principal investigator of a National Institue of Mental Health study assessing the longitudinal course of children with symptoms of mania.

Jean A. Frazier, MD, is the Director of Child Psychopharmacology and the Child and Adolescent Neuropsychiatric Research Program at Cambridge Health Alliance, where she is also Codirector of the Center for Child and Adolescent Development. Dr. Frazier is Associate Professor of Psychiatry at Harvard Medical School and is internationally known for her work with children with serious mental illness and those with developmental disabilities. She has published over 70 articles and book chapters and has won numerous awards, including the Annual Exemplary Psychiatrist Award from the National Alliance on Mental Illness and the Outstanding Psychiatrist Award for Research from the Massachusetts Psychiatric Society.

Mary A. Fristad, PhD, is Professor of Psychiatry and Psychology at The Ohio State University (OSU) and the Director of Research and Psychological Services in the OSU Division of Child and Adolescent Psychiatry. Dr. Fristad has published over 125 articles and book chapters addressing the assessment and treatment of childhood-onset depression, suicidality, and bipolar disorder. She edited the *Handbook of Serious Emotional Disturbance in Children and Adolescents* and has written a book for families entitled *Raising a Moody Child: How to Cope with Depression and Bipolar Disorder.* Dr. Fristad serves on the board of directors for five web-based education and support groups for children and families with mood disorders. She has been the principal or co-principal investigator on over two dozen federal, state, and local grants, all focusing on the assessment and/or treatment of childhood-onset mood disorders.

Barbara Geller, MD (*see* "About the Editors").

Martin Gignac, MD, FRCP, has been working as a psychiatrist and clinical research coordinator at the adolescents' unit of the Institut Philippe-Pinel de Montréal, where he is also head of the outpatient clinic for severe disruptive disorders in adolescence. In addition, he has been involved in several studies and published articles and book chapters in the field of pediatric psychopharmacology.

Joseph A. Jackson, DO, is Instructor in Psychiatry at Harvard Medical School and the Medical Director of the Developmental Disabilities Program at the Center for Child and Adolescent Development, Cambridge Health Alliance. His expertise is in working with children with multicomplex disorders, particularly those with comorbid pervasive developmental disorders and bipolar disorder.

Gagan Joshi, MD, is a clinical and research psychiatrist and the Scientific Director of the Pervasive Developmental Disorders Research Program in the Pediatric Psychopharmacology Unit at Massachusetts General Hospital and Instructor in Psychiatry at Harvard Medical School. Dr. Joshi's clinical and research interest is in pediatric bipolar disorder and pervasive developmental disorders, with particular focus on the comorbid conditions associated with these disorders. Besides conducting research, he also takes care of youth with these conditions in his clinical practice at Massachusetts General Hospital. He received the prestigious Ethel Dupont Warren Fellowship Award through the Department of Psychiatry at Harvard Medical School, the Norma Fine Fellowship, the 25th Collegium Internationale Neuro-Psychopharmalogicum Congress Young Investigators Award, and the American Academy of Child and Adolescent Psychiatry Pilot Research Award.

Paramjit T. Joshi, MD, is the Endowed Chair of the Department of Psychiatry and Behavioral Sciences at the Children's National Medical Center and Professor of Psychiatry, Behavioral Sciences, and Pediatrics at the George Washington University School of Medicine in Washington, DC. She is a Distinguished Fellow of the American Psychiatric Association and a recipient of its Bruno Lima award for outstanding contributions in the care and understanding of disaster psychiatry, as well as of the Exemplary Psychiatrist Award from the National Alliance on Mental Illness. She has held several national offices with the American Academy of Child and Adolescent Psychiatry and the American Board of Psychiatry and Neurology and currently is the President of the Society of Professors of Academic Programs of Child and Adolescent Psychiatry (2006–2008). She has taught and published extensively on mood disorders, psychopharmacology, and childhood trauma.

Robert A. Kowatch, MD, PhD, is Professor of Psychiatry and Pediatrics at Cincinnati Children's Hospital Medical Center. Dr. Kowatch has authored or coauthored more than 50 articles, 14 book chapters, and one book. He has published in the areas of the diagnosis and treatment of children and adolescents with bipolar disorder, sleep disorders, and depression. His articles have been published in the *Journal of the American Academy of Child and Adolescent Psychiatry, Neuropsychopharmacology, Archives of General Psychiatry,* and the *Journal of Child Neurology,* among others. He is a member of the American Academy of Child and Adolescent Psychiatry, the Society for Biological Psychiatry, and the American College of Neuropharmacology, and his research interests are in the diagnosis, treatment, and neurobiology of child and adolescent mood disorders.

Joan L. Luby, MD, is an infant preschool psychiatrist and Associate Professor of Child Psychiatry at the Washington University School of Medicine in St. Louis, where she is the founder and director of the Early Emotional Development Program. Dr. Luby has been awarded grants from the National Institute of Mental Health and the National Alliance for Schizophrenia and Depression, which have supported her program of research on the phenomenology of early-onset mood disorders. Findings from these studies have been widely published in both child and adult psychiatric journals, and she has been the recipient of several awards, including the Gerald Klerman award for outstanding research in depression. Dr. Luby has committed her career to the study and clinical assessment and treatment of preschool children. She currently chairs the Infancy Committee of the American Academy of Child and Adolescent Psychiatry.

Molly McGrath, LCSW, is a research clinician with the Early Emotional Development Program at Washington University. She has contributed to the work on the Pediatric Depression Study and the Treatment of Early Age Mania study. As a teaching assistant at Washington University's George Warren Brown School of Social Work, Ms. McGrath lectures and facilitates discussions in courses on the foundations of social work practice. She also serves as a mental health consultant providing resources, referrals, behavioral observations, and inservice training for staff at an Early Head Start facility in the St. Louis area.

David J. Miklowitz, PhD, is Professor of Psychology and Psychiatry at the University of Colorado at Boulder and a Senior Clinical Research Fellow in the Department of Psychiatry at Oxford University. His research focuses on family environmental factors and family psychoeducational treatments for adult- and childhood-onset bipolar disorder. He developed the family psychoeducational intervention known as "family-focused treatment" for adults and youth with bipolar disorder. Dr. Miklowitz has received awards from the University of California, Los Angeles; the International Congress on Schizophrenia Research; the National Alliance for Research on Schizophrenia and Depression; the University of Colorado; the International Society for Bipolar Disorders. He has received funding for his research from the National Institute of Mental Health, the John D. and Catherine T. MacArthur Foundation, the Robert Sutherland Foundation, and the Danny Alberts Foundation. Dr. Miklowitz has published more than 170 research articles and book chapters on bipolar disorder and schizophrenia, and five books, including *The Bipolar Disorder Survival Guide*.

Kimberley L. Mullen, MA, is a doctoral candidate in clinical psychology at the University of Colorado at Boulder and has contributed to the research on family-focused treatment (FFT) for adolescents diagnosed with bipolar disorder. She currently works at the Denver Veterans Affairs Medical Center, where she provides clinical services and conducts research on the application of FFT for families of returning Iraq or Afghanistan veterans with posttraumatic stress disorder.

Nick C. Patel, PharmD, PhD, is Assistant Professor of Pharmacy at the University of Georgia, and of Psychiatry at the Medical College of Georgia. His research interests are the pharmacological treatment of child and adolescent mood disorders and neuropsychopharmacology using magnetic resonance spectroscopy. He has authored or coauthored numerous articles in these areas.

Jennifer Pautsch, MA, is Study Coordinator for the Early Intervention in Depression Study, which is piloting PCIT-ED, the parent–child interaction therapy–emotional development study sponsored by the National Institute of Mental Health. She also oversees the clinical research mental health assessments in a multidisciplinary clinical preschool research program at Washington University School of Medicine, headed by Joan Luby. The research team is investigating major depressive disorder in a large, community-based preschool sample. Ms. Pautsch has coauthored multiple articles on preschool mood disorders and a treatment program targeting mood dysregulation in preschool-age children.

Mani N. Pavuluri, MD, PhD, is Associate Professor in Psychiatry and Founding Director of the Pediatric Mood Disorders Clinic and the Pediatric Translational Research in Affective and Cognitive Neurocircuitry and Treatment Lab at the University of Illinois at Chicago. Dr. Pavuluri's work has been funded by the National Institutes of Health, the National Institute of Child Health and Human Development, GlaxoSmithKline, Johnson & Johnson, AstraZeneca, and Abbott Pharmaceuticals. Her main area of interest is the interaction between affect dysregulation and cognitive function in pediatric bipolar disorder and medication effects on the brain.

Mark A. Riddle, MD, is Professor of Psychiatry and Pediatrics and Director of the Division of Child and Adolescent Psychiatry at the Johns Hopkins University School of Medicine, Baltimore, Maryland. He also serves as Vice-President for Psychiatric Sciences at the Kennedy Krieger Institute, a Johns Hopkins-affiliated organization for individuals with developmental disabilities. Dr. Riddle's research, teaching and clinical practice focus on pediatric psychopharmacology and medication side effects. His publications include over 200 research articles, reviews, chapters, and edited volumes.

Adelaide S. Robb, MD, is Associate Professor of Psychiatry and Pediatrics and Medical Director of Inpatient Psychiatry at the Children's National Medical Center, where she also teaches the psychopharmacology course for child psychiatry fellows and is active in research and clinical practice. She is an investigator on National Institute of Mental Health-, foundation-, and industry-sponsored trials of pharmaceutical treatments for bipolar disorder and other psychiatric disorders in children and adolescents and has authored multiple book chapters and articles.

Russell E. Scheffer, MD, is Professor and Chair of the Department of Psychiatry and Behavioral Sciences as well as Professor of Pediatrics at the Kansas University Medical Center–Wichita. Dr. Scheffer receives or has received research support and/or served as a speaker for Abbott Labs, AstraZeneca, BMS Pfizer, and Shire.

Melissa Meade Stalets, MA, is an infant mental health specialist for an early intervention program in Illinois, where she provides consultation and training to direct-service providers and collaborates with social service and other agencies to promote healthy social/emotional development among young children. Previously, she engaged in research at Southern Illinois University School of Medicine, The Ohio State University and, most recently, in the Early Emotional Development Program at Washington University School of Medicine. She has authored and coauthored multiple articles on preschool mood disorders and has authored a treatment program targeting mood dysregulation in preschool-age children.

Rebecca Tillman, MS, is a senior statistical data analyst at Washington University in St. Louis. Ms. Tillman has authored more than a dozen articles on diagnostic characteristics, phenomenology, longitudinal course, family psychopathology, and molecular genetics of child bipolar disorder.

Benedetto Vitiello, MD, a psychiatrist with expertise in psychopharmacology and treatment research, has been with the National Institute of Mental Health since 1989, and is currently Chief of the Child and Adolescent Treatment and Preventive Interventions Research Branch. He is Adjunct Professor of Psychiatry at Johns Hopkins University, and his research activity has focused on clinical trials in children and adolescents and ethical aspects of research participation.

Karen Dineen Wagner, MD, PhD, is the Marie B. Gale Professor and Vice Chair in the Department of Psychiatry and Behavioral Sciences and Director of the Division of Child and Adolescent Psychiatry at the University of Texas Medical Branch in Galveston. Dr. Wagner is an internationally recognized expert in the pharmacological treatment of childhood mood disorders. She received an honorary doctorate (Doctor of Science) from the State University of New York in 2004 for her contributions to the field of child psychiatry. She has served in leadership positions in professional organizations and as a member of the National Institute of Mental Health Advisory Council.

John T. Walkup, MD, is Associate Professor of Psychiatry and Behavioral Sciences, Division of Child and Adolescent Psychiatry, Johns Hopkins Medical Institutions in Baltimore, Maryland. He currently serves as the Deputy Director of the Division of Child and Adolescent Psychiatry and is the principal investigator of the National Institute of Mental Health-funded Johns Hopkins Research Unit of Pediatric Psychopharmacology and Psychosocial Interventions. He is the current Chair of the Medical Advisory Board of the Tourette Syndrome Association. Dr. Walkup is the author of a number of articles and book chapters on psychopharmacology, Tourette syndrome, obsessive–compulsive disorder, and other anxiety disorders.

Timothy E. Wilens, MD, is Associate Professor of Psychiatry at Harvard Medical School in Boston, Massachusetts. In addition, he is Director of Substance Abuse Services in the Clinical and Research Program in Pediatric Psychopharmacology at Massachusetts General Hospital. Dr. Wilens has written more than 190 peer-reviewed articles and has published more than 70 book chapters and 300 abstracts and presentations for national and international scientific meetings.

Janet Wozniak, MD, is a clinical and research psychiatrist and the Director of the Pediatric Bipolar Disorder Research Program in the Pediatric Psychopharmacology Unit at Massachusetts General Hospital, as well as Assistant Professor of Psychiatry at Harvard Medical School. Widely regarded as a national expert on the topic of pediatric bipolar disorder and attention-deficit/hyperactivity disorder, Dr. Wozniak has collaborated on research studies on these conditions for over 15 years. She is the author of dozens of scientific articles, and her 1995 paper on childhood mania is one of the 10 most cited papers ever to be published in the *Journal of the American Academy of Child and Adolescent Psychiatry*. Dr. Wozniak cares for hundreds of children and adolescents with these conditions in her clinical practice at Massachusetts General Hospital.

Contents

Part II. COMORBID DISORDERS AND SPECIAL POPULATIONS

Part III. OTHER ISSUES

CHAPTER 1

Introduction

MELISSA P. DELBELLO *and* BARBARA GELLER

TREATMENT OF PEDIATRIC BIPOLAR DISORDER: A DECADE OF PROGRESS AND CONTROVERSY

During the past decade there has been enormous progress in our understanding of the phenomenology, neurobiology, and treatment of children and adolescents with bipolar disorder. In particular, the number of controlled treatment studies of mania in children and adolescents is rapidly increasing, thereby greatly improving our understanding of effective treatment options for bipolar disorder in youth. Clinicians no longer need to extrapolate data from studies of bipolar adults to treat children and adolescents with bipolar disorder. Indeed, consistent with the differences in phenomenology and neurobiology between youth and adults with bipolar disorder, emerging data suggest possible developmental differences in treatment response. The considerable growth of data-based evidence has also enabled clinicians to develop age-specific treatment algorithms and to identify developmental differences in tolerability and safety.

Despite considerable progress in evidence-based treatments for pediatric bipolar disorder, the imminent decisions of the United States Food and Drug Administration (FDA) regarding the potential approval of several pharmacological agents for use in adolescent mania has lead to reexamination of the diagnostic debate that surrounds pediatric bipolar disorder. Until recently, lithium was the only treatment approved by the FDA for use in adolescents with bipolar disorder, and no treatment has been approved for children with bipolar disorder. However, now risperidone is approved by

1

the FDA for mania in youth. This is the first FDA approval that was based on data. Despite the controversy, the negative impact on development that is often associated with childhood and adolescent bipolar disorder is indisputable, and the functional and symptomatic improvements that have been observed following effective treatments are unquestionable. The next decade of research will clarify some of the remaining questions. For example, future research is necessary to determine whether youth with bipolar disorder develop into adults with bipolar disorder, which biological markers determine the optimal treatment for a specific individual, and what are the most effective early intervention and prevention strategies for children and adolescents with risk factors for developing bipolar disorder. Advances in these and other related areas will allow the development of novel treatment strategies and, ultimately, will improve the outcomes of children and adolescents with and at risk for developing bipolar disorder.

ORGANIZATION OF THE BOOK

This book is organized into three main parts. Part I provides an overview of the clinical characteristics of pediatric bipolar disorder and potential approaches to identifying biological and clinical predictors of treatment response. It also examines specific pharmacological and nonpharmacological treatments for bipolar disorder in children and adolescents. Part II discusses treatment strategies for specific clinical populations, including children and adolescents with bipolar disorder and comorbid psychiatric disorders and children at high risk for developing bipolar disorder. Part III reviews other topics related to treatment, including common side effects of pharmacological agents used to treat bipolar youth, as well as ethical concerns regarding the treatment of childhood and adolescent bipolar disorder.

In Chapter 2, Rebecca Tillman and Barbara Geller discuss the potential utility of applying biological tools and clinical symptoms to predict medication response for a specific individual with bipolar disorder. Additionally, the authors review the different approaches used by investigators to define "the pediatric bipolar phenotype." They also discuss naturalistic studies examining the generally poor outcomes of youth with bipolar disorder, justifying the need for systematic treatment studies that are discussed in the remaining chapters. In Chapter 3, Nick C. Patel and Melissa P. DelBello further examine the possibility of using novel neuroimaging techniques to develop targeted treatment intervention strategies for children and adolescents with bipolar disorder. In particular, magnetic resonance spectroscopy (MRS) and functional magnetic resonance imaging (fMRI) may facilitate implementations of more effective treatments earlier in the illness course for an individual patient by identifying neurochemical and neurofunctional predictors of treatment response, respectively. In this chapter, the authors also highlight examples of the progress that has been made using neuro-imaging to identify markers and, ultimately, predictors of treatment response.

The next five chapters provide a detailed examination of specific pharmacological and nonpharmacological biological treatment options for children and adolescents with bipolar disorder. In Chapter 4, Robert L. Findling and Mani N. Pavuluri summarize the history and neurobiology of lithium, as well as the data-based evidence for lithium as a treatment for youth with bipolar disorder. Despite the relatively recent increase in novel pharmacological options, Chapter 4 serves as a reminder of the crucial need for additional data-based studies examining lithium, one of the oldest treatments for bipolar disorder, for children and adolescents with bipolar disorder. In Chapter 5, Jean A. Frazier, Hallie R. Bregman, and Joseph A. Jackson provide a historical perspective on the use of antipsychotics for bipolar disorder, discuss whether antipsychotics are necessary to effectively treat youth with bipolar disorder and psychosis, and review the evidence supporting the use of second-generation ("atypical") antipsychotics as mood stabilizers in children and adolescents with bipolar disorder. Although atypical antipsychotics may prove to be the most effective treatment options for children and adolescents with bipolar disorder, they are not without side effects. The authors discuss common side effects associated with antipsychotics and examine strategies for maximizing the tolerability of these agents. In Chapter 6, Robert A. Kowatch reviews efficacy and tolerability data and recommended dosing for antiepileptic agents in children and adolescents with bipolar disorder. Kowatch also discusses potential drug interactions and adverse events and reviews guidelines for laboratory monitoring of and contraindications for use of these medications. In contrast to studies of adults with bipolar disorder, controlled studies do not support the efficacy of antiepileptic agents for children and adolescents. Nonetheless, the results of open-label studies suggest that antiepileptic agents may be useful to treat specific symptoms, including depression and aggression, in youth with bipolar disorder. In Chapter 7, Adelaide S. Robb and Paramjit T. Joshi describe novel pharmacological approaches and provide a comprehensive review of the literature of thyroid hormone dysfunction and supplementation in patients with bipolar disorder. The authors also explore other potential hormonal targets for treatment development in bipolar disorder. Recent studies support the role of abnormalities in second-messenger systems in the pathophysiology of bipolar disorder. Robb and Joshi discuss the role of calcium-channel blockers and other medications that affect second-messenger systems as treatment options. Finally, the authors examine other novel pharmacological treatment approaches. In Chapter 8, Russell E. Scheffer reviews the biological rationale for investigating omega-3 fatty acids in patients with bipolar disorder and examines clinical scenarios for which omega-3 fatty acids may be indicated. Scheffer also explores the possibility of using other complementary and alternative medicines, including Saint-John's-wort and S-adenosyl-L-methionine (SAM-e).

The next two chapters examine the importance of including psychosocial interventions in the treatment plan for children and adolescents with bipolar disorder. First, in Chapter 9, David J. Miklowitz, Kimberley L. Mullen, and Kiki D. Chang explore the relationships among kindling, psychosocial stress, and the onset of mood disorders as the rationale for using psychosocial interventions that include families of patients. Next, the authors review the role of psychosocial interventions and incorporating families in treatments for patients with bipolar disorder. Finally, they discuss implementing family-focused treatment in individuals with and at familial risk for developing bipolar disorder. In Chapter 10, Kristen H. Davidson and Mary A. Fristad review the theoretical basis for and goals of psychoeducational psychotherapy and the evidence to support using this approach to treat children and adolescents. In particular, they describe multifamily psychoeducational group therapy, which they developed, implemented, and validated as a treatment for youth with bipolar disorder.

Part II of the book approaches treatment by focusing on specific subpopulations of youth with bipolar disorder. Comorbidity is the rule rather than the exception in children and adolescents with bipolar disorder. However, youth with co-occurring disorders may be more challenging to treat than those without psychiatric comorbidities. In Chapter 11, Karen Dineen Wagner examines pharmacotherapy for children and adolescents with co-occurring bipolar disorder and attention-deficit/hyperactivity disorder (ADHD). Additionally, Wagner reviews the literature examining whether stimulants treat or exacerbate manic symptoms. Although the author concludes that current evidence suggests that stimulants may be effective in conjunction with mood stabilizers for youth with ADHD and bipolar disorder, additional studies are needed to determine whether stimulants precipitate the onset of mania in children and adolescents. In Chapter 12, Timothy E. Wilens and Martin Gignac examine the complex relationships between bipolar disorder and substance use disorders. The authors propose several potential mechanisms to explain the high rates of comorbidity between these illnesses. Nonetheless, substance use negatively affects illness course in adolescents with bipolar disorder. Additionally, because the onset of bipolar disorder generally occurs prior to the onset of substance use disorder, there may be a unique "window of opportunity" to prevent the onset of substance use disorder in youth with bipolar disorder. The authors also examine multimodal approaches to treating co-occurring substance use and bipolar disorder in adolescents. In Chapter 13, Gagan Joshi and Janet Wozniak examine other comorbid psychiatric disorders that occur in children and adolescents with bipolar disorder, including conduct disorder, oppositional defiant disorder, anxiety disorders, and pervasive developmental disorders. Specifically, they review epidemiology and clinical studies that report rates of comorbidities and describe proposed mechanisms for the comorbid disorders. Although these disorders commonly co-occur with bipolar disorder in youth, there are very few evidence-based treatments for these subgroups. The authors review the small body of literature of treatment studies and examine practical strategies for treating youth with bipolar disorder and psychiatric comorbidities.

In Chapter 14, Joan L. Luby and colleagues review the growing literature describing preschool bipolar disorder. They also describe a novel parent–child interaction therapy as a treatment for preschool bipolar disorder. Finally, they review the studies that present data on treating young children with bipolar disorder with psychopharmacological agents. In Chapter 15, Kiki D. Chang discusses the new era of treatment for children and adolescents with bipolar disorder, which includes early intervention and preventative strategies. He reviews potential clinical characteristics and biomarkers that might serve as markers for early intervention strategies. Additionally, he examines the pros and cons of antidepressant and stimulant use in youth at risk for developing bipolar disorder and explores pharmacological and psychotherapeutic treatments for this population. In Chapter 16, Shannon Rae Barnett, Mark A. Riddle, and John T. Walkup discuss treatment of the depressed phase of bipolar disorder. Most treatments have been based on studies of adults with bipolar disorder. The authors examine the differences and similarities between bipolar depression in youth and adults. They also review the use of mood stabilizers, antipsychotics, antidepressants, stimulants, and psychotherapy, as well as other options, in patients with bipolar depression and discuss whether antidepressants induce cycling in patients with bipolar disorder.

In Part III of this book, two of the most significant side effects of psychotropic medications used to treat children and adolescents with bipolar disorder are discussed. First, in Chapter 17, Paramjit T. Joshi and Adelaide S. Robb describe polycystic ovary syndrome (PCOS), which is a potential side effect of some of the medications used to treat bipolar youth. The authors review the definition, prevalence, and clinical characteristics of PCOS. They also discuss potential etiological factors associated with PCOS. Next, in Chapter 18, Christoph U. Correll provides a comprehensive overview of the metabolic side effects associated with pharmacological agents used to treat bipolar disorder. Additionally, the author discusses strategies for monitoring and treating the metabolic side effects of these psychotropic medications. Finally, in Chapter 19, Benedetto Vitiello examines several ethical concerns related to the treatment of children and adolescents with bipolar disorder. Specifically, he explores the role of the parent or legal guardian in treatment and the ethics of using "off-label" medications to treat bipolar disorder in youth. Vitiello also discusses ethical concerns related to children and adolescents participating as research subjects in treatment studies and precautions taken in most studies to address these concerns.

In conclusion, we hope that the information provided in this book will enable clinicians, parents, and other individuals involved in the treatment of children and adolescents with and at risk for developing bipolar disorder to implement state-of-the-art clinical care for these individuals. Despite the past decade of enormous growth in evidence-based treatment strategies for children and adolescents with bipolar disorder, gaps in our knowledge of how to provide optimal treatments for some children and adolescents with bipolar disorder still exist. Specifically, ongoing studies are examining treatments for bipolar depression and prevention of recurrent episodes, as well as treatment and prevention strategies for youth with bipolar disorder and comorbid disorders. While we await the results of these studies, it is only through systematic trials of adequate doses and durations of therapeutic interventions, whether pharmacological, nonpharmacological biological, or psychotherapeutic, that will we be able to minimize the side effects associated with medications and decrease the morbidity and mortality associated with childhood and adolescent bipolar disorder.

PART I

DIAGNOSIS
AND TREATMENTS

CHAPTER 2

Diagnosis, Prognosis, and Personalized Medicine

REBECCA TILLMAN *and* BARBARA GELLER

WAITING FOR PERSONALIZED MEDICINE

Across medical specialties, the current goal is personalized care in which testing for specific genetic and environmental pathways will allow targeted prevention and treatment that takes into account both efficacy and adversity. Achieving this goal will be the coup de grace to the "final common pathway" approach, needed when biological pathogenesis is unknown. For example, at one time there was a final common pathway for "low blood," the syndrome of feeling tired, looking pale, and having painful lower extremities on going up stairs. As medical knowledge advanced (see Figure 2.1), multiple genetic and environmental etiologies made specific diagnoses possible, and these replaced the cluster of symptoms that formed the syndrome of "low blood," or anemia. Although psychiatry remains in the cluster of symptoms stage for final common pathway syndromes such as bipolar disorders, ongoing research will hopefully provide the way to diseases, that is, syndromes, for which pathogeneses are known.

Specific biological markers, such as genetic variants, will in the future permit personalized choice of the best treatments. One example of what personalized medicine can bring is illustrated in Table 2.1. Chung et al. (2004) reasoned that Stevens–Johnson syndrome (SJS) was an autoimmune disease and therefore examined genetic variants (alleles) of human leukocyte antigens (HLA) in participants who were receiving carbamazepine

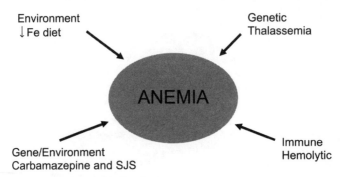

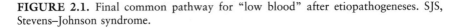

FIGURE 2.1. Final common pathway for "low blood" after etiopathogeneses. SJS, Stevens–Johnson syndrome.

(CBZ) for epilepsy. The three groups studied were those on CBZ who developed SJS, those on CBZ who did not have SJS, and healthy controls. The HLA-B*1502 allele occurred in 100% of participants who developed SJS but in only 3.0% of those who did not and in 8.6% of healthy controls. These findings may one day inform a clinically useful test for adversity prior to giving CBZ , as it could predict who would get the serious SJS side effect.

An example from child psychiatry is work from Yang, Wang, Li, and Faraone (2004) that reported that the A/A phenotype of the norepinephrine transporter gene G1287A was associated with poor response to methylphenidate. One day, these results may be useful as a strategy to decide which attention-deficit/hyperactivity disorder (ADHD) drug to use as a first choice.

Additionally, neuroimaging techniques, such as functional magnetic resonance imaging and magnetic resonance spectroscopy, may help identify

TABLE 2.1. Frequency of HLA Alleles in Patients with Stevens–Johnson Syndrome

HLA allele	CBZ–SJS (%)	CBZ–tolerant (%)	Normal (%)
B*1502	100.0	3.0	8.6
Cw*0801	93.2	16.8	14.0
A*1101	81.8	50.5	57.0
DRB1*1202	75.0	11.9	19.4
B*1502, Cw*0801	93.2	3.0	7.5
B*1502, A*1101	81.8	2.0	6.5
B*1502, DRB1*1202	75.0	1.0	5.4
B*1502, Cw*0801, A*1101, DRB1*1202	66.0	0.0	3.2

Note. Adapted from Chung et al. (2004). Copyright 2004 by Nature Publishing Group. Adapted by permission from Macmillan Publishers Ltd. CBZ, carbamazepine; SJS, Stevens–Johnson syndrome.

neurofunctional and neurochemical predictors of treatment response, as well as treatment effects (DelBello, Cecil, Adler, Daniels, & Strakowski, 2006). For example, Figure 2.2 demonstrates a significant difference between choline levels in medial ventral prefrontal cortex between remitters and nonremitters to olanzapine in adolescents with bipolar I disorder.

DO WE NEED CATEGORICAL SYNDROMES, DISEASES WITH PATHOGENESES, OR DIMENSIONS TO TREAT?

Even in branches of medicine in which there are known pathogenetic factors, for example, infectious diatheses, treatment is often both specific to the causative factor, such as an antibiotic, and nonspecific to dimensional symptoms that cut across diagnostic categories. Pain is one example of a dimension that is treated somewhat similarly whether it is due to a fractured femur or to postabdominal surgery. Cardinal biological tests (for diseases with known pathogeneses) or cardinal clinical symptoms (for psychiatric syndromes) are those that occur only in a particular disease or syndrome. Figure 2.3 presents dimensions (fever, increased white blood cell count) and cardinal biology (pathology specimen for appendicitis and throat culture for "strep" throat) for two co-occurring infectious diseases.

How these models from medicine might apply to child psychiatry is presented in Figure 2.4. Aggression/irritability (A/I) and hyperactivity (HA) are the two most common dimensions that bring children to treatment.

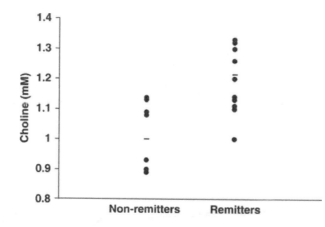

FIGURE 2.2. Baseline medial ventral prefrontal choline levels in first-hospitalization manic adolescents who were nonremitters (n = 8) and remitters (n = 11) to olanzapine treatment. Adapted from DelBello, Cecil, Adler, Daniels, and Strakowski (2006). Copyright 2006 by Nature Publishing Group. Adapted by permission from Macmillan Publishers Ltd.

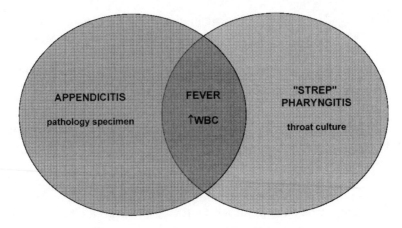

FIGURE 2.3. Dimensional overlap versus cardinal biology for co-occurring infections.

Like most dimensions, for example fear or pain, they are nonspecific in that they occur in multiple diagnostic categories. For example, A/I was found to have been present in 20–60% of young adults with various diagnoses when they were children (Kim-Cohen et al., 2003). But dimensions can be highly sensitive, meaning that they would pick up most cases. For bipolar I disorder, mixed or manic type, across the age span, most cases of bipolar I disorder would be detected if the dimension of A/I was used as a screen. But so would cases of many other diagnoses, such as antisocial per-

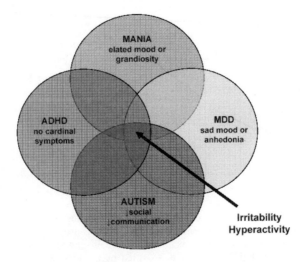

FIGURE 2.4. Dimensional overlap versus cardinal symptoms for co-occurring child diagnoses.

sonality disorder, oppositional defiant disorder (ODD), major depressive disorder (MDD), and so forth (Geller et al., 2006). By way of analogy, using sore throat as a screen for "strep" throat would detect most cases of "strep," but only 5% of sore throats are due to "strep." In all likelihood, less than 5% of children presenting with A/I will have bipolar I disorder (Craney & Geller, 2003).

Treatment geared to the dimension of A/I has been conducted, and some examples of double-blind, placebo-controlled studies for child psychiatry are presented in Table 2.2.

What these data tell us is that treatment for A/I is nonspecific for any diagnosis, so that response of symptoms to lithium or a neuroleptic, for example, does not help with differential diagnosis.

It is useful in child psychiatry, as in other branches of medicine, to consider impairment from symptoms, syndromes, and dimensions in developing comprehensive treatment plans.

VARIOUS DEFINITIONS
OF CHILD BIPOLAR I DISORDER PHENOTYPES

Figure 2.5 presents various schemas that have been published to demonstrate that, in research, what you find depends on the net that you cast. Essentially, the Geller, Tillman, Craney, and Bolhofner (2004), Biederman, Faraone, Chu, and Wozniak (1999), and Dickstein et al. (2005) phenotypes overlap with respect to using DSM-IV criteria for bipolar I disorder. Differ-

TABLE 2.2. Double-Blind Placebo-Controlled Studies of Aggression/Irritability (A/I) in Child Psychiatry

Author (year)	n	Diagnosis	Targeted dimension	Drug	Outcome
Campbell et al. (1995)	50	Conduct disorder	A/I	Lithium	More effective than placebo
Malone, Delaney, Luebbert, Cater, and Campbell (2000)	40	Conduct disorder	A/I	Lithium	More effective than placebo
Aman, DeSmedt, Derivan, Lyons, and Findling (2002)	118	Conduct disorder, oppositional defiant disorder, or disruptive behavior disorder not otherwise specified	A/I	Risperidone	More effective than placebo
McCracken et al. (2002)	101	Autistic disorder	A/I	Risperidone	More effective than placebo

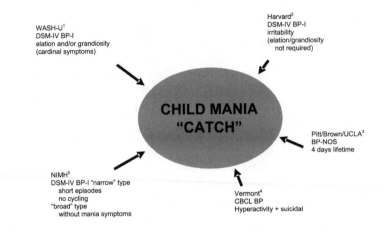

FIGURE 2.5. Research findings depend on phenotypic net cast. [1]Geller, Tillman, Craney, and Bolhofner (2004); [2]Biederman, Faraone, Chu, and Wozniak (1999); [3]Birmaher et al. (2006); [4]Hudziak, Althoff, Derks, Faraone, and Boomsma (2005); [5]Dickstein et al. (2005).

ences are that the Geller et al. (2004) phenotype required euphoria and/or grandiosity (cardinal symptoms of mania) to avoid diagnosing mania only by symptoms that overlap with those for ADHD (e.g., hyperactivity, distractibility). This is analogous to DSM-IV requiring sad mood or anhedonia (cardinal symptoms of depression) to diagnose MDD. In this schema, almost all children had both elation and irritable mood concurrently, which is similar to prevalence of these symptoms in adults with bipolar I disorder (Goodwin & Jamison, 1990). The Biederman et al. (1999) group does not use a cardinal symptom approach. Dickstein et al. (2005) use elated mood as a necessary criterion and do not enter children who have daily cycling (daily mood changes).

Hudziak, Althoff, Derks, Faraone, and Boomsma (2005) reported on a pattern from the Child Behavior Checklist (CBCL) that included hyperactive and suicidal symptoms that they have labeled the CBCL bipolar phenotype. Studies have shown that this pattern identifies participants with bipolar I disorder in the Biederman, Monuteaux, Kendrick, Klein, and Faraone (2005) group but does not identify clinical bipolar I in many other studies (Carlson & Kelly, 1998; Dienes, Chang, Blasey, Adleman, & Steiner, 2002; Geller, Warner, Williams, & Zimerman, 1998; Hazell, Lewin, & Carr, 1999; Kahana, Youngstrom, Findling, & Calabrese, 2003; Volk & Todd, 2007; Youngstrom, Youngstrom, & Starr, 2005). Birmaher et al. (2006) have reported a syndrome of bipolar disorder, not otherwise specified, defined as at least 4 days lifetime of bipolar symptoms.

Table 2.3 presents a comparison of cardinal symptoms across studies by the methods used. These data suggest that directly interviewing or ob-

TABLE 2.3. Cardinal Symptoms in Child Bipolar I Disorder by Methods

Author (year)	n	Version of SADS	Child interviewed	% elated	% grandiose
Geller et al. (2000)	93	WASH-U-KSADS	Yes	89.3	86.0
Findling et al. (2001)	90	K-SADS-P/L, K-SADS-E	Yes	85.6	83.3
Axelson et al. (2006)	220	K-SADS-P, K-SADS-P/L	Yes	86.4	57.3
TEAM (still recruiting)	306	WASH-U-KSADS	Yes	97.1	95.8
Wozniak et al. (1995)	43	K-SADS-E	No	14.0	N/A
Biederman, Faraone, et al. (2005)	197	K-SADS-E	No	27.9	60.9

Note. TEAM, NIMH-funded multisite Treatment of Early Age Mania (TEAM) study.

serving children is necessary to identify elated mood and grandiosity, as the prevalence of these two symptoms was substantially higher in studies that included direct child interviews in addition to separate interviews of the parents about the children.

How much these phenotypes overlap with each other and with various comorbidities such as ADHD and ODD is the basis for much ongoing research (e.g., DelBello, Zimmerman, Mills, Getz, & Strakowski, 2004; Rucklidge, 2006).

PROGNOSIS FROM NATURAL HISTORY AND FROM TREATMENT STUDIES

Table 2.4 shows the data from several longitudinal studies that followed patients naturalistically; that is, these patients were seen for usual clinical care by their own practitioners, but research data was collected at intervals. All studies report long episode duration, and high rates of relapse after recovery have also been reported (Biederman, Faraone, et al., 2005; Birmaher et al., 2006; Geller et al., 2004). Thus the prognosis for untreated children with mania is poor and is the reason for considering aggressive pharmacological and nondrug interventions.

Figures 2.6 and 2.7 show relapse rates during treatment studies. Findling et al. (2005) studied participants (mean age = 10.8 ± 3.5 years) who were stabilized on both lithium and valproate and then randomized to either lithium or valproate for approximately 18 months. By the end of the

TABLE 2.4. Baseline Episode Duration and "Longitudinal Stability" of Child DSM-IV Bipolar I Disorder

Author (year)	Episode measure	Ascertainment	Diagnosis blind and controlled	Duration (weeks)
Geller et al. (2004)	Prospective	Consecutive new cases from designated pediatric and psychiatric sites	Yes	mean 79.2 (SD = 66.7)
Biederman, Faraone, et al. (2005)	Retrospective	Consecutively referred to child psychiatry service	No	mean 180.1 (SD not given)
Birmaher et al. (2006)	Retrospective and prospective	Convenience sample	No	median 52.0
Tohen et al. (2007)	Prospective	Convenience sample	No	mean 44.3 (SD = 107.0)
TEAM (still recruiting)	Retrospective	Convenience sample in TEAM drug study	No	mean 252.2 (SD = 134.8)[a]

Note. TEAM, NIMH-funded multisite Treatment of Early Age Mania (TEAM) study.
[a]4.8 (SD = 2.6) years.

study, about 63% had relapsed and another 20% had discontinued (10% for noncompliance, 8.3% for side effects, and 1.7% for other reasons), which suggests that the outcome with monitored treatment may not be better than the naturalistic outcome.

In a sample of older adolescents followed clinically, Strober, Morrell, Lampert, and Burroughs (1990) reported significantly higher relapse rates in patients who discontinued their lithium. Better prognosis in compliant patients has also been reported for adults with bipolar I disorder (e.g., Schou, 1997) and is encouraging, with the caveat that better compliance may be a marker for differences in other features that may also augur for a better prognosis.

Recently, DelBello, Hanseman, Adler, Fleck, and Strakowski (2007) reported that only 35% of participants in a follow-up study of adolescents (mean age = 15.2 ± 1.9 years) showed at least 75% compliance. These data on compliance underscore the need for nondrug interventions that enhance compliance.

IMPORTANCE OF NONPHARMACOLOGICAL INTERVENTIONS

In the controlled, blindly rated natural history follow-up study of children with cardinal symptom mania, maternal warmth, a concept akin to expressed emotion, was a robust predictor at both 2-year and 4-year intervals

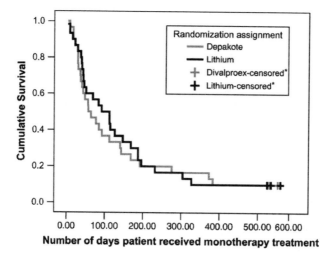

FIGURE 2.6. Blind, controlled study of relapse over 1.5 years on lithium or valproate in children. Adapted from Findling et al. (2005). Copyright 2005 by Lippincott Williams & Wilkins. Adapted by permission. *Completed 72 weeks of treatment.

(see Figure 2.8; Geller, Craney, et al., 2002; Geller et al., 2004). These data are consistent with reports on the importance of expressed emotion in adults with bipolar I disorder and make a strong case for not limiting therapy to drugs (e.g., Honig, Hofman, Hilwig, Noorthoorn, & Ponds, 1995; Miklowitz, Goldstein, Nuechterlein, Snyder, & Mintz, 1988; Ramana & Bebbington, 1995).

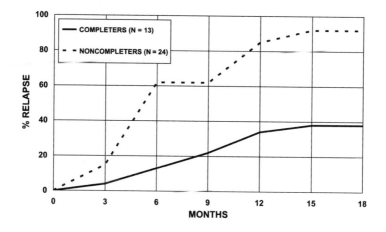

FIGURE 2.7. Open, nonrandomized lithium for bipolar disorder in adolescents. Adapted from Strober, Morrell, Lampert, and Burroughs (1990). Copyright 1990 by American Psychiatric Publishing, Inc. Adapted by permission from the *American Journal of Psychiatry.*

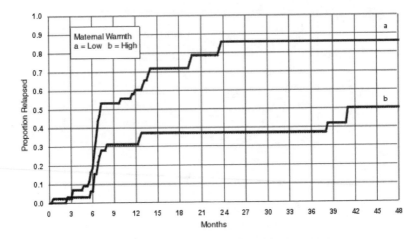

FIGURE 2.8. Relapse after recovery in participants with cardinal symptom bipolar disorder by maternal warmth. Adapted from Geller, Tillman, Craney, and Bolhofner (2004). Copyright 2004 by the American Medical Association. Adapted by permission. Cox proportional hazard modeling for maternal warmth, controlling for gender, age and mixed mania, was significant ($\chi^2 = 13.6$, $p = .0002$, $df = 1$). Hazard ratio was 3.7 (95% confidence interval = 1.8–7.4). Kaplan–Meier estimate of relapse was 50.3% (95% confidence interval = 28.9–71.6%) for the 32 participants with high maternal warmth and 85.9% (95% confidence interval = 73.9–98.0%) for the 43 participants with low maternal warmth.

DEFINITIONS OF EPISODE DURATION AND OF CYCLING PATTERNS

One of the more difficult issues in the field has been how to define episode duration and how to define daily mood switches (also called *daily rapid cycling* or *ultradian cycling*). Historically, earlier literature used the term *rapid cycling* to describe the occurrence of four or more episodes per year. This terminology, however, became confusing, because the term *rapid cycling* was also used to denote daily (ultradian) or every few days (ultrarapid) mood switches.

The disparities in how these episode-duration and rapid-cycling terms were used for bipolar I disorder in children are presented in Table 2.5. It can be noted that Wagner et al. (2006) found 17.1 ± 18.9 episodes per year, whereas Birmaher et al. (2006), Geller et al. (2004), Tohen et al. (2007), and the ongoing NIMH-funded multisite Treatment of Early Age Mania (TEAM) study found episode durations from 309.8 ± 749.6 days to 4.8 ± 2.6 years. Although it is possible that these are differences in the phenomenology of episode duration between samples, it is also possible that terminology is the reason for these discrepancies.

Table 2.6 presents a suggestion for clarity (Geller, Tillman, & Bolhofner,

TABLE 2.5. Current (Baseline) Episode Duration, n Lifetime Episodes, and % Daily (Ultradian) Cycling in Children with Full DSM-IV Criteria for Bipolar I Disorder

Author (year)	n	Age ± SD (years)	Prospective	Recruitment	SADS series tool	Blinded and controlled assessment	Current episode duration	% first episode	n lifetime episodes	% subjects with daily cycling
Geller et al. (2004)	86	10.8 ± 2.7	Yes	Consecutive new case	WASH-U	Yes	79.2 ± 66.7 weeks	81.4	1.2 ± 0.4	77.9
Biederman, Faraone, et al. (2005)	197	8.4 (SD N/A)	No	Consecutive referrals	E	No	N/A	N/A	N/A	N/A
Birmaher et al. (2006)	152	13.2 ± 3.0	Partly	Convenience	P/L	No	median 52.0 weeks	N/A	N/A	N/A[a]
Wagner et al. (2006)	115	Range 7–18	No	Convenience	P/L	No	N/A	N/A	17.1 ± 18.9[b]	N/A
TEAM (still recruiting)	306	10.2 ± 2.7	No	Convenience	WASH-U	No	4.8 ± 2.6 years	91.5	1.1 ± 0.3	98.7

Note. Adapted from Geller, Tillman, and Bolhofner (2007). Copyright by Mary Ann Liebert, Inc. Adapted by permission. TEAM, ongoing NIMH-funded multisite Treatment of Early Age Mania (TEAM) study; WASH-U-KSADS, Washington University in St. Louis Kiddie Schedule for Affective Disorders and Schizophrenia (Geller et al., 2001); KSADS-E, Kiddie Schedule for Affective Disorders and Schizophrenia—Epidemiologic Version (Orvaschel & Puig-Antich, 1987); KSADS-P/L, Kiddie Schedule for Affective Disorders and Schizophrenia—Present and Lifetime Version (Kaufman et al., 1997).

[a]These investigators reported 82.3% with mood lability, which may be measuring the same concept as daily cycling (Axelson et al., 2006).
[b]Number of episodes within past year in active drug group.

TABLE 2.6. Proposed Definitions of Episodes and Cycling Phenomena

Phenomenon	Definition
Episode	Onset to offset of full DSM-IV criteria for bipolar I disorder[a]
Ultra-rapid cycling[b]	Mood switches every few days during an episode
Ultradian cycling[b]	Mood switches multiple times daily during an episode

Note. Adapted from Geller, Tillman, and Bolhofner (2007). Copyright by Mary Ann Liebert, Inc. Adapted by permission.
[a]Episodes are defined using Frank et al. (1991) criteria.
[b]These terms are from Kramlinger and Post (1996).

2007). In this schema, episode duration would refer to the time frame from onset to offset of DSM-IV bipolar I symptoms. The term *rapid cycling* would no longer be used to denote multiple episodes per year. Rather, the word *cycling* would be used to denote switches every few days (e.g., 2 days high, 2 days low) or to denote daily mood switches (e.g., euphoric to euthymic, euphoric to depressed). Daily mood switches were reported to occur 3.7 ± 2.1 times per day during episodes with a mean duration of 3.6 ± 2.5 years (Geller, Zimerman, et al., 2002). Although 77.9–98.7% of bipolar I in children presents with daily mood switches (ultradian cycling; see Table 2.5), this phenomenon occurs in about 20% of adults with bipolar I (Goodwin & Jamison, 1990).

SUMMARY

The increasing consensus on the existence of and poor prognosis for bipolar I disorder in children across investigative groups warrants the attention to the treatment issues discussed in this chapter.

REFERENCES

Aman, M. G., DeSmedt, G., Derivan, A., Lyons, B., & Findling, R. L. (2002). Double-blind, placebo-controlled study of risperidone for the treatment of disruptive behaviors in children with subaverage intelligence. *American Journal of Psychiatry, 159*(8), 1337–1346.
Axelson, D., Birmaher, B., Strober, M., Gill, M. K., Valeri, S., Chiappetta, L., et al. (2006). Phenomenology of children and adolescents with bipolar spectrum disorders. *Archives of General Psychiatry, 63*(10), 1139–1148.
Biederman, J., Faraone, S. V., Chu, M. P., & Wozniak, J. (1999). Further evidence of a bidirectional overlap between juvenile mania and conduct disorder in children. *Journal of the American Academy of Child and Adolescent Psychiatry, 38*(4), 468–476.
Biederman, J., Faraone, S. V., Wozniak, J., Mick, E., Kwon, A., Cayton, G. A., et al. (2005). Clinical correlates of bipolar disorder in a large, referred sample of children and adolescents. *Journal of Psychiatric Research, 39*(6), 611–622.
Biederman, J., Monuteaux, M. C., Kendrick, E., Klein, K. L., & Faraone, S. V. (2005). The CBCL

as a screen for psychiatric comorbidity in paediatric patients with ADHD. *Archives of Disease in Childhood, 90*(10), 1010–1015.

Birmaher, B., Axelson, D., Strober, M., Gill, M. K., Valeri, S., Chiappetta, L., et al. (2006). Clinical course of children and adolescents with bipolar spectrum disorders. *Archives of General Psychiatry, 63*(2), 175–183.

Campbell, M., Adams, P. B., Small, A. M., Kafantaris, V., Silva, R. R., Shell, J., et al. (1995). Lithium in hospitalized aggressive children with conduct disorder: A double-blind and placebo-controlled study. *Journal of the American Academy of Child and Adolescent Psychiatry, 34*(4), 445–453.

Carlson, G. A., & Kelly, K. L. (1998). Manic symptoms in psychiatrically hospitalized children: What do they mean? *Journal of Affective Disorders, 51*(2), 123–135.

Chung, W. H., Hung, S. I., Hong, H. S., Hsih, M. S., Yang, L. C., Ho, H. C., et al. (2004). Medical genetics: A marker for Stevens–Johnson syndrome. *Nature, 428*(6982), 486.

Craney, J. L., & Geller, B. (2003). A prepubertal and early adolescent bipolar disorder I phenotype: Review of phenomenology and longitudinal course. *Bipolar Disorders, 5*(4), 243–256.

DelBello, M. P., Cecil, K. M., Adler, C. M., Daniels, J. P., & Strakowski, S. M. (2006). Neurochemical effects of olanzapine in first-hospitalization manic adolescents: A proton magnetic resonance spectroscopy study. *Neuropsychopharmacology, 31*(6), 1264–1273.

DelBello, M. P., Hanseman, D., Adler, C. M., Fleck, D. E., & Strakowski, S. M. (2007). Twelve-month outcome of adolescents with bipolar disorder following first hospitalization for a manic or mixed episode. *American Journal of Psychiatry, 164*(4), 582–590.

DelBello, M. P., Zimmerman, M. E., Mills, N. P., Getz, G. E., & Strakowski, S. M. (2004). Magnetic resonance imaging analysis of amygdala and other subcortical brain regions in adolescents with bipolar disorder. *Bipolar Disorders, 6*(1), 43–52.

Dickstein, D. P., Rich, B. A., Binstock, A. B., Pradella, A. G., Towbin, K. E., Pine, D. S., et al. (2005). Comorbid anxiety in phenotypes of pediatric bipolar disorder. *Journal of Child and Adolescent Psychopharmacology, 15*(4), 534–548.

Dienes, K. A., Chang, K. D., Blasey, C. M., Adleman, N. E., & Steiner, H. (2002). Characterization of children of bipolar parents by parent-report CBCL. *Journal of Psychiatric Research, 36*(5), 337–345.

Findling, R. L., Gracious, B. L., McNamara, N. K., Youngstrom, E. A., Demeter, C. A., Branicky, L. A., et al. (2001). Rapid, continuous cycling and psychiatric co-morbidity in pediatric bipolar I disorder. *Bipolar Disorders, 3*(4), 202–210.

Findling, R. L., McNamara, N. K., Youngstrom, E. A., Stansbrey, R., Gracious, B. L., Reed, M. D., et al. (2005). Double-blind 18-month trial of lithium versus divalproex maintenance treatment in pediatric bipolar disorder. *Journal of the American Academy of Child and Adolescent Psychiatry, 44*(5), 409–417.

Frank, E., Prien, R. F., Jarrett, R. B., Keller, M. B., Kupfer, D. J., Lavori, P. W., et al. (1991). Conceptualization and rationale for consensus definitions of terms in major depressive disorder: Remission, recovery, relapse, and recurrence. *Archives of General Psychiatry, 48*(9), 851–855.

Geller, B., Craney, J. L., Bolhofner, K., Nickelsburg, M. J., Williams, M., & Zimerman, B. (2002). Two-year prospective follow-up of children with a prepubertal and early adolescent bipolar disorder phenotype. *American Journal of Psychiatry, 59*(6), 927–933.

Geller, B., Tillman, R., & Bolhofner, K. (2007). Proposed definitions of bipolar I disorder episodes and daily rapid cycling phenomena in preschoolers, school-age children, adolescents, and adults. *Journal of Child and Adolescent Psychopharmacology, 17*(2), 217–222.

Geller, B., Tillman, R., Bolhofner, K., Zimerman, B., Strauss, N. A., & Kaufmann, P. (2006). Controlled, blindly rated, direct-interview family study of a prepubertal and early-adolescent bipolar I disorder phenotype: Morbid risk, age at onset, and comorbidity. *Archives of General Psychiatry, 63*(10), 1130–1138.

Geller, B., Tillman, R., Craney, J. L., & Bolhofner, K. (2004). Four-year prospective outcome and natural history of mania in children with a prepubertal and early adolescent bipolar disorder phenotype. *Archives of General Psychiatry, 61*(5), 459–467.

Geller, B., Warner, K., Williams, M., & Zimerman, B. (1998). Prepubertal and young adolescent bipolarity versus ADHD: Assessment and validity using the WASH-U-KSADS, CBCL and TRF. *Journal of Affective Disorders, 51*(2), 93–100.

Geller, B., Zimerman, B., Williams, M., Bolhofner, K., Craney, J. L., DelBello, M. P., et al. (2000). Diagnostic characteristics of 93 cases of a prepubertal and early adolescent bipolar disorder phenotype by gender, puberty and comorbid attention deficit hyperactivity disorder. *Journal of Child and Adolescent Psychopharmacology, 10*(3), 157–164.

Geller, B., Zimerman, B., Williams, M., DelBello, M. P., Bolhofner, K., Craney, J. L., et al. (2002). DSM-IV mania symptoms in a prepubertal and early adolescent bipolar disorder phenotype compared to attention-deficit hyperactive and normal controls. *Journal of Child and Adolescent Psychopharmacology, 12*(1), 11–25.

Goodwin, F. K., & Jamison, K. R. (Eds.). (1990). *Manic-depressive illness*. New York: Oxford University Press.

Hazell, P. L., Lewin, T. J., & Carr, V. J. (1999). Confirmation that Child Behavior Checklist clinical scales discriminate juvenile mania from attention deficit hyperactivity disorder. *Journal of Paediatrics and Child Health, 35*(2), 199–203.

Honig, A., Hofman, A., Hilwig, M., Noorthoorn, E., & Ponds, R. (1995). Psychoeducation and expressed emotion in bipolar disorder: Preliminary findings. *Psychiatry Research, 56*(3), 299–301.

Hudziak, J. J., Althoff, R. R., Derks, E. M., Faraone, S. V., & Boomsma, D. I. (2005). Prevalence and genetic architecture of Child Behavior Checklist—juvenile bipolar disorder. *Biological Psychiatry, 58*(7), 562–568.

Kahana, S. Y., Youngstrom, E. A., Findling, R. L., & Calabrese, J. R. (2003). Employing parent, teacher, and youth self-report checklists in identifying pediatric bipolar spectrum disorders: An examination of diagnostic accuracy and clinical utility. *Journal of Child and Adolescent Psychopharmacology, 13*(4), 471–488.

Kaufman, J., Birmaher, B., Brent, D., Rao, U., Flynn, C., Moreci, P., et al. (1997). Schedule for Affective Disorders and Schizophrenia for School-Age Children—Present and Lifetime Version (K-SADS-PL): Initial reliability and validity data. *Journal of the American Academy of Child and Adolescent Psychiatry, 36*(7), 980–988.

Kim-Cohen, J., Caspi, A., Moffitt, T. E., Harrington, H., Milne, B. J., & Poulton, R. (2003). Prior juvenile diagnoses in adults with mental disorder: Developmental follow-back of a prospective-longitudinal cohort. *Archives of General Psychiatry, 60*(7), 709–717.

Kramlinger, K. G., & Post, R. M. (1996). Ultra-rapid and ultradian cycling in bipolar affective illness. *British Journal of Psychiatry, 168*(3), 314–323.

Malone, R. P., Delaney, M. A., Luebbert, J. F., Cater, J., & Campbell, M. (2000). A double-blind placebo-controlled study of lithium in hospitalized aggressive children and adolescents with conduct disorder. *Archives of General Psychiatry, 57*(7), 649–654.

McCracken, J. T., McGough, J., Shah, B., Cronin, P., Hong, D., Aman, M. G., et al. (2002). Risperidone in children with autism and serious behavioral problems. *New England Journal of Medicine, 347*(5), 314–321.

Miklowitz, D. J., Goldstein, M. J., Nuechterlein, K. H., Snyder, K. S., & Mintz, J. (1988). Family factors and the course of bipolar affective disorder. *Archives of General Psychiatry, 45*(3), 225–231.

Orvaschel, H., & Puig-Antich, J. (1987). *Schedule for Affective Disorders and Schizophrenia for School-Age Children: Epidemiologic version*. Fort Lauderdale, FL: Nova University.

Ramana, R., & Bebbington, P. (1995). Social influences on bipolar affective disorders. *Social Psychiatry and Psychiatric Epidemiology, 30*(4),152–160.

Rucklidge, J. J. (2006). Impact of ADHD on the neurocognitive functioning of adolescents with bipolar disorder. *Biological Psychiatry, 60*(9), 921–988.

Schou, M. (1997). The combat of non-compliance during prophylactic lithium treatment. *Acta Psychiatrica Scandinavica*, 95(5), 361–363.

Strober, M., Morrell, W., Lampert, C., & Burroughs, J. (1990). Relapse following discontinuation of lithium maintenance therapy in adolescents with bipolar I illness: A naturalistic study. *American Journal of Psychiatry*, 147(4), 457–461.

Tohen, M., Kryzhanovskaya, L., Carlson, G., DelBello, M., Wozniak, J., Kowatch, R., et al. (2007). Olanzapine versus placebo in the treatment of adolescents with bipolar mania. *American Journal of Psychiatry*, 164(10), 1547–1556.

Volk, H. E., & Todd, R. D. (2007). Does the Child Behavior Checklist juvenile bipolar disorder phenotype identify bipolar disorder? *Biological Psychiatry*, 62(2), 115–120.

Wagner, K. D., Kowatch, R. A., Emslie, G. J., Findling, R. L., Wilens, T. E., McCague, K., et al. (2006). A double-blind, randomized, placebo-controlled trial of oxcarbazepine in the treatment of bipolar disorder in children and adolescents. *American Journal of Psychiatry*, 163(7), 1179–1186.

Wozniak, J., Biederman, J., Kiely, K., Ablon, J. S., Faraone, S. V., Mundy, E., et al. (1995). Mania-like symptoms suggestive of childhood-onset bipolar disorder in clinically referred children. *Journal of the American Academy of Child and Adolescent Psychiatry*, 34(7), 867–876.

Yang, L., Wang, Y. F., Li, J., & Faraone, S. V. (2004). Association of norepinephrine transporter gene with methylphenidate response. *Journal of the American Academy of Child and Adolescent Psychiatry*, 43(9), 1154–1158.

Youngstrom, E., Youngstrom, J. K., & Starr, M. (2005). Bipolar diagnoses in community mental health: Achenbach Child Behavior Checklist profiles and patterns of comorbidity. *Biological Psychiatry*, 58(7), 569–575.

CHAPTER 3

Neuropharmacology

NICK C. PATEL *and* MELISSA P. DELBELLO

Pediatric bipolar disorder is characterized by recurrent episodes of mania and depression, which may have a negative impact on a child's ability to function and lead to poor psychosocial functioning (Adleman, Barnea-Goraly, & Chang, 2004). Stabilization of acute mood episodes and prevention of relapse and recurrence are among the primary treatment goals for children and adolescents with bipolar disorder. Lithium, anticonvulsants such as valproate and lamotrigine, and atypical antipsychotics are considered first-line treatments for patients with bipolar disorder (Kowatch et al., 2005; Suppes et al., 2005). Although these medications all have been shown to improve symptoms associated with bipolar disorder, the exact mechanisms by which these medications exert mood-stabilizing effects remain unknown (DelBello & Strakowski, 2004). An appreciation of the *in vivo* neurochemical activity of mood-stabilizing medications may help clarify the neuropathophysiology of bipolar disorder. In addition, approximately half of bipolar patients respond to monotherapy of any single agent. Most patients require combinations of medications in order to achieve optimal mood stabilization (Bhangoo et al., 2003; Frye et al., 2000). Clinical predictors of treatment response have been identified, including polarity of episodes, co-occurring psychiatric disorders, and family history of treatment response (Gelenberg & Pies, 2003). However, these predictors may have limited utility for individual patients in the clinical setting. Biological markers for treatment response may be more useful in individualizing treatment planning.

Magnetic resonance spectroscopy (MRS) is a noninvasive neuroimaging technique that provides *in vivo* information regarding the concentrations of specific neurometabolites in localized regions of the brain. MRS allows for the determination of the *in vivo* neurochemical effects of medications commonly used in bipolar patients. Furthermore, MRS allows for the identification of biological markers for treatment response. Garnering such information may contribute toward targeted treatment interventions with a higher probability of response and a subsequent improvement in patient psychosocial functioning.

OVERVIEW OF MRS

MRS is a noninvasive technique that has been more recently used in studies examining the neuropathophysiology of bipolar disorder in the pediatric and adult populations. A major advantage of MRS when used in this context is that no ionizing radiation is used, which allows for serial measurements of neurometabolites in an individual. MRS studies in patients with bipolar disorder have used proton (^{1}H), lithium (^{7}Li), or phosphorus (^{31}P) spectroscopies, with the most used being ^{1}H MRS. The fundamental goal of ^{1}H MRS is to detect signals from small concentrations of neurometabolites, measured in parts per million (ppm), in a large concentration of water contained in a specific region of interest in the brain over a narrow frequency range (Figure 3.1). Practical and precise localization, the best field homogeneity possible, and effective water suppression are critical with ^{1}H MRS. Other isotopes can be evaluated (carbon [^{13}C], fluorine [^{19}F], and

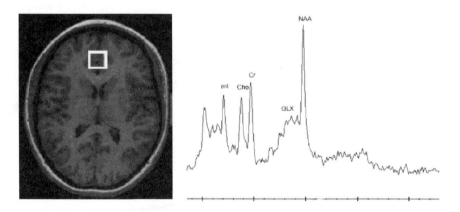

FIGURE 3.1. Proton magnetic resonance spectrum acquired within the medial prefrontal cortex of an adolescent male with bipolar disorder. Cho, choline; Cr, creatine/creatine phosphate; GLX, glutamate/glutamine/GABA; mI, *myo*-inositol; NAA, *N*-acetyl aspartate.

sodium [^{23}Na]). Details of the concepts and applications of MRS for each isotope have been reviewed elsewhere (Kato, Inubushi, & Kato, 1998; Post, Speer, Hough, & Xing, 2003; Soares, Krishnan, & Keshavan, 1996; Strakowski, DelBello, Adler, Cecil, & Sax, 2000).

The neurometabolites generally observed using ^{1}H MRS include N-acetyl aspartate (NAA), *myo*-inositol (mI), choline-containing compounds (Cho), creatine/creatine phosphate (Cr), and glutamate/glutamine/γ-aminobutyric acid (GLX; Figure 3.1). The major metabolite peaks observed using ^{31}P MRS include α-, β-, and γ-adenine triphosphate (ATP), phosphocreatine (PCr), phosphodiester compounds (PDE), inorganic phosphate (Pi), and phosphomonoester compounds (PME; Figure 3.2). The PME and PDE peaks are from membrane phospholipids and reflect membrane metabolism. ^{7}Li MRS has been used to measure brain tissue lithium concentrations *in vivo*. Studies using ^{7}Li MRS have investigated the pharmacokinetics of lithium in the human brain and evaluated brain lithium concentrations in relation to serum lithium concentrations, clinical response, and side effects in patients with bipolar disorder.

PROTON MRS

N-Acetyl Aspartate

NAA is an amino acid localized to neurons and has been accepted as a putative marker of neuronal integrity (Tsai & Coyle, 1995). NAA has been shown to increase during brain development in childhood and to decrease with older age (Charles et al., 1994; van der Knapp et al., 1990). A de-

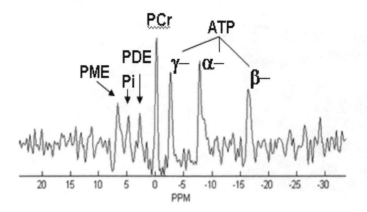

FIGURE 3.2. Phosphorus magnetic resonance spectrum acquired within the anterior cingulate cortex. ATP, adenine triphosphate; PCr, phosphocreatine; PDE, phosphodiester compounds; Pi, inorganic phosphate; PME, phosphomonoester compounds.

crease in NAA may suggest the loss, the impaired functioning, or the decreased viability of neurons. Because NAA is reduced by mitochondrial respiratory chain inhibitors and produced in the mitochondria, a decrease in NAA may reflect impaired mitochondrial energy production (DelBello & Strakowski, 2004).

Decreased concentrations of NAA have been observed in several regions of the brain in adults with bipolar disorder, including the dorsolateral prefrontal cortex (DLPFC; Winsberg et al., 2000), prefrontal gray matter (Cecil, DelBello, Morey, & Strakowski, 2002), and hippocampus (Bertolino et al., 2003; Deicken, Pegues, Anzalone, Feiwell, & Soher, 2003). In youths with bipolar disorder in themselves and their families, decreased NAA in the DLPFC (Chang et al., 2003; Sassi et al., 2005) has been reported, albeit not consistently (Gallelli et al., 2005). Decreased NAA has also been observed in the cerebellar vermis (Cecil, DelBello, Sellars, & Strakowski, 2003). In contrast, no abnormalities in NAA were reported in the frontal and temporal cortices (Castillo, Kwock, Courvoisie, & Hooper, 2000) or anterior cingulate cortex (ACC; Davanzo et al., 2001; Davanzo et al., 2003). Despite conflicting preliminary data, perhaps due to differences in patient selection and study methodologies, neuronal dysfunction or degeneration may indeed occur early in the course of illness within specific prefrontal regions.

Lithium is considered a first-line treatment option in bipolar disorder, and it has been studied in pediatric bipolar mania and depression (Kafantaris, Coletti, Dicker, Padula, & Kane, 2003; Kowatch et al., 2000; Patel, DelBello, Bryan, et al., 2006). It has been suggested that lithium may possess neurotrophic effects, resulting in increases in brain NAA. Some ^{1}H MRS studies of adult patients with bipolar disorder have supported this notion (Brambilla et al., 2005; Moore, Bebchuk, et al., 2000; Sharma, Venkatasubramanian, Barany, & Davis, 1992; Silverstone et al., 2003), whereas others have not (Kato, Hamakawa, et al., 1996; Ohara et al., 1998). Specifically, lithium treatment was associated with increased NAA in the DLPFC, frontal and temporal lobes, and basal ganglia (BG), suggesting that the neurotrophic effects of lithium may be specific to localized brain regions in patients with bipolar disorder. There are limited data evaluating the treatment effects of lithium on NAA concentrations in pediatric patients with bipolar disorder. In the ACC, lithium treatment (7 days) was not associated with an increase in NAA (Davanzo et al., 2001). Similarly, lithium exposure did not correlate with NAA/Cr ratios in the DLPFC of youths with bipolar disorder (Gallelli et al., 2005).

Few ^{1}H MRS studies examining the treatment effects of other psychotropic medications commonly used in patients with bipolar disorder on NAA exist. Valproate, which is effective in the treatment of pediatric bipolar mania (Kowatch et al., 2000; Wagner et al., 2002), has been shown to have no significant effect on NAA (Gallelli et al., 2005; Silverstone et al.,

2003). In fact, Cecil et al. (2002) reported that a longer duration of valproate exposure was associated with lower NAA concentrations in the orbital frontal gray matter of adults with bipolar disorder, suggesting valproate may not have neurotrophic effects. On the contrary, treatment (4 weeks) with the atypical antipsychotic olanzapine in first-hospitalization adolescents with mania resulted in an increase in frontal gray matter NAA, suggesting that olanzapine may have neuroprotective effects or may normalize mitochondrial dysfunction in bipolar disorder (DelBello, Cecil, Adler, Daniels, & Strakowski, 2006). Lamotrigine, an anticonvulsant effective for adolescent bipolar depression (Chang, Saxena, & Howe, 2006), also may have neurogenic effects, as it increased NAA/Cr ratios in the DLPFC over an 8-week period (Chang et al., 2005). There are no data available examining the effects of carbamazapine and other atypical antipsychotics on NAA concentrations in bipolar disorder.

Myo-Inositol

For several decades, inositol metabolism has been postulated to play a significant role in the etiology and treatment effects of bipolar disorder. mI is a sugar involved in cellular second-messenger signaling pathways, including the phosphoinositide cycle. It is through this major second-messenger system that lithium is thought to exert its mood-stabilization effects in bipolar disorder. Depletion of mI may dampen the phosphoinositide cycle in overactive neural networks of patients with bipolar disorder (Allison & Stewart, 1971; Berridge, 1989).

Available ^{1}H MRS data in adults with bipolar disorder do not support an alteration in brain mI concentrations (Cecil et al., 2002; Dager et al., 2004; Moore, Breeze, et al., 2000; Silverstone et al., 2002; Winsberg et al., 2000). In contrast, elevated mI has been observed in the medial prefrontal cortex of euthymic children with bipolar disorder compared with healthy controls (Cecil et al., 2003; DelBello, Adler, & Strakowski 2006). Elevated mI/Cr ratios have also been reported in the ACC of children with bipolar mania compared with children with intermittent explosive disorder and healthy controls (Davanzo et al., 2001; Davanzo et al., 2003). One study showed that children at risk for developing bipolar disorder had higher mI concentrations in ventral prefrontal gray matter than healthy controls (Cecil et al., 2003). Elevated mI in youths with or at risk for bipolar disorder may indeed be localized specifically to the ACC and ventral prefrontal region. Such abnormalities in mI have not been observed in the DLPFC of euthymic children with bipolar disorder who are on medication (Chang et al., 2003), symptomatic children with bipolar disorder who are on medication (Gallelli et al., 2005), or children at risk for bipolar disorder (Gallelli et al., 2005).

Compared with other medications used for the treatment of bipolar disorder, lithium has by far been the most extensively studied medication with regard to its effects on brain mI. No difference in mI concentrations in prefrontal and temporal regions of the brain were observed between adult patients with bipolar disorder receiving lithium and healthy controls (Brambilla et al., 2005; Moore, Breeze, et al., 2000; Silverstone et al., 2002). Similarly, Chang et al. (2003) reported no significant difference in DLPFC mI/Cr ratios in euthymic youths with bipolar disorder compared with healthy controls. In this particular study, 36% of youths with bipolar disorder had had exposure to lithium. These data suggest that normalization of alterations in mI may occur with lithium.

There are a limited number of ^{1}H MRS studies that examine the temporal effects of lithium on mI in adults and children. To date, there are no ^{1}H MRS studies that evaluate the temporal effects of lithium in adults with acute mania. Such studies in adults with bipolar depression have produced conflicting results. In one study, lithium administration over 3–4 weeks decreased frontal lobe mI compared with baseline (Moore et al., 1999); it is important to note that when appropriate statistical procedures were used, this decrease was not significant. Increased mI concentrations in regional gray matter were reported following 5–7 months of lithium treatment in another study of adult bipolar depression (Friedman et al., 2004). These discrepant results may be explained by the duration of exposure to lithium, as changes in enzyme activity may occur with continued lithium treatment (Kaya, Resmi, Ozerdem, Guner, & Tunca, 2004). In adult healthy volunteers, treatment with lithium did not affect mI (Brambilla et al., 2004; Silverstone, Hanstock, Fabian, Staab, & Allen, 1996; Silverstone, Rotzinger, Pukhovsky, & Hanstock, 1999), suggesting that lithium effects on mI may be specific to bipolar patients.

Acute lithium treatment in children with mania or mixed mania resulted in a significant reduction in ACC mI/Cr ratios from baseline to week 1 (Davanzo et al., 2001). This reduction was specifically present in responders, suggesting that a decrease in ACC mI/Cr ratio may indeed predict improvement in manic symptoms. A recent study of open-label lithium in adolescents with bipolar depression evaluated the acute (1 week) and chronic (6 weeks) effects of lithium on medial and left and right lateral ventral prefrontal mI (Patel, DelBello, Cecil, et al., 2006). In contrast to the findings in pediatric bipolar mania, mI concentrations in these prefrontal regions at weeks 1 and 6 were not different from those at baseline. These results indicate that in adolescents with bipolar depression, the mechanism by which lithium exerts antidepressant activity may not be consistent with the inositol depletion hypothesis (Berridge, 1989). Interestingly, mI concentrations at week 6 were significantly higher than those at week 1 in the medial and right lateral ventral prefrontal cortices (Patel, DelBello, Cecil, et al., 2006), suggesting that the acute effects may not be sustained with continued administration.

The effects of other psychotropic medications on brain mI concentration have not been extensively studied. Normalization of mI concentrations in frontal, prefrontal, and temporal regions of the brain has been reported in adults (Cecil et al., 2002; Moore, Breeze, et al., 2000; Silverstone et al., 2002) and children (Chang et al., 2003) previously exposed to or on valproate. However, chronic valproate treatment has not been shown to significantly affect regional gray matter or ACC mI in adults (Friedman et al., 2004; Moore, Breeze, et al., 2000). In an unpublished study of children with bipolar disorder, no significant difference was observed in mI/Cr ratios in the ACC before and after divalproex treatment (Davanzo et al., 2002). Treatment with olanzapine also did not significantly affect prefrontal mI of adolescents with bipolar disorder who were experiencing a manic or mixed episode (DelBello, Cecil, et al., 2006). In contrast, an increase in DLPFC mI/Cr ratios was reported with lamotrigine treatment in adolescents with bipolar depression (Chang et al., 2005). There are no data available examining the effects of carbamazapine and other atypical antipsychotics on mI concentrations in bipolar disorder.

Choline

The Cho peak mainly consists of phosphorylcholine and glycerophosphorylcholine and represents a potential biomarker for membrane phospholipid metabolism. Increases in Cho may indicate membrane catabolism, which may be reflective of neurodegenerative conditions (Moore & Galloway, 2002).

Evidence from ^{1}H MRS studies in adult patients with bipolar disorder suggests that Cho is elevated in the BG during euthymia (Hamakawa, Kato, Murashita, & Kato, 1998; Kato, Hamakawa, et al., 1996), and in the ACC and BG during a depressive episode (Hamakawa et al., 1998; Moore, Breeze, et al., 2000). In the study by Moore, Breeze, et al. (2000), severity of depressive symptoms positively correlated with ACC Cho concentrations. One study of adults with bipolar mania has reported a trend of decreased Cho in the medial prefrontal gray matter (Cecil et al., 2002); however, others have reported no alterations in Cho in the DLFPC (Michael et al., 2003) and hippocampus (Blasi et al., 2004). In euthymic pediatric patients with bipolar disorder, no differences in Cho concentrations across various brain regions have been observed as compared with healthy controls (Castillo et al., 2000; Cecil et al., 2003; Chang et al., 2003; Chang et al., 2005; Sassi et al., 2005). Decreased ACC Cho/Cr ratios have been reported in children with bipolar mania (Davanzo et al., 2003), although this finding has not been consistent (Davanzo et al., 2001). Alterations in Cho in bipolar patients may be regional, although additional studies are needed for replication.

Because lithium inhibits choline transport, which results in increased intracellular choline, a decrease in the Cho peak should be observed with lithium administration. Indeed, cross-sectional ^{1}H MRS studies in adult bipolar disorder have shown similar or decreased Cho in patients versus healthy controls, supporting the normalization or decreasing effect of lithium on Cho concentrations (Brambilla et al., 2005; Ohara et al., 1998; Kato, Hamakawa, et al., 1996; Wu et al., 2004). The aforementioned longitudinal study by Moore et al. (1999) also showed decreased frontal Cho with lithium administration. Increased Cho in the ACC and BG has been observed in patients treated with lithium (Sharma et al., 1992; Soares et al., 1999), but these results may be limited by the small sample sizes. In children and adolescents, lithium administration during a manic or depressive episode did not affect Cho in the prefrontal region (Davanzo et al., 2001; Patel, DelBello, Cecil, et al., 2006).

There are limited data evaluating the effects of valproate and other psychotropic medications on Cho in bipolar disorder. Similar to lithium, valproate may decrease Cho concentrations, as demonstrated in one ^{1}H MRS study of the temporal lobe of euthymic patients with bipolar disorder (Wu et al., 2004). However, in a separate sample of euthymic adults with bipolar disorder, this same group of investigators did not find any difference between patients on valproate and healthy controls (Wu et al., 2004). Antidepressant use may also normalize ACC Cho (Moore, Breeze, et al., 2000). In contrast, olanzapine-induced increases in prefrontal Cho have been reported in adolescents with bipolar disorder who were experiencing a manic or mixed episode (DelBello, Cecil, et al., 2006). The authors suggest that an increase in prefrontal Cho may initiate intracellular events that subsequently lead to the dampening of overactive second-messenger systems or membrane effects (DelBello, Cecil, et al., 2006). In the same study, higher baseline medial prefrontal Cho predicted symptom remission, identifying a potential biomarker for successful treatment with olanzapine. No data are available that examine the effects of carbamazapine, lamotrigine, or other atypical antipsychotics on Cho in youths with bipolar disorder.

Creatine/Creatine Phosphate

The Cr peak, which consists of both phosphorylated and dephosphorylated creatine, is assumed to be stable, possibly allowing it to be used as an internal reference in ^{1}H MRS studies. Although Cr is often used in reporting concentrations of other neurometabolites as ratios in studies of patients with bipolar disorder, the stability of the Cr peak in this population has yet to be determined (Glitz, Manji, & Moore, 2002). To address this methodological issue, concentrations of neurometabolites may be determined using water as an internal reference through the use of appropriate fitting techniques, such as the LC Model program (Provencher, 1993).

Although nonsignificant differences in Cr in the BG (Hamakawa et al., 1998) and prefrontal (Cecil et al., 2002; Michael et al., 2003) and frontal (Dager et al., 2004; Friedman et al., 2004; Hamakawa, Kato, Shioiri,

Inubushi, & Kato, 1999) structures have been observed across mood states in adults with bipolar disorder, one study of euthymic patients has reported decreased Cr in the hippocampus (Deicken et al., 2003), and another study has reported increased Cr in the thalamus (Deicken, Eliaz, Feiwell, & Schuff, 2001). Hamakawa et al. (1999) reported lower frontal cortex Cr concentrations in adults with bipolar depression as compared with euthymic adults with bipolar disorder. In euthymic youths with bipolar disorder, trends of decreased Cr in the cerebellar vermis (Cecil et al., 2003) and DLPFC (Sassi et al., 2005) have been reported. In contrast, no alterations in medial prefrontal cortex Cr in euthymic children with bipolar disorder(Cecil et al., 2003) and ACC Cr in children with bipolar mania (Davanzo et al., 2003) were seen. Alterations in Cr concentrations may represent abnormal cellular energy metabolism in patients with bipolar disorder and may suggest that the use of Cr peaks as a standard may not be appropriate in ^1H MRS studies of bipolar disorder.

Very few studies have evaluated medication effects on Cr in bipolar disorder. Antipsychotic treatment has been shown to be associated with higher BG Cr concentrations, whereas benzodiazepine treatment has been associated with lower BG Cr concentrations (Hamakawa et al., 1998). Lithium and valproate did not alter regional gray matter Cr in adult patients with bipolar depression (Friedman et al., 2004). Similarly, lithium and olanzapine did not significantly affect prefrontal Cr in adolescents with depression and mania, respectively (DelBello, Cecil, et al., 2006; Patel, DelBello, Cecil, et al., 2006). No data are available that examine the effects of carbamazapine, lamotrigine, and other atypical antipsychotics on Cr concentrations in bipolar disorder.

Glutamate/Glutamine/GABA

The GLX peak includes glutamate, glutamine, and γ-aminobutyric acid (GABA) and is considered a marker of glutamatergic neurotransmission. Neurotoxicity is represented by sustained increases in glutamate. Increased GLX has been reported in prefrontal white matter (Cecil et al., 2002) and DLFPC (Michael et al., 2003) of adult patients with bipolar disorder experiencing acute mania. Higher GLX and lactate concentrations were also found in the ACC gray matter of adult patients with bipolar depression compared with healthy controls (Dager et al., 2004). In pediatric bipolar disorder, increased GLX was observed in the frontal and temporal lobes of euthymic patients (Castillo et al., 2000), but no alterations in ACC GLX were found in patients with mania (Davanzo et al., 2001; Davanzo et al., 2003). These findings suggest that neurotoxicity may occur early in the course of this illness and may be specific to certain regions. Alternatively, abnormal cellular metabolism secondary to mitochondrial dysfunction may potentially explain these findings (Dager et al., 2004).

There are limited data evaluating the effects of psychotropic medications on GLX in bipolar disorder. In one study of adults with bipolar depression, lithium induced decreases in GLX concentrations in regional gray matter, but valproate did not (Friedman et al., 2004). No effect on GLX has been reported with lithium and olanzapine treatment in children with bipolar mania (Davanzo et al., 2001; DelBello, Cecil, et al., 2006), or with lithium treatment in adolescents with bipolar depression (Patel, DelBello, Cecil, et al., 2006). There are no data available examining the effects of carbamazapine, lamotrigine, and other atypical antipsychotics on GLX concentrations in bipolar disorder.

PHOSPHORUS MRS

Despite the utility of phosphorus magnetic resonance spectroscopy (^{31}P MRS) in the investigation of phospholipid metabolism, this technique continues to be limited in sensitivity and spatial resolution. A limited number of ^{31}P MRS studies of patients with bipolar disorder exist, with most of these coming from two particular research groups. In summary, ^{31}P MRS studies of PME in bipolar disorder have suggested the possibility of state-dependent abnormalities in phospholipid metabolism. Specifically, patients in the manic and depressive phases of the illness have been shown to have increased PME in the frontal lobe, as compared with euthymic patients (Kato, Shioiri, Takahashi, & Inubushi, 1991; Kato, Takahashi, Shioiri, & Inubushi, 1992; Kato, Takahashi, Shioiri, & Inubushi, 1993). Lower frontal and temporal PME concentrations have been observed in euthymic patients with bipolar disorder compared with healthy controls (Deicken, Fein, & Weiner, 1995; Deicken, Weiner, & Fein, 1995; Kato, Takahashi, Shioiri, & Inubushi, 1992; Kato, Takahashi, et al., 1993; Kato, Shioiri, et al., 1994).

Lithium inhibits inositol monophosphatase, resulting in increased inositol monophosphate, as well as an increase in the PME peak. It has been reported that lithium-associated increases in PME concentrations may normalize with continued lithium administration (Renshaw, Summers, Renshaw, Hines, & Leigh, 1986). ^{31}P MRS studies of lithium-treated patients in manic and depressive states have reported increased PME (Kato et al., 1991; Kato, Takahashi, et al., 1993; Kato, Takahashi, et al., 1994; Kato et al., 1995). Interestingly, Kato et al. (1991) found that frontal PME concentrations in lithium-treated patients with bipolar mania were higher than those in lithium-treated euthymic patients with bipolar disorder, suggesting that elevations in PME during the manic phase may not be fully attributable to lithium. Furthermore, PME concentrations in euthymic patients and patients with bipolar mania did not correlate with brain lithium concentrations (Kato, Takahashi, et al., 1993). Lower intracellular pH has been found to be a predictor of lithium response and is thought to be related to the pathophysiology of lithium responsiveness rather than to the direct pharmacological effects of lithium (Kato, Inubushi, & Kato, 2000). PME/ PCr peak ratios did not change in healthy participants following lithium administration (Silverstone et al., 1996), possibly suggesting that lithium effects on PME may be limited to patients with bipolar disorder. Studies of patients with bipolar disorder using both ^{1}H and ^{31}P MRS techniques in the same regions in the brain may clarify mechanisms of action and predictors of response to medications.

LITHIUM MRS

Lithium magnetic resonance spectroscopy (^{7}Li MRS) can be used to measure both the steady-state concentration and the pharmacokinetics of brain Li in patients with bipolar disorder without localization to particular regions of brain (Soares, Boada, & Keshavan, 2000). ^{7}Li MRS is still at a relatively early stage of development, and little *in vivo* ^{7}Li MRS has been done, particularly in patients with bipolar disorder. Several studies have found positive correlations between brain and serum lithium concentrations, but brain concentrations were lower than serum concentrations (Gyulai et al., 1991; Kato, Takahashi, & Inubushi, 1992; Kato, Shioiri, Inubushi, & Takahashi, 1993; Kato, Inubushi, & Takahashi, 1994; Sachs et al., 1995). This particular finding suggests that some patients who have therapeutic serum lithium levels may have subtherapeutic brain lithium levels (Sachs et al., 1995). Also, 12-hour brain lithium concentration may be independent of dosing schedule of lithium (daily vs. alternate day), although patients with alternate-day lithium dosing have an increased risk of relapse (Jensen et al., 1996). Recently, Moore et al. (2002) reported that brain-to-serum lithium concentration ratio positively correlated with age. Thus, children and adolescents may need higher maintenance serum lithium concentrations to ensure therapeutic brain concentrations.

Few studies have examined brain lithium concentration as a predictor of lithium response or side effects. Brain concentrations may, in fact, be better predictors of toxicity than serum concentrations. For example, Kato, Fujii, Shioiri, Inubushi, and Takahashi (1996) showed that brain concentration of lithium was significantly associated with hand tremor, whereas serum concentration was not. Kato, Inubushi, and Takahashi (1994) also showed that treatment response to lithium is related to brain concentration.

FUNCTIONAL MAGNETIC RESONANCE IMAGING

Functional magnetic resonance imaging (fMRI) allows the comparison of oxygenated with deoxygenated blood to determine the relative activation of brain regions (Adleman et al., 2004). This technique, although relatively new, is useful for evaluating brain activation patterns in patients with psychiatric disorders during cognitive or affective tasks. However, the use of fMRI in children and adolescents poses some unique challenges, including coordination of mood state in youths with rapid cycling.

To date, fMRI studies have demonstrated differential activation in frontostriatal circuits in children with bipolar disorder (Blumberg et al., 2003; Chang et al., 2004; Rich et al., 2006). In an fMRI study of 10 adolescents with bipolar disorder and 10 healthy controls, Blumberg et al. (2003) reported increased activation in left putamen and thalamus in adolescents with bipolar disorder while they were performing a color-naming Stroop task. However, adolescents with bipolar disorder did not have the normal age-related activation increases in the rostral ventral prefrontal cortex that were observed in healthy control participants.

Chang et al. (2004) used a visuospatial working-memory task and an affective task to compare brain activation between 12 euthymic medicated boys with bipolar disorder and 10 matched healthy boys. For the visuospatial working-memory task, boys with bipolar disorder exhibited greater activation in the bilateral anterior cingulate, left putamen, left thalamus, left DLPFC, and right inferior frontal gyrus, whereas healthy control participants showed greater activation in the cerebellar vermis. Boys with bipolar disorder showed greater activation in the bilateral DLPFC, inferior frontal gyrus, and right insula than healthy boys when they were viewing negatively valenced pictures; healthy participants showed greater activation in the right posterior cingulate. When viewing positively valenced pictures, boys with bipolar disorder exhibited greater activation in the bilateral caudate and thalamus, left middle/superior frontal gyrus, and left anterior cingulate.

More recently, Rich et al. (2006) used emotional versus nonemotional face processing to compare neuronal activation in 22 youths with bipolar disorder and 21 healthy control participants. Youths with bipolar disorder showed greater activation in the left amygdala, accumbens, putamen, and ventral prefrontal cortex when rating face hostility and greater activation in the left amygdala and bilateral accumbens when rating their fear of the face.

Using fMRI, Adler et al. (2005) evaluated neuronal activation in adolescents with bipolar disorder and comorbid attention-deficit/hyperactivity disorder (ADHD) versus those without comorbid ADHD. Eleven youths with bipolar disorder and ADHD and 15 with bipolar disorder but without ADHD, all of whom were medication-free for a minimum of 2 weeks, performed a single-digit continuous-performance task alternated with a control task in a block-design paradigm. Comorbid ADHD was associated with greater activation in the posterior parietal cortex and middle temporal gyrus and with less activation in the ventrolateral prefrontal cortex and anterior cingulate. These findings preliminarily indicate variations in neuronal activation of bipolar patients when comorbid ADHD is present.

Most youths with bipolar disorder in these fMRI studies, with the exception of the study by Adler et al. (2005), were receiving medication, which makes it difficult to determine whether differences in activation are related to the pathophysiology of the disorder or to medication effects. Future fMRI studies employing methodologies designed to evaluate medication effects will help clarify whether mood-stabilizing agents, either as monotherapy or in combination, do indeed alter brain activation in patients with bipolar disorder.

CONCLUSION

MRS techniques have clearly revolutionized our ability to study the neurochemical activity of mood-stabilizing medications, furthering our understanding of the neuropathophysiology of bipolar disorder. MRS studies of children and adolescents with bipolar disorder suggest neurochemical abnormalities in the frontal lobe, specifically in the ACC and DLFPC. It may be in these regions that certain psychotropic medications, such as lithium and olanzapine, act to normalize such abnormalities.

MRS techniques will continue to be used as a research tool to understand the neurochemical effects of medications used in bipolar disorder and to predict treatment response to specific medications. Future MRS studies need to address methodological limitations that currently exist. First, few studies have evaluated patients with bipolar disorder before and after treatment with a single medication. Ideally, study designs such as that used by DelBello, Cecil, et al. (2006), will help to clarify which neurochemical changes are inherent to the neuropathophysiology associated with bipolar disorder and which result from both acute and chronic medication effects. Second, variability in study samples and brain region studies have contributed to difficulties in interpretation. For example, some ^{1}H MRS studies have included patients in different mood states. As neurochemical abnormalities may be state-dependent, future studies should strive to improve patient homogeneity. Variability of brain regions studied makes it difficult to discern whether neurochemical differences are due to differing MRS methodologies or to actual underlying regional neurochemical differences. Studies should examine brain networks, such as the anterior limbic network, that appear to function abnormally in bipolar disorder. Third, the identification of potential neurochemical predictors of successful treatment requires the longitudinal use of symptom rating scales with established reliability that are administered by trained raters. Finally, most MRS studies to date have evaluated the neurochemical effects of lithium. Emerging data are examining the effects of other medications, such as valproate, lamotrigine, and atypical antipsychotics. Future studies not only should aim to evaluate the effects of a single medication but also should evaluate other management strategies, including combination pharmacological treatment.

Technological advances will also improve the conduct of future MRS studies. More recent MRS sampling techniques, particularly whole-brain or multislice chemical-shift imaging methods, allow for the assessment of a larger region of interest with greater spatial resolution. Perhaps more important, such assessments will be able to be conducted over a shorter period of time, which is a critical factor with children and adolescents with bipolar disorder. The use of higher field strength, such as 3 Tesla or 4 Tesla, will improve the spectral resolution of neurometabolite signals.

In spite of its current limitations, MRS holds considerable promise as a tool to further our understanding of the neuropathophysiology of bipolar disorder and the mechanisms of action of mood-stabilizing medications and to identify biological markers of treatment response. Such knowledge will ultimately help guide clinicians in better tailoring pharmacological treatment regimens to individual patients in order to achieve favorable outcomes, including improved long-term prognoses.

REFERENCES

Adleman, N. E., Barnea-Goraly, N., & Chang, K. D. (2004). Review of magnetic resonance imaging and spectroscopy studies in children with bipolar disorder. *Expert Review of Neurotherapeutics, 4*, 69–77.

Adler, C. M., DelBello, M. P., Mills, N. P., Schmithorst, V., Holland, S., & Strakowski, S. M. (2005). Comorbid ADHD is associated with altered patterns of neuronal activation in adolescents with bipolar disorder performing a simple attention task. *Bipolar Disorders, 7*, 577–588.

Allison, J. H., & Stewart, M. A. (1971). Reduced brain inositol in lithium-treated rats. *Nature: New Biology, 233*, 267–268.

Berridge, M. J. (1989). The Albert Lasker Medical Awards: Inositol trisphosphate, calcium, lithium, and cell signaling. *Journal of the American Medical Association, 262*, 1834–1841.

Bertolino, A., Frye, M., Callicott, J. H., Mattay, V. S., Rakow, R., Shelton-Repella, J., et al. (2003). Neuronal pathology in the hippocampal area of patients with bipolar disorder: A study with proton magnetic resonance spectroscopic imaging. *Biological Psychiatry, 53*, 906–913.

Bhangoo, R. K., Lowe, C. H., Myers, F. S., Treland, J., Curran, J., Towbin, K. E., et al. (2003). Medication use in children and adolescents treated in the community for bipolar disorder. *Journal of Child and Adolescent Psychopharmacology, 13*, 515–522.

Blasi, G., Bertolino, A., Brudaglio, F., Sciota, D., Altamura, M., Antonucci, N., et al. (2004). Hippocampal neurochemical pathology in patients at first episode of affective psychosis: A proton magnetic resonance spectroscopic imaging study. *Psychiatry Research, 131*, 95–105.

Blumberg, H. P., Martin, A., Kaufman, J., Leung, H. C., Skudlarski, P., Lacadie, C., et al. (2003). Frontostriatal abnormalities in adolescents with bipolar disorder: Preliminary observations from functional MRI. *American Journal of Psychiatry, 160*, 1345–1347.

Brambilla, P., Stanley, J. A., Nicoletti, M. A., Sassi, R. B., Mallinger, A. G., Frank, E., et al.

(2005). 1H magnetic resonance spectroscopy investigation of the dorsolateral prefrontal cortex in bipolar disorder patients. *Journal of Affective Disorders, 86,* 61–67.

Brambilla, P., Stanley, J. A., Sassi, R. B., Nicoletti, M. A., Mallinger, A. G., Keshavan, M. S., et al. (2004). 1H MRS study of dorsolateral prefrontal cortex in healthy individuals before and after lithium administration. *Neuropsychopharmacology, 29,* 1918–1924.

Castillo, M., Kwock, L., Courvoisie, H., & Hooper, S. R. (2000). Proton MR spectroscopy in children with bipolar affective disorder: Preliminary observations. *American Journal of Neuroradiology, 21,* 832–838.

Cecil, K. M., DelBello, M. P., Morey, R., & Strakowski, S. M. (2002). Frontal lobe differences in bipolar disorder as determined by proton MR spectroscopy. *Bipolar Disorders, 4,* 357–365.

Cecil, K. M., DelBello, M. P., Sellars, M. C., & Strakowski, S. M. (2003). Proton magnetic resonance spectroscopy of the frontal lobe and cerebellar vermis in children with a mood disorder and a familial risk for bipolar disorders. *Journal of Child and Adolescent Psychopharmacology, 13,* 545–555.

Chang, K., Adleman, N., Dienes, K., Barnea-Goraly, N., Reiss, A., & Ketter, T. (2003). Decreased N-acetylaspartate in children with familial bipolar disorder. *Biological Psychiatry, 53,* 1059–1065.

Chang, K., Adleman, N. E., Dienes, K., Simeonova, D. I., Menon, V., & Reiss, A. (2004). Anomalous prefrontal–subcortical activation in familial pediatric bipolar disorder: A functional magnetic resonance imaging investigation. *Archives of General Psychiatry, 61,* 781–792.

Chang, K., Gallelli, K., Howe, M., Saxena, K., Wagner, C., Spielman, D., et al. (2005). Prefrontal neurometabolite changes following lamotrigine treatment in adolescents with bipolar depression. *Neuropsychopharmacology, 30,* S102–S103.

Chang, K., Saxena, K., & Howe, M. (2006). An open-label study of lamotrigine adjunct or monotherapy for the treatment of adolescents with bipolar depression. *Journal of the American Academy of Child and Adolescent Psychiatry, 45,* 298–304.

Charles, H. C., Lazeyras, F., Krishnan, K. R., Boyko, O. B., Patterson, L. J., Doraiswamy, P. M., et al. (1994). Proton spectroscopy of human brain: Effects of age and sex. *Progress in Neuro-Psychopharmacology and Biological Psychiatry, 18,* 995–1004.

Dager, S. R., Friedman, S. D., Parow, A., Demopulos, C., Stoll, A. L., Lyoo, I. K., et al. (2004). Brain metabolic alterations in medication-free patients with bipolar disorder. *Archives of General Psychiatry, 61,* 450–458.

Davanzo, P., Thomas, M., Barnett, S., Yue, K., Venkatraman, T., Cunanan, C., et al. (2002). *Magnetic resonance spectroscopy in bipolar children before and after valproate treatment.* Poster session presented at the annual meeting of the American Academy of Child and Adolescent Psychiatry, San Francisco.

Davanzo, P., Thomas, M. A., Yue, K., Oshiro, T., Belin, T., Strober, M., et al. (2001). Decreased anterior cingulate myo-inositol/creatine spectroscopy resonance with lithium treatment in children with bipolar disorder. *Neuropsychopharmacology, 24,* 359–369.

Davanzo, P., Yue, K., Thomas, M. A., Belin, T., Mintz, J., Venkatraman, T. N., et al. (2003). Proton magnetic resonance spectroscopy of bipolar disorder versus intermittent explosive disorder in children and adolescents. *American Journal of Psychiatry, 160,* 1442–1452.

Deicken, R. F., Eliaz, Y., Feiwell, R., & Schuff, N. (2001). Increased thalamic N-acetylaspartate in male patients with familial bipolar I disorder. *Psychiatry Research, 106,* 35–45.

Deicken, R. F., Fein, G., & Weiner, M. W. (1995). Abnormal frontal lobe phosphorous metabolism in bipolar disorder. *American Journal of Psychiatry, 152,* 915–918.

Deicken, R. F., Pegues, M. P., Anzalone, S., Feiwell, R., & Soher, B. (2003). Lower concentration of hippocampal N-acetylaspartate in familial bipolar I disorder. *American Journal of Psychiatry, 160,* 873–882.

Deicken, R. F., Weiner, M. W., & Fein, G. (1995). Decreased temporal lobe phosphomonoesters in bipolar disorder. *Journal of Affective Disorders, 33,* 195–199.

DelBello, M. P., Adler, C. M., & Strakowski, S. M. (2006). The neurophysiology of childhood and adolescent bipolar disorder. *CNS Spectrums, 11,* 298–311.

DelBello, M. P., Cecil, K. M., Adler, C. M., Daniels, J. P., & Strakowski, S. M. (2006). Neurochemical effects of olanzapine in first-hospitalization manic adolescents: A proton magnetic resonance spectroscopy study. *Neuropsychopharmacology, 31,* 1264–1273.

DelBello, M. P., & Strakowski, S. M. (2004). Neurochemical predictors of response to pharmacologic treatments for bipolar disorder. *Current Psychiatry Reports, 6,* 466–472.

Friedman, S. D., Dager, S. R., Parow, A., Hirashima, F., Demopulos, C., Stoll, A. L., et al. (2004). Lithium and valproic acid treatment effects on brain chemistry in bipolar disorder. *Biological Psychiatry, 56,* 340–348.

Frye, M. A., Ketter, T. A., Leverich, G. S., Huggins, T., Lantz, C., Denicoff, K. D., et al. (2000). The increasing use of polypharmacotherapy for refractory mood disorders: 22 years of study. *Journal of Clinical Psychiatry, 61,* 9–15.

Gallelli, K. A., Wagner, C. M., Karchemskiy, A., Howe, M., Spielman, D., Reiss, A., et al. (2005). N-acetylaspartate levels in bipolar offspring with and at high-risk for bipolar disorder. *Bipolar Disorders, 7,* 589–597.

Gelenberg, A. J., & Pies, R. (2003). Matching the bipolar patient and the mood stabilizer. *Annals of Clinical Psychiatry, 15,* 203–216.

Glitz, D. A., Manji, H. K., & Moore, G. J. (2002). Mood disorders: Treatment-induced changes in brain neurochemistry and structure. *Seminars in Clinical Neuropsychiatry, 7,* 269–280.

Gyulai, L., Wicklund, S. W., Greenstein, R., Bauer, M. S., Ciccione, P., Whybrow, P. C., et al. (1991). Measurement of tissue lithium concentration by lithium magnetic resonance spectroscopy in patients with bipolar disorder. *Biological Psychiatry, 15,* 1161–1170.

Hamakawa, H., Kato, T., Murashita, J., & Kato, N. (1998). Quantitative proton magnetic resonance spectroscopy of the basal ganglia in patients with affective disorders. *European Archives of Psychiatry and Clinical Neuroscience, 248,* 53–58.

Hamakawa, H., Kato, T., Shioiri, T., Inubushi, T., & Kato, N. (1999). Quantitative proton magnetic resonance spectroscopy of the bilateral frontal lobes in patients with bipolar disorder. *Psychological Medicine, 29,* 639–644.

Jensen, H. V., Plenge, P., Stensgaard, A., Mellerup, E. T., Thomsen, C., Aggernaes, H., et al. (1996). Twelve-hour brain lithium concentration in lithium maintenance treatment of manic-depressive disorder: Daily versus alternate-day dosing schedule. *Psychopharmacology, 124,* 275–278.

Kafantaris, V., Coletti, D. J., Dicker, R., Padula, G., & Kane, J. M. (2003). Lithium treatment of acute mania in adolescents: A large open trial. *Journal of the American Academy of Child and Adolescent Psychiatry, 42,* 1038–1045.

Kato, T., Fujii, K., Shioiri, T., Inubushi, T., & Takahashi, S. (1996). Lithium side effects in relation to brain lithium concentration measured by lithium-7 magnetic resonance spectroscopy. *Progress in Neuro-Psychopharmacology and Biological Psychiatry, 20,* 87–97.

Kato, T., Hamakawa, H., Shioiri, T., Murashita, J., Takahashi, Y., Takahashi, S., et al. (1996). Choline-containing compounds detected by proton magnetic resonance spectroscopy in the basal ganglia in bipolar disorder. *Journal of Psychiatry and Neuroscience, 21,* 248–254.

Kato, T., Inubushi, T., & Kato, N. (1998). Magnetic resonance spectroscopy in affective disorders. *Journal of Neuropsychiatry and Clinical Neurosciences, 10,* 133–147.

Kato, T., Inubushi, T., & Kato, N. (2000). Prediction of lithium response by 31P-MRS in bipolar disorder. *International Journal of Neuropsychopharmacology, 3,* 83–85.

Kato, T., Inubushi, T., & Takahashi, S. (1994). Relationship of lithium concentrations in the brain measured by lithium-7 magnetic resonance spectroscopy to treatment response in mania. *Journal of Clinical Psychopharmacology, 14,* 330–335.

Kato, T., Shioiri, T., Inubushi, T., & Takahashi, S. (1993). Brain lithium concentrations measured with lithium-7 magnetic resonance spectroscopy in patients with affective disorders:

Relationship to erythrocyte and serum concentrations. *Biological Psychiatry*, *33*, 147–152.

Kato, T., Shioiri, T., Murashita, J., Hamakawa, H., Inubushi, T., & Takahashi, S. (1994). Phosphorus-31 magnetic resonance spectroscopy and ventricular enlargement in bipolar disorder. *Psychiatry Research*, *55*, 41–50.

Kato, T., Shioiri, T., Murashita, J., Hamakawa, H., Takahashi, Y., Inubushi, T., et al. (1995). Lateralized abnormality of high energy phosphate metabolism in the frontal lobes of patients with bipolar disorder detected by phase-encoded 31P-MRS. *Psychological Medicine*, *25*, 557–566.

Kato, T., Shioiri, T., Takahashi, S., & Inubushi, T. (1991). Measurement of brain phosphoinositide metabolism in bipolar patients using in vivo 31P-MRS. *Journal of Affective Disorders*, *22*, 185–190.

Kato, T., Takahashi, S., & Inubushi, T. (1992). Brain lithium concentration by 7Li- and 1H- magnetic resonance spectroscopy in bipolar disorder. *Psychiatry Research*, *45*, 53–63.

Kato, T., Takahashi, S., Shioiri, T., & Inubushi, T. (1992). Brain phosphorous metabolism in depressive disorders detected by phosphorus-31 magnetic resonance spectroscopy. *Journal of Affective Disorders*, *26*, 223–230.

Kato, T., Takahashi, S., Shioiri, T., & Inubushi, T. (1993). Alterations in brain phosphorous metabolism in bipolar disorder detected by in vivo 31P and 7Li magnetic resonance spectroscopy. *Journal of Affective Disorders*, *27*, 53–59.

Kato, T., Takahashi, S., Shioiri, T., Murashita, J., Hamakawa, H., & Inubushi, T. (1994). Reduction of brain phosphocreatine in bipolar II disorder detected by phosphorus-31 magnetic resonance spectroscopy. *Journal of Affective Disorders*, *31*, 125–133.

Kaya, N., Resmi, H., Ozerdem, A., Guner, G., & Tunca, Z. (2004). Increased inositol-monophosphatase activity by lithium treatment in bipolar patients. *Progress in Neuro-Psychopharmacology and Biological Psychiatry*, *28*, 521–527.

Kowatch, R. A., Fristad, M., Birmaher, B., Wagner, K. D., Findling, R. L., & Hellander, M. (2005). Treatment guidelines for children and adolescents with bipolar disorder. *Journal of the American Academy of Child and Adolescent Psychiatry*, *44*, 213–235.

Kowatch, R. A., Suppes, T., Carmody, T. J., Bucci, J. P., Hume, J. H., Kromelis, M., et al. (2000). Effect size of lithium, divalproex sodium, and carbamazepine in children and adolescents with bipolar disorder. *Journal of the American Academy of Child and Adolescent Psychiatry*, *39*, 713–720.

Michael, N., Erfurth, A., Ohrmann, P., Gossling, M., Arolt, V., Heindel, W., et al. (2003). Acute mania is accompanied by elevated glutamate/glutamine levels within the left dorsolateral prefrontal cortex. *Psychopharmacology*, *168*, 344–346.

Moore, C. M., Breeze, J. L., Gruber, S. A., Babb, S. M., Frederick, B. B., Villafuerte, R. A., et al. (2000). Choline, myo-inositol and mood in bipolar disorder: A proton magnetic resonance spectroscopic imaging study of the anterior cingulate cortex. *Bipolar Disorders*, *2*, 207–216.

Moore, C. M., Demopulos, C. M., Henry, M. E., Steingard, R. J., Zamvil, L., Katic, A., et al. (2002). Brain-to-serum lithium ratio and age: An in vivo magnetic resonance spectroscopy study. *American Journal of Psychiatry*, *159*, 1240–1242.

Moore, G. J., Bebchuk, J. M., Hasanat, K., Chen, G., Seraji-Bozorgzad, N., Wilds, I. B., et al. (2000). Lithium increases N-acetyl-aspartate in the human brain: In vivo evidence in support of bcl-2's neurotrophic effects? *Biological Psychiatry*, *48*, 1–8.

Moore, G. J., Bebchuk, J. M., Parrish, J. K., Faulk, M. W., Arfken, C. L., Strahl-Bevacqua, J., et al. (1999). Temporal dissociation between lithium-induced changes in frontal lobe myo-inositol and clinical response in manic-depressive illness. *American Journal of Psychiatry*, *156*, 1902–1908.

Moore, G. J., & Galloway, M. P. (2002). Magnetic resonance spectroscopy: Neurochemistry and treatment effects in affective disorders. *Psychopharmacology Bulletin*, *36*, 5–23.

Ohara, K., Isoda, H., Suzuki, Y., Takehara, Y., Ochiai, M., Takeda, H., Igarashi, Y., et al. (1998). Proton magnetic resonance spectroscopy of the lenticular nuclei in bipolar I affective disorder. *Psychiatry Research, 84,* 55–60.

Patel, N. C., DelBello, M. P., Bryan, H. S., Adler, C. M., Kowatch, R. A., Stanford, K., et al. (2006). Open-label lithium for the treatment of adolescents with bipolar depression. *Journal of the American Academy of Child and Adolescent Psychiatry, 45,* 289–297.

Patel, N. C., DelBello, M. P., Cecil, K. M., Adler, C. M., Bryan, H. S., Stanford, K. E., et al. (2006). Lithium treatment effects on *myo*-inositol in adolescents with bipolar depression. *Biological Psychiatry, 60,* 998–1004.

Post, R. M., Speer, A. M., Hough, C. J., & Xing, G. (2003). Neurobiology of bipolar illness: Implications for future study and therapeutics. *Annals of Clinical Psychiatry, 15,* 85–94.

Provencher, S. W. (1993). Estimation of metabolite concentrations from localized in vivo proton NMR spectra. *Magnetic Resonance in Medicine, 30,* 672–679.

Renshaw, P. F., Summers, J. J., Renshaw, C. E., Hines, K. G., & Leigh, J. S., Jr. (1986). Changes in the 31P-NMR spectra of cats receiving lithium chloride systemically. *Biological Psychiatry, 21,* 694–698.

Rich, B. A., Vinton, D. T., Roberson-Nay, R., Hommer, R. E., Berghorst, L. H., McClure, E. B., et al. (2006). Limbic hyperactivation during processing of neutral facial expressions in children with bipolar disorder. *Proceedings of the National Academy of Sciences of the USA, 103,* 8900–8905.

Sachs, G. S., Renshaw, P. F., Lafer, B., Stoll, A. L., Guimaraes, A. R., Rosenbaum, J. F., et al. (1995). Variability of brain lithium levels during maintenance treatment: A magnetic resonance spectroscopy study. *Biological Psychiatry, 38,* 422–428.

Sassi, R. B., Stanley, J. A., Axelson, D., Brambilla, P., Nicoletti, M. A., Keshavan, M. S., et al. (2005). Reduced NAA levels in the dorsolateral prefrontal cortex of young bipolar patients. *American Journal of Psychiatry, 162,* 2109–2115.

Sharma, R., Venkatasubramanian, P. N., Barany, M., & Davis, J. M. (1992). Proton magnetic resonance spectroscopy of the brain in schizophrenic and affective patients. *Schizophrenia Research, 8,* 43–49.

Silverstone, P. H., Hanstock, C. C., Fabian, J., Staab, R., & Allen, P. S. (1996). Chronic lithium does not alter human myo-inositol or phosphomonoester concentrations as measured by 1H and 31P MRS. *Biological Psychiatry, 40,* 235–246.

Silverstone, P. H., Rotzinger, S., Pukhovsky, A., & Hanstock, C. C. (1999). Effects of lithium and amphetamine on inositol metabolism in the human brain as measured by 1H and 31P MRS. *Biological Psychiatry, 46,* 1634–1641.

Silverstone, P. H., Wu, R. H., O'Donnell, T., Ulrich, M., Asghar, S. J., & Hanstock, C. C. (2002). Chronic treatment with both lithium and sodium valproate may normalize phosphoinositol cycle activity in bipolar patients. *Human Psychopharmacology, 17,* 321–327.

Silverstone, P. H., Wu, R. H., O'Donnell, T., Ulrich, M., Asghar, S. J., & Hanstock, C. C. (2003). Chronic treatment with lithium, but not sodium valproate, increases cortical N-acetyl-aspartate concentrations in euthymic bipolar patients. *International Clinical Psychopharmacology, 18,* 73–79.

Soares, J. C., Boada, F., & Keshavan, M. S. (2000). Brain lithium measurements with (7)Li magnetic resonance spectroscopy (MRS): A literature review. *European Neuropsychopharmacology, 10,* 151–158.

Soares, J. C., Boada, F., Spencer, S., Wells, K. F., Mallinger, A. G., Frank, F., et al. (1999). NAA and choline measures in the anterior cingulate of bipolar disorder patients. *Biological Psychiatry, 45,* 119S.

Soares, J. C., Krishnan, K. R., & Keshavan, M. S. (1996). Nuclear magnetic resonance spectroscopy: New insights into the pathophysiology of mood disorders. *Depression, 4,* 14–30.

Strakowski, S. M., DelBello, M. P., Adler, C., Cecil, D. M., & Sax, K. W. (2000). Neuroimaging in bipolar disorder. *Bipolar Disorders, 2,* 148–164.

Suppes, T., Dennehy, E. B., Hirschfeld, R. M., Altshuler, L. L., Bowden, C. L., Calabrese, J. R., et al. (2005). The Texas implementation of medication algorithms: Update to the algorithms for treatment of bipolar I disorder. *Journal of Clinical Psychiatry, 66,* 870–886.

Tsai, G., & Coyle, J. T. (1995). N-acetylaspartate in neuropsychiatric disorders. *Progress in Neurobiology, 46,* 531–540.

van der Knaap, M. S., van der Grond, J., van Rijen, P. C., Faber, J. A., Valk, J., & Willemse, K. (1990). Age-dependent changes in localized proton and phosphorus MR spectroscopy of the brain. *Radiology, 176,* 509–515.

Wagner, K. D., Weller, E. B., Carlson, G. A., Sachs, G., Biederman, J., Frazier, J. A., et al. (2002). An open-label trial of divalproex in children and adolescents with bipolar disorder. *Journal of the American Academy of Child and Adolescent Psychiatry, 41,* 1224–1230.

Winsberg, M. E., Sachs, N., Tate, D. L., Adalsteinsson, E., Spielman, D., & Ketter, T. A. (2000). Decreased dorsolateral prefrontal N-acetyl aspartate in bipolar disorder. *Biological Psychiatry, 47,* 475–481.

Wu, R. H., O'Donnell, T., Ulrich, M., Asghar, S. J., Hanstock, C. C., & Silverstone, P. H. (2004). Brain choline concentrations may not be altered in euthymic bipolar disorder patients chronically treated with either lithium or sodium valproate. *Annals of General Hospital Psychiatry, 3,* 13.

CHAPTER 4

Lithium

ROBERT L. FINDLING
and MANI N. PAVULURI

LITHIUM AND ITS EVOLUTION

Lithium, a monovalent cation, was discovered in 1817 (Manji & Lenox, 1998). Lithium was initially utilized for a multitude of ailments until its serendipitous discovery as a treatment for mania (Cade, 1949). Clinical trials in adult patients with bipolar disorder have established the efficacy of lithium in acute mania and bipolar depression and as a maintenance therapy (reviewed in Goodwin & Jamison, 1990; Janicak, Davis, Preskorn, & Ayd, 2001; Suppes, Baldessarini, Faedda, & Tohen, 1991). Despite the burgeoning literature indicating the chronicity and perniciousness of pediatric bipolar disorder (Findling et al., 2001; Geller et al., 2002; Wozniak et al., 1995), only a few lithium treatment studies have been done in the pediatric population. Although the Food and Drug Administration (FDA) "grandfathered" the indication of lithium for bipolar disorder in children who are 12 years old and older, presently there are no methodologically stringent studies to definitively support the use of lithium in pediatric mania.

The purpose of this chapter is to review what is known about the neurobiological effects of lithium and to provide the reader with a summary of what is known about the effectiveness and safety of lithium in children and adolescents with bipolar disorders.

43

MECHANISM OF ACTION
AND NEUROBIOLOGY OF LITHIUM'S EFFECT

Lithium and Signal Transduction

Lithium primarily acts at a molecular level on the intracellular second-messenger systems. At therapeutic concentrations, lithium induces receptor-stimulated cleavage or hydrolysis of a membrane phospholipid, phosphatidylinositol biphosphate (PIP_2), which consequently triggers a cascade of reactions in the intracellular signaling pathway. Further, lithium dampens the ability of cell stimulation by depleting the cellular pools of PIP_2 by directly depleting inositol (Allison & Stewart, 1971; Hallcher & Sherman, 1980). In short, *in vitro* studies demonstrated that lithium both reduces neuronal excitability and enhances membrane stabilization. It is hypothesized that these are the primary mechanisms of action behind the therapeutic effects of lithium.

Recent human studies of *in vivo* magnetic resonance spectroscopy (MRS) demonstrate that lithium lowers *myo*-inositol levels in frontal cortex within 5 days of treatment (Moore, Bebchuk, & Manji, 1997; Moore et al., 1999). Further, coadministration of *myo*-inositol attenuates some of lithium's effects on signal transduction pathways (Lenox, McNamara, Watterson, & Watson, 1996; Manji, Bersudsky, Chen, Belmaker, & Potter, 1996). These results support the findings from the intracellular studies that described the membrane-stabilizing properties of lithium. However, these results should be interpreted with the caveat that no such increase was noted in *myo*-inositol levels with acute or chronic exposure to lithium in adolescents with pediatric bipolar depression when compared with baseline levels. In fact, there was significant increase in *myo*-inositol after 42 days of lithium treatment when compared with the *myo*-inositol levels at day 7 (Patel et al., 2006a). Until these studies are replicated and in larger samples, caution needs to be exercised in translating the *in vitro* and animal findings to humans.

Lithium and Neurotransmission

Preclinical studies and information from adult human studies have provided information regarding the effects of lithium on neurotransmission and insights into the basis of the neuropsychopharmacological effects of lithium.

Serotonin

The effect of lithium on the serotonin system occurs at multiple levels (Manji & Lenox, 1998). Serotonin effects are seen during prolonged exposure rather than after a single lithium dose (Price, Charney, Delgado, & Heninger, 1990). Some preliminary evidence suggests that lithium normalizes low platelet serotonin reuptake in patients with bipolar disorder and that this effect persists after drug discontinuation (Meltzer, Arora, & Goodnick, 1983; Poirier et al., 1988). Due to multiple receptor subtypes, widespread distribution of serotonergic fibers throughout the brain, and absence of specific pharmacological ligands, the effects of lithium on serotonin neural transmission have not yet been fully characterized.

Dopamine

Lithium is known to (1) cause a dose-dependent decrease in dopamine formation (Ahluwalia, Grewaal, & Singhal, 1981; Engel & Berggren, 1980); (2) alter coupling efficacy between G-proteins and dopamine receptors; (3) reduce dopamine-sensitive adenylate cyclase activity, and (4) reduce dopamine-mediated increases in acetylcholine. Another potentially relevant finding is lithium's ability to block supersensitive dopamine receptors that are induced by antipsychotic medication (Staunton, Magistretti, Shoemaker, & Bloom, 1982). Another well-studied observation is lithium's attenuation of stimulant-induced locomotor activation in animal models of mania (Goodnick & Gershon, 1985; Staunton et al., 1982). This last finding provides some theoretical evidence to support the judicious prescribing of psychostimulants to patients with bipolar disorder and comorbid attention-deficit/hyperactivity disorder (ADHD) after these patients have received mood-stabilizing therapy.

Norepinephrine

Lithium has been reported to reduce β-adrenergic receptor mediated adenylate cyclase response and cyclic adenosine monophosphate (cAMP) accumulation. Additionally, lithium has been reported to have effects on presynaptic α_2 autoreceptors (Manji & Lenox, 1998). There is also evidence to suggest that the effect of lithium on norepinephrine may be related to lithium dose and the chronicity of treatment (Ahluwalia & Singhal, 1980).

Gamma-Aminobutyric Acid

Lowered baseline levels of gamma-aminobutyric acid (GABA) in plasma and cerebrospinal fluid have been reported to normalize in adult patients with bipolar disorder who receive lithium treatment (Berrettini, Nurnberger, Hare, Simmons-Alling, & Gershon, 1986).

Lithium and Neuroprotection

Although spectroscopic studies and structural imaging studies may be conducted in patients with pediatric bipolar disorder, studies of intracellular genetic changes, including those pertaining to neuroprotective factors, are limited to animal and postmortem brain studies. Information regarding lithium's putative neuroprotective effects is summarized next.

Gene Expression

In vitro, lithium has been shown to have neuroprotective qualities (Nonaka, Katsube, & Chuang, 1998) and also to aid in the process of neurogenesis (Hao et al., 2004; Williams, Cheng, Mudge, & Harwood, 2002). For example, lithium administration has been shown to prevent stress-induced loss of dendrites (Wood, Young, Reagan, Chen, & McEwen, 2004). Lithium has also been shown to reduce excitotoxicity caused by glutamatergic activity. Manji, McNamara, Chen, and Lenox (1999) demonstrated that lithium's neurotrophic and cytoprotective effects in rodent brains *in vivo* occur as a result of lithium's ability to induce bcl-2 gene expression. The bcl-2 mediates several endogenous growth factors (e.g., nerve growth factor [NGF], brain-derived neurotrophic factor [BDNF]).

Spectroscopic Studies

Lithium concentration can be directly measured in the brain with ^{7}Li nuclear magnetic resonance (NMR) (Gonzalez et al., 1993; Renshaw & Wicklund, 1988). Recently, Moore et al. (2002) used ^{7}Li MRS to measure *in vivo* brain lithium levels in children, adolescents, and adults with bipolar disorder and reported that children and adolescents may need higher maintenance serum lithium concentrations than adults to ensure that brain lithium concentrations reach therapeutic levels.

Structural Imaging Studies

Further evidence for the neurotropic effects of lithium comes from several human studies that have used magnetic resonance imaging (MRI). In these studies, lithium was found to induce an increase in gray matter volume (Moore, Bebchuk, Wilds, Chen, & Manji, 2000; Sassi et al., 2002). Preliminary results from a sample of pediatric patients with bipolar disorder reported larger amygdala volumes (as a result of increases in gray matter volume) among those patients exposed to lithium or valproate when compared with those not exposed to such treatments (Chang et al., 2005).

CLINICAL APPLICATIONS

Pharmacokinetic Study

As it is an element, lithium is not metabolized (Schou, 1988). In adults, lithium is absorbed in the gastrointestinal tract, with maximum plasma concentrations occurring about 2 to 4 hours after oral dosing. The volume of distribution of lithium approximates that of total body water. The excretion of lithium occurs in a biphasic manner with a rapid initial excretion phase followed by a more slow excretion phase. In young adults, the half-life of lithium is approximately 20–24 hours (Marcus, 1994).

Lithium is primarily excreted in the urine. The rate of renal excretion is related to an individual's glomerular filtration rate (GFR). Thus patients with higher GFRs excrete lithium more rapidly than those with lower GFRs (Goodnick & Schorr-Cain, 1991). Because GFRs are generally more rapid in children than in adults and because developmentally based differences in gastrointestinal absorption may also occur (Kearns et al., 2003), it is possible that the pharmacokinetics (PK) of lithium may be different in children than in adults. Unfortunately, there are not a lot of data about the biodisposition of lithium in children or adolescents.

The PK of lithium was described in 9 children between the ages of 9 and 11 years by Vitiello et al. (1988). In this study, the children were treated with a single 300 mg dose of lithium. Intensive blood and salivary sampling was done 36 hours postdose. The authors found that the PK parameter estimates observed in these participants were similar to those that had been previously described in adults, thus supporting the use of similar dosing intervals in children and adolescents to those typically employed in adults. The authors also noted that the small sample size precluded definitive comparative statements to be made between children and adults.

The monitoring of serum lithium levels is an important aspect of lithium therapy because of the narrow therapeutic index of lithium. Unfortunately, serum level measurement requires phlebotomy, a procedure that is oftentimes not well received by children or teenagers. For this reason, during the course of this study, Vitiello and colleagues (1988) examined whether salivary lithium levels could be used in place of serum lithium levels during lithium therapy. The authors found that salivary levels and serum levels of lithium were not well correlated. For this reason, the authors concluded that the use of salivary lithium levels was not a rational strategy for therapeutic drug monitoring of lithium in children receiving this compound.

Metabolism and Drug Interactions

Both lithium and sodium are reabsorbed at the renal proximal convoluted tubule, as well as at the collecting ducts and distal tubules (Dousa & Hechter, 1970a, 1970b). For this reason, changes in a patient's hydration status and drugs that affect renal function may alter lithium concentrations. For this reason, sodium or water restriction or dehydration is not advised when a patient is prescribed lithium.

Thiazide diuretics (Goodnick & Schorr-Cain, 1991) and angiotensin converting enzyme (ACE) inhibitors may cause an increase in lithium levels. Perhaps more pertinent to children and teenagers, nonsteroidal anti-inflammatory drugs (NSAIDs) can also substantially increase lithium levels. It should be noted that caffeine-containing agents and theophylline may decrease lithium levels (Finley, Warner, & Peabody, 1995).

Dosing Studies

When prescribing lithium to children and adolescents with bipolar illness, a key goal is to maximize therapeutic benefits while minimizing side effects. This is particularly important because lithium has a narrow therapeutic index. In adults, this goal is generally accomplished by achieving target lithium levels within the range of 0.6–1.2 mEq/L (Schou, Juel-Nielsen, Strömgren, & Voldby, 1954; Schou, 1986). In order to attain therapeutic lithium levels in adults, the starting dose of lithium that is oftentimes prescribed is 900 mg/day, which is given in divided doses. Subsequent dosing adjustments are then made in adults based on the presence or absence of side effects, the degree of symptom amelioration, and serum lithium levels.

Although there are no methodologically stringent data that have tested the assumption that the lithium levels used in therapeutic drug monitoring in adults are applicable to children and adolescents, in the absence of data to the contrary, this is the dosing strategy that seems to be employed most frequently by practitioners. For clinicians caring for a very ill child with mania, there is a need to promptly achieve adequate lithium levels in hopes of providing timely symptom amelioration.

However, when considering the initiation of lithium in children and adolescents, large between-patient differences in body size exist. Thus the use of a single starting dose is not a rational treatment strategy for the initiation of lithium in pediatric patients.

Two studies have attempted to identify scientifically supported strategies for promptly achieving therapeutic lithium levels in children. In the first such study, Weller, Weller, and Fristad (1986) enrolled 15 children between the ages of 6 and 12 years and treated them with a dose of approximately 30 mg/kg/day in thrice-daily divided doses. The authors found that this dosing paradigm was generally effective in safely achieving therapeutic levels in these medically healthy children. The limitations of this study include its small number of participants and the absence of older adolescents.

In the second study, Geller and Fetner (1989) examined the utility of using the nomogram of Cooper, Bergner, and Simpson (1973) in predicting initial lithium dosing in 6 children between the ages of 9 and 12 years. In this study, the authors administered a 600 mg dose of lithium that was followed by a 24-hour postdose lithium level measurement. The authors noted that using this strategy was useful in determining initial lithium dosing in this study cohort.

The use of nomogram-based dosing requires being able to accurately measure lithium levels to the second decimal place. Unfortunately, such measurement is not available to many practitioners. In addition, many patients for whom lithium therapy may be considered are outpatients; for this reason, practical considerations exist in performing the required 24-hour postdose sampling procedures. Therefore, the use of nomogram-based dosing does not appear to be commonly implemented in clinical practice.

In summary, due to the limitations of employing both these dosing strategies to many patients presenting for clinical care, there remains a compelling need to develop other scientifically supported dosing paradigms for the initiation of lithium in children and adolescents. At present, we employ the following dosing strategy in our clinical practices. Patients are initially prescribed lithium at a dose of 20 mg/kg per day, or 900 mg/day (whichever is less). The lithium total daily dose is given in twice- or thrice-divided doses with the ultimate goal of achieving drug levels of approximately 0.6–1.2 mEq/L. The initial dose is then gradually increased in order to achieve the desired blood levels. Doses are not increased if: (1) blood levels exceed 1.2 mEq/L, (2) side effects preclude dose increases, or (3) adequate symptom reduction occurs.

Treatment Studies and Case Reports

A relatively large number of publications have considered the treatment effects and tolerability of lithium in children and adolescents with pediatric bipolar disorder. As can be seen in Table 4.1, only a small number of the publications were prospective clinical trials. What follows is a summary of selected clinical trials that have been published within the past decade that have examined the use of lithium in children and/or adolescents with bipolar illness.

Geller and colleagues (1998) studied 25 adolescents ages 12–18 years with bipolar disorders. The patients met diagnostic symptom criteria for bipolar I disorder (BP I), bipolar II disorder (BP II), or major depressive disorder (MDD) with high risk for developing future bipolar illness (e.g., delusions, medication-related bipolar switching, psychomotor retardation, or bipolar illness in a first-degree relative). All patients also suffered from a comorbid substance dependence disorder. These participants were then randomized to receive 6 weeks of either lithium or placebo. The dosing in this trial used the Cooper nomogram and target lithium levels of 0.9–1.3 mEq/L. The outcome measures that were employed were percent positive urine toxicology screens and global assessment of functioning. Significant between-group differences for the number of positive toxicology screens and global assessment of functioning responder scores were found. It should be noted that this was not an acute mania trial and that mood symptomatology was not a primary outcome measure. The most commonly reported lithium-

TABLE 4.1. Selected Reports of Lithium Treatment in Pediatric Bipolar Disorder

Author (year)	Study design	Sample size	Patient ages (years)	Diagnoses	Comments
Annell (1969)	CR	$n = 12$	9–18	Varied	Generally favorable response.
Berg et al. (1974)	CR	$n = 1$	14	MD	Patient required higher than usual doses to achieve therapeutic blood levels.
Biermann & Pflug (1974)	CR	$n = 1$	13	CYC	Lithium treatment prevented relapse.
Brumback & Weinberg (1977)	CR	$n = 6$	4–13	MD	2 responded, 3 developed depression, 1 developed EEG changes.
Carlson & Strober (1978)	CR	$n = 6$	12–16	MD	3 responded to Li, 3 had "less dramatic responses."
Carlson et al. (1992)	RCT	$n = 7$	5–9	Disruptive behavior + mood disorder	Combination Li + MPH may be reasonable option.
Davanzo et al. (2003)	CR	$n = 25$	5–12	BD	Improvement noted in hospitalized children.
Davis (1979)	CR	$n = 4$	9–12	MD	"Responded well" to lithium.
DeLong & Nieman (1983)	RCT	$n = 11$	6–13	MD	Open-label Li responders were randomized to either Li or PCB and then crossed over to the alternate treatment. Li > PCB.
DeLong & Aldershof (1987)	CR	$n = 59$	3–20 ($M = 10.9$)	MD	Clinical benefit reported. Well tolerated.
Dugas et al. (1975)	CR	$n = 43$	5–21	Varied	Benefit noted for patients with manic depressive illness.

Study	Design	n	Age	Population	Findings
Dyson & Barcai (1970)	CR	$n = 2$	8, 13	Children of Li-responding parents with affective symptoms	Li associated with clinical improvements.
Feinstein & Wolpert (1973)	CR	$n = 1$	6	MD	Mood stabilization reported.
Findling et al. (2003)	OLP	$n = 90$	5–17	BP I or BP II	Combination Li + DVPX effective.
Findling et al. (2005)	RCT (maintenance discontinuation)	$n = 60$	5–17	BP I or BP II	Li = DVPX as monotherapy.
Geller et al. (1998)	RCT	$n = 25$	12–18	Substance abuse disorder + BP or MDD (with familial predictors of BP)	Li superior to PCB on global function and number of positive urine drug screens.
Gram & Rafaelsen (1972)	RCT	$n = 2$	10, 22	Affective symptoms and parental MD	Benefit from Li.
Hagino et al. (1995)	CR	$n = 20$	4–6	Varied	Side effects common.
Hassanyeh & Davison (1980)	CR	$n = 7$	12–15	MD	6/7 patients responded to lithium.
Horowitz (1977)	CR	$n = 8$	15–18	MD	All patients remitted with Li.
Hsu (1986)	CR	$n = 8$	15–17	Mania	Half of the patients responded to Li.
Jones & Berney (1987)	CR	$n = 4$	14–17	BD with rapid cycling	2/4 patients benefited from Li.
Kafantaris et al. (1998)	OLP	$n = 48$	12–18	Manic or mixed episode	Psychosis may diminish response.
Kafantaris et al. (2003)	OLP	$n = 100$	12–18	Mania	Li beneficial and well tolerated. Almost ½ also treated with antipsychotic.

(continued)

51

TABLE 4.1. (*continued*)

Author (year)	Study design	Sample size	Patient ages (years)	Diagnoses	Comments
Kafantaris et al. (2004)	RCT (maintenance discontinuation)	n = 40	12–18	Mania	Clinical worsening seen in patients both randomized to PCB and maintained on Li.
Kelly et al. (1976)	CR	n = 1	5	MD	Salutary effect seen.
Kowatch et al. (2000)	OLP	n = 13	8–18	BP I or BP II	Substantial benefit.
Kowatch et al. (2003)	OLP	n = 14	7–18	BD	Combination therapy may be useful.
Kutcher et al. (1990)	CR	n = 20	M = 17.5	BD	Patients without PD are more responsive than those with PD.
Licamele & Goldberg (1989)	CR	n = 1	7	AD + ADHD	Combination treatment with MPH beneficial.
McKnew et al. (1981)	RCT	n = 2	9, 12	Offspring of MD patients with BD	Crossover design. Li beneficial.
McNeil et al. (1978)	CR	n = 1	16	MD	Treatment "successful."
Patel et al. (2006b)	OLP	n = 27	12–18	Depressive symptoms in BP I	Approximately 50% response rate.
Pavuluri et al. (2004)	RCT[a]	n = 37	5–18	Manic or mixed	Li + Risp = DVPX + Risp; both beneficial.
Pavuluri et al. (2006)	OLP	n = 40	4–17	Manic or mixed preschool-onset BD	Li augmentation with Risp beneficial.
Rogeness et al. (1982)	CR	n = 1	17	MD	"Dramatic" improvement observed.
State et al. (2004)	CR	n = 29	12–19	Mania	Li = DVPX. Those with ADHD had reduced acute response.

Study	Design	n	Age	Diagnosis	Findings
Strober et al. (1988)	CR	$n = 50$	Adolescent	BD	Prepubertal onset less responsive than adolescent onset.
Strober et al. (1990)	CR	$n = 37$	13–17	BP I	Patients who remained on treatment were less likely to relapse.
Strober et al. (1998)	CR	$n = 30$	13–17	Mania	ADHD may diminish response.
Sylvester et al. (1984)	CR	$n = 2$	10, 12	Mania with psychosis	Lithium useful.
Tomasson & Kuperman (1990)	CR	$n = 1$	13	BD	Lithium helpful.
Tumuluru et al. (2003)	CR	$n = 5$	3–5	BD	Improvement noted with Li.
van Krevelen & van Voorst (1959)	CR	$n = 1$	14	Mania	Lithium response "favorable."
Varanka et al. (1988)	CR	$n = 10$	6–12	Mania with psychosis	Improvement noted.
Warneke (1975)	CR	$n = 1$	14	MD	"Dramatic benefit."
White & O'Shanick (1977)	CR	$n = 1$	15	MD	"Marked improvement."

Note. AD, affective disorder; ADHD, attention-deficit/hyperactivity disorder; BD, bipolar disorder; BP I, bipolar I disorder; BP II, bipolar II disorder; CR, case report; CYC, cyclothymia; DVPX, divalproex; EEG, electroencephalogram; Li, lithium; MD, manic depression; MDD, major depressive disorder; MPH, methylphenidate; OLP, open-label prospective study; PCB, placebo; PD, personality disorder; RCT, randomized controlled trial; Risp, risperidone.
[a]Consecutive assignment.

related side effects in this study included thirst, polyuria/polydipsia, nausea, vomiting, and dizziness.

Kowatch and colleagues (2000) took 42 children and adolescents with a manic, hypomanic, or mixed episode associated with either BP I or BP II. These youths were than randomized to a 6-week treatment protocol to receive lithium, divalproex sodium, or carbamazepine. The dosing for lithium used the weight-based paradigm of Weller et al. (1986), treating youths at 30 mg/kg/day divided into thrice-daily doses and adjusting lithium doses to achieve serum levels of 0.8–1.2 mEq/L. In this study, all three medications were found to have approximately equal effectiveness. The patients prescribed lithium generally experienced substantial benefit from treatment. No participant discontinued the lithium due to adverse events, and the most common lithium side effects that were noted included nausea, increased appetite, polyuria, and diarrhea.

Despite the fact that many of the participants received benefit from the treatments provided in this study, many of these participants did not achieve symptom remission. For this reason, 11 of the 14 lithium-treated youths were then enrolled into a 16-week open-label extension study (Kowatch, Sethuraman, Hume, Kromelis, & Weinberg, 2003). During this subsequent trial, participants were able to receive adjunctive mood-stabilizing medications. Of the 6 lithium responders who entered this trial, 3 stayed on lithium monotherapy. However, 3 of these initial responders ultimately received adjunctive therapy with either carbamazepine or divalproex sodium in order to achieve optimal mood stabilization. Of the 5 lithium nonresponders who entered this trial, 4 completed the study while receiving lithium and divalproex sodium in combination. The authors also noted that lithium plus divalproex sodium, when given together, may be a useful treatment strategy for achieving and sustaining therapeutic benefit in youths with bipolar illness. The authors also noted that for a substantial proportion of young patients with bipolar disorder, more than one mood stabilizer might be necessary in order to achieve optimal thymoleptic effects.

Kafantaris, Coletti, Dicker, Padula, and Kane (2003) described the results of a 4-week open-label trial of lithium in a group of 100 adolescents between the ages of 12 and 18 years, all of whom were suffering from a manic or mixed episode. Based on this group's prior findings that adolescents with mania and psychosis may respond less well to lithium (Kafantaris, Coletti, Dicker, Padula, & Pollack, 1998) and that adjunctive treatment with antipsychotics may be needed for optimal treatment of bipolar adolescents with psychosis (Kafantaris, Dicker, Colletti, & Kane, 2001; Kafantaris et al., 2001), youths with psychotic features or severe aggression and/or agitation were treated with adjunctive antipsychotics (mostly either risperidone or haloperidol; n = 46). In this study, the nomogram of Cooper et al. (1973) was used to determine initial dosing. Lithium treatment was then adjusted so that lithium levels ranged from 0.6–1.2 mEq/L. At the end of the study, the mean dose of lithium was 1,355 mg/day with a mean lithium serum level of 0.93 mEq/L. Substantial improvements in symptoms of both mania and depression were noted in the study cohort.

Approximately half of these patients met response criteria, and 26 of the participants were considered to be remitted of manic symptoms. Overall, the medication was generally well tolerated. Only 3 patients discontinued trial participation due to side effects (2 for gastrointestinal side effects and 1 for intermittent diplopia). The most commonly reported side effects were weight gain, polydipsia, polyuria, headache, tremor, and gastrointestinal symptoms (pain, nausea, vomiting, anorexia, diarrhea). The authors observed that almost half the patients on adjunctive antipsychotics required combination treatment beyond 4 weeks (Kafantaris et al., 2001) suggesting that psychosis requires combination treatment beyond this period of time.

In this study cohort, patients who were considered responders to lithium monotherapy were subsequently able to be randomized to receive either lithium or placebo for 2 subsequent weeks in a double-blind fashion (Kafantaris et al., 2004). Nineteen patients received lithium, and 21 were randomized to receive placebo. The authors found that there were no significant differences between the two groups in regard to manic symptoms at the end of the study, with a significant increase in manic symptoms occurring in both groups. The investigators noted that the lack of between-group differences may have been due to the short stabilization period (4 weeks), brief length of study (2 weeks), higher rates of manic symptoms in those treated with lithium, small sample size, a possible nocebo effect, the natural fluctuation of mood symptoms, and the fact that lithium was abruptly discontinued. Despite these methodological considerations, the authors concluded that lithium monotherapy may be insufficient to prevent mild worsening of symptoms early in the course of recovery.

Based on the findings that many youths with bipolar illness might not fully respond to drug monotherapy, Findling and colleagues (2003) treated 90 children and adolescents between the ages of 5 and 17 with combination lithium and divalproex sodium. Substantial symptomatic improvement that was larger in magnitude than what had been described in previously published drug monotherapy studies was found. In addition, higher rates of symptomatic remission than had been seen in a study of rapid-cycling adults treated with both lithium and divalproex sodium in combination (Calabrese et al., 2005) was also noted. The combination pharmacological regimen was reasonably well tolerated. The most common side effects were gastrointestinal effects, polyuria, and tremor. The most frequent side effects putatively ascribed to lithium that led to study discontinuation included ataxia and increased thyrotropin levels (Gracious et al., 2004).

In order to assess the effectiveness of lithium versus divalproex as a maintenance therapy for pediatric-age patients with bipolar disorder, Findling and colleagues (2005) randomized 60 youths who achieved symptomatic remission with acute treatment with a combination of lithium and divalproex sodium and randomized these youths to drug monotherapy for up to 18 months. The authors found that lithium was equal to divalproex sodium in maintaining mood stabilization. However, the median time to relapse was 114 days for youths randomized to lithium monotherapy. Of note, the authors found that concurrent use of medications to treat ADHD was not associated with an accelerated time to study discontinuation. Only 3 participants randomized to lithium monotherapy completed the entire 18-month-long trial, and the most common mood state that led to discontinuation was mania/mood cycling. In contrast, for a group of adults with the rapid-cycling variant of bipolar illness who had participated in a clinical trial of a similar design (Calabrese et al., 2005), depression was the most common mood state associated with study discontinuation.

Findling and colleagues (2006) subsequently treated 38 of the patients who relapsed in the monotherapy maintenance trial with the reinitiation of combination lithium plus divalproex therapy. Thirty-four of the patients (89%) responded to reinitiation of combination treatment, but 4 required the subsequent addition of antipsychotic therapy in order to achieve optimal clinical stabilization. The authors concluded that most youths with bipolar disorder who stabilize on combination therapy and who subsequently relapse on monotherapy can be safely and effectively restabilized with combination therapy.

Pavuluri and coinvestigators (2004) conducted a 6-month open trial that compared the effectiveness of risperidone plus divalproex sodium therapy with that of risperidone plus lithium therapy ($n = 20$). In this study, 37 children or adolescents between the ages of 5 and 18 suffering from a mixed or manic episode participated. The authors noted that both treatment arms had similar degrees of effectiveness and that either combination drug therapy regimen was associated with salutary effects, with reductions in both manic and depressive symptomatology. The participants tolerated the lithium-plus-risperidone combination regimen reasonably well, with only 2 participants discontinuing study participation as a result of enuresis and fatigue. The most common side effects noted in these participants were weight gain, sedation, gastrointestinal symptoms, tremor, polyuria, and cognitive blunting. These authors also noted high rates of response in those patients treated with lithium and risperidone, further adding support to the strategy of using lithium in combination with another thymoleptic drug in the treatment of pediatric bipolar illness.

Pavuluri and colleagues (2006) treated a group of patients with lithium monotherapy. Those patients who were not responders could then receive risperidone augmentation treatment. In a 12-month trial of 38 participants presenting in a manic or mixed state (all of whom were of preschool age at illness onset), 17 responded to lithium monotherapy, 21 received augmentation with risperidone. The response rate in those youths treated with lithium plus risperidone was 85.7%. Significant predictors of inadequate response to lithium monotherapy, subsequently requiring combination pharmacotherapy, were: (1) severity of ADHD at baseline, (2) a history of sexual or physical abuse, and (3) preschool age. Two participants withdrew from the study due to lithium intolerance. Side effects were similar regardless of whether the participants stayed on lithium monotherapy or required augmentation with risperidone. Weight gain, nausea and vomiting, increased appetite, stomach pain, and sedation were the most common side effects. Overall, lithium, alone or in combination with risperidone, was found to be safe and well tolerated in participants with very early onset bipolar disorder.

Finally, Patel and colleagues (2006b) conducted an open-label study in 27 teenagers between the ages of 12 and 18 with a Children's Depression Rating Scale—Revised (Poznanski & Mokros, 1995) total score of 40 or greater and a Young Mania Rating Scale (Young, Biggs, Ziegeler, & Mayer, 1978) score of less than 20. In this group of youths with prominent depressive symptomatology, approximately half of the patients were found to respond to treatment, with less than 10% of participants discontinuing due to lithium-related side effects.

Lithium Formulations

Lithium is commercially available as lithium carbonate in tablets and capsules. It is also available as lithium citrate syrup. It appears that most patients and families prefer to have lithium administered as tablets or capsules for the sake of convenience. However, if children are unable to swallow tablets or capsules, patients may be prescribed lithium citrate syrup.

Monitoring Lithium and Related Side Effects

As lithium has a relatively low therapeutic index, careful attention to serum levels is vital in the clinical management of patients for whom lithium is prescribed. Lithium levels are generally measured 12 hours after the last dose.

Early signs of lithium toxicity include ataxia, dysarthria, and reduced motor coordination. Symptoms of mild toxicity include listlessness, slurred speech, and coarse tremors. At moderate levels of lithium toxicity, symptoms include more prominent coarse tremors, ataxia, confusion, and delirium. Severe symptoms of toxicity can include seizures, coma, or even death (Jefferson, Greist, & Ackerman, 1987).

During lithium dose titration, frequent monitoring of lithium levels is necessary in order to minimize the risk of overmedication. Once lithium doses are stable, levels may be checked less frequently. We generally recommend that after a patient has been treated on a stable dose of lithium with adequate therapeutic levels for 3 consecutive months, lithium levels may be checked every 3 months, but no less frequently than this.

A summary of the most common lithium-related side effects and possible means to address these side events are summarized in this section and in Table 4.2. It should be noted that most of the literature about the side effects of lithium consists of studies in adults. For that reason, whether or not certain side effects occur more or less frequently in children and adolescents than in adults generally remains an empirical question deserving future study.

Renal Side Effects

The syndrome of polyuria–polydypsia occurs in a substantial number of lithium-treated patients. In children this may lead to enuresis. This side effect can be quite problematic and may lead to lithium discontinuation.

Lithium reversibly reduces the kidney's ability to concentrate urine. It is important to note that the proximal reabsorption of sodium and lithium in the kidneys occurs via a similar mechanism; therefore, states of sodium depletion, such as salt restriction, may increase retention of lithium and increase the chance for toxicity.

TABLE 4.2. Lithium Side Effects and Solutions

Side effect	Intervention
Nausea, vomiting, abdominal pain	Prescribe SR preparations or lithium citrate. Administer with food.
Diarrhea	Reduce the dose and/or prescribe an immediate release preparation; stop the drug if diarrhea persists.
Thirst	Do not restrict drinking (to avoid dehydration).
Enuresis	Limit fluid drinking for 1–2 hours before sleep (This does not mean overt fluid restriction, as that should be avoided.); lower the dose if possible.
Signs of toxicity	Lower dose or discontinue lithium.
Hypothyroidism (high TSH, low T3 and/or T4)	Consider synthetic thyroid supplements. Consider referral to an endocrinologist.
Tremor	Lower dose or prescribe propranolol.
Cognitive dulling	SR preparation, dose adjustment.
Syncope, palpitations, electrocardiogram changes (sinoatrial block and tachycardia)	Consultation with a cardiologist.
Teratogenicity/Ebstein's anomaly	Education, monitoring during pregnancy; consider treatment with other agents.

Note. SR = slow release; TSH = thryotropin; T3= triiodothyronine; T4 = thyroxine.

Clinically relevant nephrotoxicity and kidney dysfunction may also occur as a result of long-term lithium administration; the rate at which these seemingly uncommon events occur in children and adolescents prescribed lithium is not definitely known. Nephrotic syndrome/proteinuria is a rare and idiosyncratic event that may occur as a result of lithium therapy (Markowitz et al., 2000).

Although creatinine clearance assessment is the "gold standard" by which renal function is measured, the practical issues of collecting urine for this assessment generally preclude creatinine clearance being monitored routinely during the course of lithium treatment. More commonly, renal function is assessed by initially and then periodically measuring creatinine and blood urea nitrogen (BUN) and obtaining routine urinalyses to assess the presence of protienuria.

Strategies to manage polyuria–polydypsia include adequate fluid replacement, lithium dosing adjustments, and referral to a pediatric nephrologist if concerns about renal function or lithium-related nephrotic syndrome are present.

Thyroid-Related Side Effects

Clinically, patients may develop goiter with or without hypothyroidism. The rate at which thyroid dysfunction occurs during lithium therapy in children and adolescents is not known. However, in our clinical experience of pediatric patients taking lithium, an increase in thyrotropin levels (thyroid-stimulating hormone; TSH) is not uncommon (Gracious et al., 2004).

Lithium interferes with the production of thyroid hormones at multiple steps, including iodine uptake, tyrosine iodination, and release of triiodothyronine (T_3) and thyroxine (T_4; Johnson, 1988; Lazarus, 1986).

In view of lithium's potential for causing hypothyroidism, it is important to perform baseline thyroid measurements. In follow-up, patients should be observed for development of goiter and should have thyroid functioning assessed. We generally recommend that TSH levels not exceed 10 mU/L.

Development of thyroid abnormalities does not necessitate a change in lithium therapy but, rather, assessment and treatment of the thyroid problem, usually in consultation with an endocrinologist. Thyroid dysfunction can generally be treated by addition of thyroid hormone (e.g., synthetic T_4). No intervention may be necessary if there is only a change in TSH level without low T_3 and T_4. Given the critical role of thyroid hormone in children's growth, thyroid function should be carefully monitored during treatment with lithium. For this reason, we recommend having thyroid levels checked prior to treatment, monthly during the first 3 months of therapy and then every 3 months thereafter (Amdisen & Andersen, 1982; Lindstedt, Nilsson, Walinder, Skott, & Ohman, 1977; Rogers & Whybrow, 1971).

Parathyroid Side Effects

Lithium may lead to hyperparathyroidism at therapeutic levels. Lithium increases the threshold for the calcium-sensing set point, thereby releasing excessive parathyroid hormone. If there are preexisting parathyroid abnormalities, lithium may unmask them, resulting in adenoma or hyperplasia (Mallette, Khouri, Zengotita, Hollis, & Malini, 1989; McHenry et al., 1991).

Neurological Side Effects

Neurological side effects that may occur at therapeutic doses during lithium therapy include a 7–16 Hz tremor that may be similar in appearance to an essential tremor. Although propranolol has been described as being useful for treating this tremor in adults (Gelenberg & Jefferson, 1995), there are few data about the use of this intervention in young people. If tremors do occur, a reduction in lithium might be a reasonable strategy rather than initiating propranolol. It does not appear that lithium-related tremors commonly lead to medication discontinuation.

Headaches may also occur, but they do not seem to substantially interfere with lithium treatment. Dysarthria and ataxia have also been described and can be problematic for some patients. There is some evidence to suggest that preschool-age patients may be more vulnerable than older patients (Hagino et al., 1995). Cognitive dulling has also been reported; however, the cognitive effects of lithium in children and teenagers have not been adequately studied (Pachet & Wisniewski, 2003).

Cardiac Side Effects

Lithium may lead to changes in electrocardiograms (EKGs). These effects can lead to benign flattening of T waves. More serious consequences may include sino-atrial block and/or tachycardia. Fortunately, serious cardiac consequences do not appear to be common at therapeutic lithium doses when this drug is prescribed to children without preexisting cardiac illness. Should EKG changes of potential clinical relevance occur, or should cardiac-related symptoms become present, consultation with a pediatric cardiologist should be considered. Our practice is generally to obtain an EKG prior to treatment initiation, after 2 months' therapy, and yearly thereafter (Hsu et al., 2005).

Dermatological Side Effects

Acne, psoriasis, and folliculitis–pruritis–hyperkeratitis may occur. Hair loss and alopecia are other possible lithium-related side effects (Wagner & Teicher, 1991).

Gastrointestinal Side Effects

Weight gain, diarrhea, nausea, and/or abdominal pain appear to occur in a substantial number of patients. In clinical practice, we recommend that a patient's weight be assessed prior to and during lithium therapy. These side effects typically do not seem to lead to medication discontinuation (Dunner, 2000).

Hematological Side Effects

A relative increase in white blood cell counts, particularly neutrophils and eosinophils, may occur during lithium therapy. This is generally a benign phenomenon for which clinical intervention is usually not needed (Oyewumi, McNight, & Cernovsky, 1999).

Lithium and Pregnancy

One of the physiological changes that occurs during pregnancy is an increase in the GFR. Therefore, women may require higher doses of lithium during pregnancy. In addition, as a result of fluid fluctuations during the peripartum period, lithium levels need to be monitored very carefully in order to avoid toxicity (Yonkers et al., 2004).

Lithium and Teratogenicity

Ebstein's anomaly, a tricuspid valve abnormality, is a rare and potentially serious malformation that may occur in newborns exposed to lithium during the first trimester *in utero* (Yonkers et al., 2004). Therefore, families and teenage girls should be educated about this possibility.

CONCLUSIONS

Lithium has complex neurobiological effects, and, for this reason, the means by which lithium exerts its therapeutic action has yet to be adequately defined. At present, lithium is the most extensively studied agent for the treatment of pediatric bipolar disorder. Unfortunately, much more still needs to be learned about the use of lithium in pediatric patients suffering from bipolar illness. PK and dosing studies that more rigorously define the biodisposition and appropriate dosing of lithium are needed. Acute and maintenance efficacy studies of appropriate methodological rigor need to be performed. In addition, we need to learn much more about the long-term safety of lithium in this vulnerable patient population.

Despite the complexities associated with the clinical management of lithium in pediatric patients and the relative dearth of rigorous scientific evidence about its use in children and adolescents, based on the extant data, lithium appears to be a valuable treatment for children and adolescents with bipolar illness. However, pediatric patients suffering from bipolar illness deserve the conducting of more research with lithium.

DISCLOSURE

Robert L. Findling receives or has received research support from, acted as a consultant to, and/or served as a speaker for Abbott, AstraZeneca, Bristol-Myers Squibb, Celltech-Medeva, Forest, GlaxoSmithKline, Johnson & Johnson, Lilly, New River, Novartis, Otsuka, Pfizer, Sanofi-Synthelabo, Shire, Solvay, and Wyeth. Mani N. Pavuluri receives or has received research support from, acted as a consultant to, and/or served as a speaker for GlaxoSmithKline, Abbott Pharmaceuticals, Johnson & Johnson, and AstraZeneca.

REFERENCES

Ahluwalia, P., Grewaal, D. S., & Singhal, R. L. (1981). Brain GABAergic and dopaminergic systems following lithium treatment and withdrawal. *Progress in Neuro-Psychopharmacology, 5,* 527–530.

Ahluwalia, P., & Singhal, R. L. (1980). Effect of low-dose lithium administration and subsequent withdrawal on biogenetic amines in rat brain. *British Journal of Pharmacology, 71,* 601–607.

Allison, J. H., & Stewart M. A. (1971). Reduced brain inositol in lithium-treated rats. *Nature: New Biology, 233,* 267–268.

Amdisen, A., & Andersen, C. (1982). Lithium treatment of thyroid function: A survey of 237 patients in long-term lithium treatment. *Pharmachopsychiatria, 15,* 149–155.

Annell, A.-L. (1969). Lithium in the treatment of children and adolescents. *Acta Psychiatrica Scandinavica,* Suppl. 270, 19–30.

Berg, I., Hullin, R., Allsopp, M., O'Brien, P., & MacDonald, R. (1974). Bipolar manic-depressive psychosis in early adolescence: A case report. *British Journal of Psychiatry, 125,* 416–417.

Berrettini, W. H., Nurnberger, J. I., Jr., Hare, T. A., Simmons-Alling, S., & Gershon, E. S. (1986). CSF GABA in euthymic manic-depressive patients and controls. *Biological Psychiatry, 21*(8–9), 844–846.

Biermann, I., & Pflug, B. (1974). Ein Fall kindlicher Zyklothymie mit besonderer familiärer Belastung [A case of childhood cyclothmia associated with familial loading]. *Acta Paedopsychiatrica, 40,* 196–203.

Brumback, R. A., & Weinberg, W. A. (1977). Mania in childhood: II. Therapeutic trial of lithium carbonate and further description of manic-depressive illness in children. *American Journal of Diseases of Children, 131,* 1122–1126.

Cade, J. (1949). Lithium salts in the treatment of psychotic excitement. *Medical Journal of Australia, 2,* 349–352.

Calabrese, J. R., Shelton, M. D., Rapport, D. J., Youngstrom, E. A., Jackson, K., Bilali, S., et al. (2005). A 20-month, double-blind, maintenance trial of lithium vs. divalproex in rapid-cycling bipolar disorder. *American Journal of Psychiatry, 162,* 2152–2161.

Carlson, G. A., Rapport, M. D., Kelly, K. L., & Pataki, C. S. (1992). The effects of methylphenidate and lithium on attention and activity level. *Journal of the American Academy of Child and Adolescent Psychiatry, 31*, 262–270.

Carlson, G. A, & Strober, M. (1978). Manic-depressive illness in early adolescence. A study of clinical and diagnostic characteristics in six cases. *Journal of the American Academy of Child Psychiatry, 17*, 138–153.

Chang, K., Karchemskiy, A., Barnea-Goraly, N., Garrett, A., Simeonova, D., & Reis, A. (2005). Reduced amygdalar gray matter volume in familial pediatric bipolar disorder. *Journal of the American Academy of Child and Adolescent Psychiatry, 44*(6), 565–573.

Cooper, T. B., Bergner, P. E., & Simpson, G. M. (1973). The 24-hour serum lithium level as a prognosticator of dosage requirements. *American Journal of Psychiatry, 130*, 601–603.

Davanzo, P., Gunderson, B., Belin, T., Mintz, J., Pataki, C., Ott, D., et al. (2003). Mood stabilizers in hospitalized children with bipolar disorder: A retrospective review. *Psychiatry and Clinical Neurosciences, 57*, 504–510.

Davis, R. E. (1979). Manic-depressive variant syndrome in childhood: a preliminary report. *American Journal of Psychiatry, 136*, 702–706.

DeLong, G. R., & Aldershof, A. L. (1987). Long-term experience with lithium treatment in childhood: Correlation with clinical diagnosis. *Journal of the American Academy of Child and Adolescent Psychiatry, 26*, 389–394.

DeLong, G. R., & Nieman, G. W. (1983). Lithium-induced behavior changes in children with symptoms suggesting manic-depressive illness. *Psychopharmacology Bulletin, 19*, 258–265.

Dousa, T., & Hetcher, O. (1970a). Lithium and brain adenyl cyclase. *Lancet, 1*, 834–835.

Dousa, T., & Hetcher, O. (1970b). The effect of NaCl on vasopressin-sensitive adenyl cyclase. *Life Sciences, 9*, 765–770.

Dugas, M., Guériot, C., & Frohwirth, C. (1975). Le lithium a-t-il un interet en psychiatrie chez l'enfant? [Has lithium a value in child psychiatry?] *Revue de Neuropsychiatrie infantile, 23*, 365–372.

Dunner, D. L. (2000). Optimizing lithium treatment. *Journal of Clinical Psychiatry, 9*, 76–81.

Dyson, W. L., & Barcai, A. (1970). Treatment of children of lithium-responding parents. *Current Therapeutic Research, Clinical and Experimental, 12*, 286–290.

Engel, J., & Berggren, U. (1980). Effects of lithium on behavior and central monoamines. *Acta Psychiatrica Scandinavica, 61*, 133–143.

Feinstein, S. C., & Wolpert, E. A. (1973). Juvenile manic-depressive illness. Clinical and therapeutic considerations. *Journal of the American Academy of Child Psychiatry, 12*, 123–136.

Findling, R. L., Gracious, B. L., McNamara, N. K., Youngstrom, E. A., Demeter, C. A., & Calabrese, J. R. (2001). Rapid, continuous cycling and psychiatric comorbidity in pediatric bipolar I disorder. *Bipolar Disorders, 3*, 202–210.

Findling, R. L., McNamara, N. K., Gracious, B. L., Youngstrom, E. A., Stansbrey, R. J., Reed, M. D., et al. (2003). Combination lithium and divalproex sodium in pediatric bipolarity. *Journal of the American Academy of Child and Adolescent Psychiatry, 42*, 895–901.

Findling, R. L., McNamara, N. K., Stansbrey, R., Gracious, B. L., Whipkey, R. E., Demeter, C. A., et al. (2006). Combination lithium and divalproex sodium in pediatric bipolar symptom restabilization. *Journal of the American Academy of Child and Adolescent Psychiatry, 45*, 142–148.

Findling, R. L., McNamara, N. K., Youngstrom, E. A., Stansbrey, R. J., Gracious, B. L., Reed, M. D., et al. (2005). Double-blind 18-month trial of lithium versus divalproex maintenance treatment in pediatric bipolar disorder. *Journal of the American Academy of Child and Adolescent Psychiatry, 44*, 409–417.

Finley, P. R., Warner, M. D., & Peabody, C. A. (1995). Clinical relevance of drug interactions with lithium. *Clinical Pharmacokinetics, 29*, 172–191.

Gelenberg, A. J., & Jefferson, J. W. (1995). Lithium tremor. *Journal of Clinical Psychiatry, 56*, 283–287.

Geller, B., Cooper, T. B., Zimerman, B., Frazier, J., Williams, M., & Heath, J. (1998). Double-blind and placebo-controlled study of lithium for adolescent bipolar disorders with secondary substance dependency. *Journal of the American Academy of Child and Adolescent Psychiatry*, 37, 171–178.

Geller, B., Craney, J. L., Bolhofner, K., Nickelsburg, M. J., Williams, M., & Zimerman, B. (2002). Two-year prospective follow-up of children with a prepubertal and early adolescent bipolar disorder phenotype. *American Journal of Psychiatry*, 159, 927–933.

Geller, B., & Fetner, H. H. (1989). Children's 24-hour serum lithium level after a single dose predicts initial dose and steady-state plasma level. *Journal of Clinical Psychopharmacology*, 9, 155.

Gonzáles, R. G., Guimarães, A. R., Sachs, G. S., Rosenbaum, J. F., Garwood, M., & Renshaw, P. F. (1993). Measurement of human brain lithium in vivo by MR spectroscopy, *American Journal of Neuroradiology*, 14, 1027–1037.

Goodnick, P. J., & Gershon, E. S. (1985). Lithium. In A. Lajtha (Ed.), *Handbook of neurochemistry* (pp. 103–149). New York: Plenum.

Goodnick, P. J., & Schorr-Cain, C. B. (1991). Lithium pharmacokinetics. *Psychopharmacology Bulletin*, 27, 475–491.

Goodwin, F., & Jamison, K. (1990). *Manic depressive illness*. New York: Oxford University Press.

Gracious, B. L., Findling, R. L., Seman, C., Youngstrom, E. A., Demeter, C. A., & Calabrese, J. R. (2004). Elevated thyrotropin in bipolar youths prescribed both lithium and divalproex sodium. *Journal of the American Academy of Child and Adolescent Psychiatry*, 43, 215–220.

Gram, L. F., & Rafaelsen, O. J. (1972). Lithium treatment of psychotic children and adolescents: A controlled clinical trial. *Acta Psychiatrica Scandinavica*, 48, 253–260.

Hagino, O. R., Weller, E. B., Weller, R. A., Washing, D., Fristad, M. A., & Kontras, S. B. (1995). Untoward effects of lithium treatment in children aged four through six years. *Journal of the American Academy of Child and Adolescent Psychiatry*, 34, 1584–1590.

Hallcher, L. M., & Sherman, W. R. (1980). The effects of lithium ion and other agents on the activity of *myo*-inositol-1-phosphatase from bovine brain. *Journal of Biological Chemistry*, 255, 10896–10901.

Hao, Y., Creson, T., Zhang, L., Li, P., Du, F., Yuan, P., et al. (2004). Mood stabilizer valproate promotes ERK pathway-dependent cortical neuronal growth and neurogenesis. *Journal of Neuroscience*, 24, 6590–6599.

Hassanyeh, F., & Davison, K. (1980). Bipolar affective psychosis with onset before age 16 years: Report of 10 cases. *British Journal of Psychiatry*, 137, 530–539.

Horowitz, H. A. (1977). Lithium and the treatment of adolescent manic depressive illness. *Diseases of the Nervous System*, 38, 480–483.

Hsu, C. H., Liu, P. Y., Chen, J. H., Yeh, T. L., Tsai, H. Y., & Lin, L. J. (2005). Electrocardiographic abnormalities as predictors for over-range lithium levels. *Cardiology*, 103, 101–106.

Hsu, L. K. G. (1986). Lithium-resistant adolescent mania. *Journal of the American Academy of Child Psychiatry*, 25, 280–283.

Janicak, P. G., Davis, J. M., Preskorn, S. H., & Ayd, F. J., Jr. (2001). *Principles and practice of psychopharmocotherapy* (3rd ed.). Philadelphia: Lippincott Williams & Wilkins.

Jefferson, J. W., Greist, J. H., & Ackerman, D. L. (1987). *Lithium encyclopedia for clinical practice* (2nd ed.). Washington, DC: American Psychiatric Press.

Johnson, F. N. (1988). Lithium treatment of aggression, self-mutilation, and affective disorders in the context of medical handicaps. *Contemporary Pharmacotherapy*, 1, 9–18.

Jones, P. M., & Berney, T. P. (1987). Early onset rapid cycling bipolar affective disorder. *Journal of Child Psychology and Psychiatry*, 28, 731–738.

Kafantaris, V., Coletti, D. J., Dicker, R., Padula, G., & Kane, J. M. (2003). Lithium treatment of acute mania in adolescents: A large open trial. *Journal of the American Academy of Child and Adolescent Psychiatry*, 42, 1038–1045.

Kafantaris, V., Coletti, D. J., Dicker, R., Padula, G., Pleak, R. R., Alvir, J. M. J., et al. (2004). Lithium treatment of acute mania in adolescents: A placebo-controlled discontinuation study. *Journal of the American Academy of Child and Adolescent Psychiatry, 43,* 984–993.

Kafantaris, V., Coletti, D. J., Dicker, R., Padula, G., & Pollack, S. (1998). Are childhood psychiatric histories of bipolar adolescents associated with family history, psychosis, and response to lithium treatment? *Journal of Affective Disorders, 51,* 153–164.

Kafantaris, V., Dicker, R., Coletti, D. J., & Kane, J. M. (2001). Adjunctive antipsychotic treatment is necessary for adolescents with psychotic mania. *Journal of Child and Adolescent Psychopharmacology, 11,* 409–413.

Kearns, G. L., Abdel-Rahman, S. M., Alander, S. W., Blowey, D. L., Leeder, J. S., & Kauffman, R. E. (2003). Developmental pharmacology—drug disposition, action, and therapy in infants and children. *New England Journal of Medicine, 349,* 1157–1167.

Kelly, J. T., Koch, M., & Buegel, D. (1976). Lithium carbonate in juvenile manic-depressive illness. *Diseases of the Nervous System, 37,* 90–92.

Kowatch, R. A., Sethuraman, G., Hume, J. H., Kromelis, M., & Weinberg, W. A. (2003). Combination pharmacotherapy in children and adolescents with bipolar disorder. *Biological Psychiatry, 53,* 978–984.

Kowatch, R. A., Suppes, T., Carmody, T. J., Bucci, J. P., Hume, J. H., Kromelis, M., et al. (2000). Effect size of lithium, divalproex sodium, and carbamazepine in children and adolescents with bipolar disorder. *Journal of the American Academy of Child and Adolescent Psychiatry, 39,* 713–720.

Kutcher, S. P., Marton, P., & Korenblum, M. (1990). Adolescent bipolar illness and personality disorder. *Journal of the American Academy of Child and Adolescent Psychiatry, 29,* 355–358.

Lazarus, J. H. (1986). *Endocrine and metabolic effects of lithium.* New York: Plenum.

Lenox, R. H., McNamara, R. K., Watterson, J. M., & Watson, D. G. (1996). Myristoylated alanine-rich C kinase substrate (MARCKS): A molecular target for the therapeutic action of mood stabilizers in the brain? *Journal of Clinical Psychiatry, 57*(Suppl. 13), 23–33.

Licamele, W. L., & Goldberg, R. L. (1989). The concurrent use of lithium and methylphenidate in a child. *Journal of the American Academy of Child and Adolescent Psychiatry, 28,* 785–787.

Lindstedt, G., Nilsson, L., Walinder, J., Skott, A., & Ohman, R. (1977). On the prevalence diagnosis and management of lithium-induced hypothyroidism in psychiatric patients. *British Journal of Psychiatry, 130,* 452–458.

Mallette, L. E., Khouri, K., Zengotita, H., Hollis, B. W., & Malini, S. (1989). Lithium treatment increases intact and midregion parathyroid hormone and parathyroid volume. *Journal of Clinical Endocrinology and Metabolism, 68,* 654–660.

Manji, H. K., Bersudsky, Y., Chen, G., Belmaker, R., & Potter, W. Z. (1996). Modulation of protein kinase c isozymes and substrates by lithium: The role of *myo*-inositol. *Neuropsychopharmacology, 15,* 370–381.

Manji, H. K., & Lenox, R. H. (1998). Lithium: A molecular transducer of mood stabilization in the treatment of bipolar disorder. *Neuropsychopharmacology, 19,* 161–166.

Manji, H. K., McNamara, R., Chen, G., & Lenox, R. H. (1999). Signalling pathways in the brain: Cellular transduction of mood stabilisation in the treatment of manic-depressive illness. *Australian and New Zealand Journal of Psychiatry, 33,* 65–83.

Marcus, W. (1994). Lithium: A review of its pharmacokinetics, health effects, and toxicology. *Journal of Environmental Pathology, Toxicology, and Oncology, 13,* 73–79.

Markowitz, G. S., Radhakrishnan, J., Kambham, N., Valeri, A. M., Hines, W. H., & D'Agati, V. D. (2000). Lithium nephrotoxicity: A progressive combined glomerular and tubulointerstitial nephropathy. *Journal of the American Society of Nephrology, 11,* 1439–1448.

McHenry, C. R., Racke, F., Meister, M., Warnaka, P., Sarasua, M., Nemeth, E. F., & Malangoni, M. A. (1991). Lithium effects on dispersed bovine parathyroid cells grown in tissue culture. *Surgery, 110,* 1061–1066.

McKnew, D. H., Cytryn, L., Buchsbaum, M. S., Hamovit, J., Lamour, M., Rapoport, J. L., et al. (1981). Lithium in children of lithium-responding parents. *Psychiatry Research*, *4*, 171–180.

McNeil, G., Elkins, A., & Goldings, H. (1978). Juvenile manic-depressive illness successfully treated with lithium carbonate. *Journal of the Maine Medical Association*, *69*, 120–121.

Meltzer, H. Y., Arora, R. C., & Goodnick, P. (1983). Effect of lithium carbonate on serotonin uptake in blood platelets of patients with affective disorders. *Journal of Affective Disorders*, *5*, 215–221.

Moore, C. M., Demopulos, C. M., Henry, M. E., Steingard, R. J., Zamvil, L., Katic, A., et al. (2002). Brain-to-serum lithium ratio and age: An *in vivo* lithium magnetic resonance spectroscopy study. *American Journal of Psychiatry*, *159*, 1240–1242.

Moore, G. J., Bebchuk, J. M., & Manji, H. K. (1997). Proton MRS in manic-depressive illness: Monitoring of lithium induced modulation of brain *myo*-inositol. Paper presented at the annual meeting of the Society of Neuroscience, New Orleans, LA.

Moore, G. J., Bebchuk, J. M., Parrish, J. K., Faulk, M. W., Arfken, C. L., Strahl-Bevacqua, J., et al. (1999). Temporal dissociation between lithium-induced changes in frontal lobe *myo*-inositol and clinical response in manic-depressive illness. *American Journal of Psychiatry*, *156*, 1902–1908.

Moore, G. J., Bebchuk, J. M., Wilds, I. B., Chen, G., & Manji, H. K. (2000). Lithium induced increase in human brain grey matter. *Lancet*, *356*, 1241–1242.

Nonaka, S., Katsube, N., & Chuang, D. M. (1998). Lithium protects rat cerebellar granule cells against apoptosis induced by anticonvulsants, phenytoin and carbamazepine. *Journal of Pharmacology and Experimental Therapeutics*, *286*, 539–547.

Oyewumi, L. K., McNight, M., & Cernovsky, Z. Z. (1999). Lithium dosage and leukocyte counts in psychiatric patients. *Journal of Psychiatry and Neuroscience*, *24*(3), 215–221.

Pachet, A. K., & Wisniewski, A. M. (2003). The effects of lithium on cognition: An updated review. *Psychopharmacology*, *170*, 225–234.

Patel, N. C., DelBello, M. P., Bryan, H. S., Adler, C. M., Kowatch, R. A., Stanford, K., et al. (2006b). Open-label lithium for the treatment of adolescents with bipolar depression. *Journal of the American Academy of Child and Adolescent Psychiatry*, *45*, 289–297.

Patel, N. C., DelBello, M. P., Cecil, K. M., Adler, C. M., Bryan, H. S., Stanford, K. E., et al. (2006a). Lithium treatment effects on *myo*-inositol in adolescents with bipolar depression. *Biological Psychiatry*, *60*, 998–1004.

Pavuluri, M. N., Henry, D. B., Carbray, J. A., Sampson, G., Naylor, M. W., & Janicak, P. (2004). Open-label prospective trial of risperidone in combination with lithium or divalproex sodium in pediatric mania. *Journal of Affective Disorders*, *1*, 103–111.

Pavuluri, M. N., Henry, D., Sampson, G., Carbray, J., Naylor, M., & Janicak, P. G. (2006). Risperidone augmentation of lithium in youth with a history of preschool onset bipolar disorder. *Journal of Child and Adolescent Psychopharmacology*, *16*, 336–350.

Poirier, M. F., Galzin, A. M., Pimoule, C., Schoemaker, H., Le Quan Bui, K. H., Meyer, P., et al. (1988). Short-term lithium administration to healthy volunteers produces long lasting pronounced changes in platelet serotonin uptake but not imipramine binding. *Psychopharmacology*, *94*, 521–526.

Poznanski, E., & Mokros, H. (1995). *Children's Depression Rating Scale—Revised*. Los Angeles: Western Psychological Services.

Price, L. H., Charney, D. S., Delgado, P. L., & Heninger, G. R. (1990). Lithium and serotonin function: Implications for the serotonin hypothesis of depression. *Psychopharmacology*, *100*, 3–12.

Renshaw, P. F., & Wicklund, S. (1988). In vivo measurement of lithium in humans by nuclear magnetic resonance spectroscopy. *Biological Psychiatry*, *23*, 465–475.

Rogeness, G. A., Riester, A. E., & Wicoff, J. S. (1982). Unusual presentation in manic depressive disorder in adolescence. *Journal of Clinical Psychiatry*, *43*, 37–39.

Rogers, M., & Whybrow, P. (1971). Clinical hypothyroidism occurring in lithium treatment: Two case histories and a review of thyroid function in 19 patients. *American Journal of Psychiatry, 128,* 150–155.

Sassi, R. B., Nicoletti, M., Brambilla, P., Mallinger, A., Frank, E., Kupfer, D. J., et al. (2002). Increased gray matter volume in lithium-treated bipolar disorder patients. *Neuroscience Letters, 329,* 243–245.

Schou, M. (1986). Lithium treatment: A refresher course. *British Journal of Psychiatry, 149,* 541–547.

Schou, M. (1988). Lithium treatment of manic-depressive illness: Past, present, and perspectives. *Journal of the American Medical Association, 259,* 1834–1836.

Schou, M., Juel-Nielsen, N., Strömgren, E., & Voldby, H. (1954). The treatment of manic psychoses by the administration of lithium salts. *Journal of Neurology, Neurosurgery, and Psychiatry, 17,* 250–260.

State, R. C., Frye, M. A., Altshuler, L. L., Strober, M., DeAntonio, M., Hwang, S., et al. (2004). Chart review of the impact of attention-deficit/hyperactivity disorder comorbidity on response to lithium or divalproex sodium in adolescent mania. *Journal of Clinical Psychiatry, 65,* 1057–1063.

Staunton, D. A., Magistretti, P. J., Shoemaker, W. J., & Bloom, F. E. (1982). Effects of chronic lithium treatment on dopamine receptors in the rat corpus striatum: I. Locomotor activity and behavioral supersensitivity. *Brain Research, 232,* 391–400.

Strober, M., DeAntonio, M., Schmidt-Lackner, S., Freeman, R., Lampert, C., & Diamond, J. (1998). Early childhood attention deficit hyperactivity disorder predicts poorer response to acute lithium therapy in adolescent mania. *Journal of Affective Disorders, 51,* 145–151.

Strober, M., Morrell, W., Burroughs, J., Lamper, C., Danforth, H., & Freeman, R. (1988). A family study of bipolar I disorder in adolescence: Early onset of symptoms linked to increased familial loading and lithium resistance. *Journal of Affective Disorders, 15,* 255–268.

Strober, M., Morrell, W., Lampert, C., & Burroughs, J. (1990). Relapse following discontinuation of lithium maintenance therapy in adolescents with bipolar I illness: A naturalistic study. *American Journal of Psychiatry, 147,* 457–461.

Suppes, T., Baldessarini, R. J., Faedda, G. L., & Tohen, M. (1991). Risk of recurrence following discontinuation of lithium treatment in bipolar disorder. *Archives of General Psychiatry, 48,* 1082–1088.

Sylvester, C. E., Burke, P. M., McCauley, E. A., & Clark, C. J. (1984). Manic psychosis in childhood. Report of two cases. *Journal of Nervous and Mental Disease, 172,* 12–15.

Tomasson, K., & Kuperman, S. (1990). Bipolar disorder in a prepubescent child. *Journal of the American Academy of Child and Adolescent Psychiatry, 29,* 308–310.

Tumuluru, R. V., Weller, E. B., Fristad, M. A., & Weller, R. A. (2003). Mania in six preschool children. *Journal of Child and Adolescent Psychopharmacology, 13,* 489–494.

van Krevelen, V. D. A., & van Voorst, J. A. (1959). Lithium in der Behandlung einer Psychose unklarer Genese bei einem Jugendlichen [Lithium in the therapy of psychosis of unclear genesis in an adolescent.] *Acta Paedopsychiatrica, 26,* 148–152.

Varanka, T. M., Weller, R. A., Weller, E. B., & Fristad, M. A. (1988). Lithium treatment of manic episodes with psychotic features in prepubertal children. *American Journal of Psychiatry, 145,* 1557–1559.

Vitiello, B., Behar, D., Malone, R., Delaney, M. A., Ryan, P. J., & Simpson, G. M. (1988). Pharmacokinetics of lithium carbonate in children. *Journal of Clinical Psychopharmacology, 8,* 355–359.

Wagner, K. D., & Teicher, M. H. (1991). Lithium and hair loss in childhood. *Psychosomatics, 32,* 355–356.

Warneke, L. (1975). A case of manic-depressive illness in childhood. *Canadian Psychiatric Association Journal, 20,* 195–200.

Weller, E. B., Weller, R. A., & Fristad, M. A. (1986). Lithium dosage guide for prepubertal children: A preliminary report. *Journal of the American Academy of Child Psychiatry*, *25*, 92–95.

White, J. H., & O'Shanick, G. (1977). Juvenile manic-depressive illness. *American Journal of Psychiatry*, *134*, 1035–1036.

Williams, R. S., Cheng, L., Mudge, A. W., & Harwood, A. J. (2002). A common mechanism of action for three mood-stabilizing drugs. *Nature*, *417*, 292–295.

Wood, G. E., Young, L. T., Reagan, L. P., Chen, B., & McEwen, B. S. (2004). Stress-induced structural remodeling in hippocampus: Prevention by lithium treatment. *Proceedings of the National Academy of Sciences, USA*, *101*, 3973–3978.

Wozniak, J., Biederman, J., Kiely, K., Ablon, J. S., Faraone, S. V., Mundy, E., et al. (1995). Mania-like symptoms suggestive of childhood-onset bipolar disorder in clinically referred children. *Journal of the American Academy of Child and Adolescent Psychiatry*, *34*, 867–876.

Yonkers, K. A., Wisner, K. L., Stowe, Z., Leibenluft, E., Cohen, L., Miller, L., et al. (2004). Management of bipolar disorder during pregnancy and postpartum period. *American Journal of Psychiatry*, *161*, 608–620.

Young, R. C., Biggs, J. T., Ziegeler, V. E., & Mayer, D. A. (1978). A rating scale for mania: Reliability, validity and sensitivity. *British Journal of Psychiatry*, *133*, 429–435.

CHAPTER 5

Atypical Antipsychotics in the Treatment of Early-Onset Bipolar Disorder

JEAN A. FRAZIER, HALLIE R. BREGMAN,
and JOSEPH A. JACKSON

The complicated diagnostic picture of early-onset bipolar disorder (onset < 18 years of age) often presents significant treatment challenges, resulting in the use of polypharmacy (Biederman et al., 1998; Biederman et al., 1999; Pavuluri, Henry, Carbray, et al., 2004). For example, relative to the adult-onset form of illness, early-onset bipolar disorder is associated with rapid cycling, mixed mood states, chronic irritability, and higher rates of psychosis and other comorbidities, all of which are associated with poor or moderate response to traditional mood stabilizers (Carlson, Loney, Salisbury, Kramer, & Arthur, 2000). Therefore, the diagnostic complexity of children and adolescents who present along the "bipolar spectrum" has increased our need for additional pharmacotherapeutic options. As a result the atypical antipsychotics have played an expanding role in the management of youths with bipolar disorder (Biederman, Mick, Hammerness, et al., 2005; Biederman, Mick, Wozniak, et al., 2005; DelBello, Schwiers, Rosenberg, & Strakowski, 2002; Frazier et al., 2001)

Although conventional ("typical") antipsychotics have been used in the adjunctive treatment of bipolar mania in adults, their use beyond the acute phase has been limited by their serious side effects. In contrast, the more favorable side effect profiles of the *atypical* or "second-generation" antipsychotics (SGAs) signal their potential for longer term use in the treatment of mood disorders. In addition, the results of treatment studies appear to support the notion that the SGAs share mood-stabilizing properties not found among their conventional antipsychotic counterparts (Tohen et al., 2000; Tohen et al., 1999).

This chapter examines how antipsychotic medications, in particular the atypical antipsychotics, fit into the standard of care for early-onset bipolar disorder (age < 18 years). The pharmacological properties of antipsychotic medications that are relevant to mood stabilization are reviewed. The evidence supporting the use of antipsychotic agents in the acute and maintenance treatment of manic, depressive, and mixed states in youths are described. Finally, practical and safety issues relevant to prescribing antipsychotic medications to children and adolescents with bipolar disorder are addressed.

HISTORICAL PERSPECTIVE

Beginning with early reports on the efficacy of chlorpromazine in agitated states (Delay, Deniker, & Harl, 1952), antipsychotic medications have been used to treat the agitation, aggression, and psychosis associated with acute mania in adults. Beyond the tranquilization used for chemical restraint, conventional antipsychotics have demonstrated true antimanic effects (Janicak, Newman, & Davis, 1992). However, the potential benefits of conventional antipsychotics in bipolar disorder are frequently offset by serious treatment-associated side effects. Of particular concern is the high incidence (up to 40%) of acute and tardive extrapyramidal symptoms (EPS; Hunt & Silverstone, 1991). Other evidence has suggested that typical antipsychotics exacerbate major depressive episodes in patients with bipolar disorder (Krakowski, Czobor, & Volavka, 1997; Voruganti & Awad, 2004). For these reasons, the use of typical antipsychotics beyond the acute manic phase has historically been discouraged.

Clozapine was the first antipsychotic to be called "atypical" due to its unique pharmacological profile, its greater efficacy in treating negative symptoms, and its much lower propensity to cause EPS compared with "typical" antipsychotics (Shen, 1999). Evidence has since accumulated suggesting that atypical antipsychotic medications also have significant mood-stabilizing properties (Brambilla, Barale, & Soares, 2003; Shen, 1999). By design, most antipsychotic medications introduced after clozapine share these key "atypical" properties. Aripiprazole, the latest antipsychotic agent approved for clinical use in the United States, extends the concept of "atypicality" due to its unique mechanism of action at the dopamine receptor (Bowles & Levin, 2003; Shen, 1999). Finally, clozapine and later antipsychotic agents, including aripiprazole, are more broadly labeled SGAs to distinguish them from their progenitors, the "typical" or conventional antipsychotics (Fleischhacker, 2002; Shen, 1999).

SGAs are different from typical antipsychotics because of the number of rigorous clinical trials required for Food and Drug Administration (FDA) approval. Data confirming the safety and efficacy of the SGAs for the treatment of psychotic and bipolar disorders in adults have led to the displacement of the typical antipsychotic medications for both acute and long-term management of these conditions in adults (Martin, Miller, & Kotzan, 2001; Shen, 1999). Additionally, based on the strength of the adult safety and efficacy data and a handful of trials in children, atypical antipsychotics are currently recommended as one of the initial options for the treatment of mixed or manic episodes in children with bipolar disorder, regardless of the presence of psychotic symptoms (Kowatch et al., 2005; Shen, 1999). However, further research is necessary to maximize drug efficacy and patient outcomes while minimizing potential medication toxicities in youths.

MOOD-STABILIZING PROPERTIES
OF ATYPICAL ANTIPSYCHOTICS

Antipsychotic medications exert their therapeutic effects (and many adverse effects) through their binding of specific cellular receptors in the central nervous system. All antipsychotic medications bind dopamine, muscarinic, alpha1-adrenergic, and H1-histamine receptors (Shen, 1999; Stahl, 1999). In binding certain receptors, antipsychotics (typicals and atypicals) compete with endogenous receptor substrates, effectively blocking the action of the substrate at its receptor (receptor blockade). For example, antipsychotics have dopaminergic D_2 blockade, which acts in the mesolimbic tract to reduce positive symptoms of psychosis and mania (Shen, 1999; Stahl, 1999). However, blockade of D_2 receptors in the nigrostriatal and tuberoinfundibular tracts are associated with EPS and abnormal elevations of serum prolactin, respectively, side effects that are commonly seen with typical antipsychotics (Shen, 1999; Stahl, 1999). In addition, there is evidence that typical antipsychotic medications may actually induce dysphoria through dopaminergic blockade in the nucleus accumbens, which may partially be due to their relative lack of serotonergic blockade (Shen, 1999; Voruganti & Awad, 2004).

Atypical antipsychotics have the added feature of binding serotonin (5-HT) receptors (Miller et al., 1998; Shen, 1999). Blockade of the 5-HT_{2A} receptor subtype and/or 5-HT_{1A} partial agonism are believed to lower the occurrence of EPS and perhaps improve the efficacy of these drugs in treating negative symptoms of schizophrenia and bipolar disorder (Meltzer,

1999; Richelson, 1999; Shen, 1999). The competitive binding at both the dopamine and serotonin receptors may be involved in the stabilizing effects of atypical antipsychotic medications on mood (Shen, 1999; Yatham, 2002). Most atypicals bind other subtypes of dopamine receptors while binding the D_2 receptor less tightly than typical antipsychotics (Kapur & Seeman, 2000; Shen, 1999). In addition, most appear to exert antidepressant effects by altering serotonergic function. Specifically, 5-HT$_{2A}$ receptor blockade may be responsible for some of the antidepressant effects observed and may account for anecdotal reports associating SGAs with the induction of mania (Cheng-Shannon, McGough, Pataki, & McCracken, 2004; Shen, 1999). Therefore, the enhanced mood-stabilizing properties of SGAs may be due to the coexistence of both antidepressant and antimanic properties.

The lower overall side-effect burden of SGAs compared with typical agents has made them important additions to the pharmacotherapeutic options available to those suffering from bipolar disorder, particularly with respect to safety and patient compliance. Other practical considerations, such as ease of administration, wider therapeutic windows, and the lack of compulsory blood level monitoring, make these medications attractive alternatives to conventional mood stabilizers, especially in the treatment of children (Frazier et al., 2001; Frazier et al., 1999; Shen, 1999).

USE OF ANTIPSYCHOTICS IN THE TREATMENT OF EARLY-ONSET BIPOLAR DISORDER

The treatment of adults and youths with bipolar disorder has frequently included antipsychotic medications as adjunctive agents in combination with lithium or anticonvulsants, most often in the acute treatment of manic or mixed states (Brambilla et al., 2003; Pavuluri, Henry, Carbray, Naylor, & Janicak, 2005; Shen, 1999). Studies of monotherapeutic treatment with olanzapine, risperidone, ziprasidone, quetiapine, and aripiprazole for acute mania in adults with bipolar disorder have been reported. For all states of bipolar disorder, treatment studies in adults far outnumber those in youths. Therefore, the results from adult studies help to inform the treatment of early-onset bipolar disorder in the absence of comparable data in children.

As interest in treatment of bipolar disorder in children and adolescents grows, more open-label and controlled trials of these agents are being completed. To date, there have been six small open-label monotherapy trials (Barzman, DelBello, Adler, Stanford, & Strakowski, 2006; Biederman, Mick, Wozniak, et al., 2005; DelBello, Cecil, et al., 2006; DelBello et al., 2005; Frazier et al., 2001; Marchand, Wirth, & Simon, 2004) and two controlled monotherapy trials (Biederman et al., 2006; DelBello, Kowatch, et al., 2006) of SGAs in outpatient treatment of manic or mixed states in youths, one small controlled trial of quetiapine in combination with divalproex (DVP) for the acute treatment of manic and mixed states in adolescents with bipolar disorder (DelBello et al., 2002), and three open-label combination-therapy trials with DVP or lithium and quetiapine or haloperidol (Kafantaris, Dicker, Coletti, & Kane, 2001; Kafantaris, Coletti, Dicker, Padula, & Kane, 2001; Marchand et al., 2004).

Prospective studies that assess the treatment of psychotic and depressive symptoms in youths with bipolar disorder, as well as studies to evaluate maintenance therapy in this population, are limited in number. There have been two prospective studies utilizing the typical antipsychotics combined with lithium for the acute treatment of psychotic and nonpsychotic mania in adolescents with bipolar disorder (Kafantaris, Coletti, et al., 2001; Kafantaris, Dicker, et al., 2001). There have been no published studies of antipsychotic treatment for bipolar depression in youths. However, promising data were recently presented from a double-blind placebo-controlled trial of quetiapine monotherapy in adolescents with bipolar disorder and depressive symptoms (Barzman et al., 2005; Kafantaris, Coletti, et al., 2001). Evidence for the use of antipsychotics as monotherapy in the maintenance treatment of early-onset BPD is so far limited to one 9-month study that used risperidone as part of a treatment algorithm (Kafantaris, Coletti, et al., 2001; Pavuluri, Henry, Carbray, et al., 2004).

The paucity of experimental data for the treatment of bipolar disorder in children and adolescents has led to the publishing of treatment guidelines based on expert consensus (Kafantaris, Coletti, et al., 2001; Kowatch et al., 2005). Treatment response is most often assessed by treatment-associated reduction in symptom severity as measured by the Young Mania Rating Scale (YMRS; Gracious, Youngstrom, Findling, & Calabrese, 2002; Kafantaris, Coletti, et al., 2001; Young, Biggs, Ziegler, & Meyer, 1978). In the next section we briefly summarize the extant data supporting the use of typical antipsychotic medications and SGAs in the treatment of bipolar disorder in children and adolescents. Treatment-emergent adverse effects reported for individual agents are mentioned here and discussed further in a subsequent section on the prescription of these agents in early-onset bipolar disorder.

Typical Antipsychotics

There remains ongoing controversy about whether antipsychotics are necessary to treat psychosis that occurs in youths with bipolar disorder. Some literature suggests that mood stabilizers alone can be effective (Findling, McNamara, et al., 2005; Geller et al., 1998; Kafantaris, Coletti, et al., 2001; Kowatch et al., 2000; Wagner et al., 2002). However, Kafantaris and colleagues found that this may not always be true. They evaluated adjunctive haloperidol treatment with lithium in youths with bipolar disorder with psychotic features (Kafantaris, Coletti, et al., 2001); haloperidol was added after therapeutic lithium levels were obtained and then discontinued after 1 week of treatment. The patients improved on the combined treatment and experienced a quick reexacerbation of psychotic symptoms and/ or agitation when haloperidol was discontinued. Therefore, combination therapy may be necessary for a much greater period of time to maintain stability in these patients.

In another open-label treatment study, Kafantaris and colleagues treated 42 youths with bipolar disorder and psychotic features (mean age = 15.9 ± 1.9 years) with a combination of lithium and an antipsychotic (Kafantaris, Coletti, et al., 2001). The adjunctive antipsychotics included haloperidol ($n = 15$), risperidone ($n = 6$), olanzapine ($n = 3$), thiothixene ($n = 1$), and chlorpromazine ($n = 1$). Twenty-eight of the participants completed the study, and the majority of patients experienced rapid resolution of their psychoses. No significant differences were seen in response rate on any of these agents (whether typical or atypical). Half of the patients met criteria for entering the discontinuation phase of the trial during which their antipsychotic medication was stopped. Furthermore, 8 out of the 14 remaining participants who qualified for discontinuation relapsed. The authors concluded that the usual recommendation to limit antipsychotic treatment to only 4 weeks in patients with psychotic mania may be too conservative.

Atypical Antipsychotics

Clozapine

Clozapine has been evaluated systematically for both short- and long-term treatment of refractory mania in adults (Barbini et al., 1997; Kafantaris, Coletti, et al., 2001). Response rates in these studies ranged from 80 to 87%. Treatment of adults with refractory *psychotic* mania with clozapine monotherapy for 12 weeks at a mean daily dose of only 254 mg resulted in a response rate of 45% (defined by ≥ 50% reduction in YMRS score; Green et al., 2000). The data for clozapine in bipolar depression are limited to adult case reports that suggest it may have some antidepressant effects in both bipolar (Calabrese, Meltzer, & Markovitz, 1991; Kafantaris, Coletti, et al., 2001; Suppes, Phillips, & Judd, 1994) and unipolar (Naber, Holzbach, Perro, & Hippius, 1992; Ranjan & Meltzer, 1996) depression. These adult studies were important in providing some of the first information regarding the potential of clozapine and subsequent atypicals as mood stabilizers.

Evidence for the use of clozapine in the treatment of bipolar disorder in children and adolescents includes case reports and a small retrospective review describing a positive response in adolescents with refractory mania (Fuchs, 1994; Kafantaris, Coletti, et al., 2001; Kowatch et al., 1995; Masi & Milone, 1998). In addition, Masi and colleagues report the results of open label administration of clozapine (mean dose = 142.5 mg) as monotherapy or as an adjunctive agent to 10 adolescent inpatients with treatment refractory mania (Masi, Mucci, & Millepiedi, 2002). These authors found that all of the youths significantly responded to clozapine after 15–28 days of treatment (at hospital discharge). Side effects included somnolence, enuresis, sialorrhea, and increased appetite. The mean weight gain after 6 months of clozapine treatment in these same youths was 7 ± 3 kg.

Double-blind studies evaluating the safety and efficacy of clozapine in a larger number of participants is warranted and would provide valuable information regarding the use of this agent for the most refractory of children with bipolar disorder. Despite the lack of data on the treatment of youths with bipolar disorder, it is clear from studies in youths with schizophrenia that clozapine treatment remains a therapeutic option that is reserved for the treatment of refractory cases only due to its side-effect profile and requisite blood monitoring (Frazier et al., 1994; Kafantaris, Coletti, et al., 2001; Kumra et al., 1996).

Risperidone

Two blinded, randomized trials showed risperidone and haloperidol to be equally efficacious for augmentation of lithium in the acute treatment of mania in adults (Kafantaris, Coletti, et al., 2001; Sachs, Grossman, Ghaemi, Okamoto, & Bowden, 2002; Segal, Berk, & Brook, 1998). In a large multicenter, 3-week, double-blind, placebo-controlled trial, risperidone monotherapy was superior to placebo for the acute treatment of mania in adults with bipolar disorder after only 3 days of treatment based on reduction on the YMRS, and this effect was sustained for the rest of the study (Hirschfeld, Baker, Wozniak, Tracy, & Sommerville, 2003; Kafantaris, Coletti, et al., 2001). The effect of risperidone was also significant on each of the four other standard measures, including a significant reduction in depressive symptoms based on Montgomery–Asberg Depression Rating Scale (MADRS) scores.

In youths with bipolar disorder, risperidone was the second atypical antipsychotic to be assessed for its effectiveness. The first study was a systematic chart review of risperidone treatment added to ongoing pharmacological treatments ($n = 28$, mean age 10.4 ± 3.8 years). Risperidone was given at a mean dose of 1.7 mg for a mean duration of treatment of 6.1 months. Response was defined as a Clinical Global Impressions–Improvement (CGI-I) scale of ≤ 2. Eighty-two percent of patients were deemed responders. These youths showed improvements not only in mood but also in aggressive behaviors (82%) and psychotic symptoms (69%; Frazier et al., 1999; Kafantaris, Coletti, et al., 2001). Side effects included weight gain, somnolence, and sialorrhea. No EPS or tardive dyskinesia were observed. This chart review set the stage for several subsequent studies on the use of this agent in the pediatric population (Biederman, Mick, Hammerness, et al., 2005; Biederman, Mick, Wozniak, et al., 2005; Kafantaris, Coletti, et al., 2001; Pavuluri, Henry, Naylor, et al., 2004).

The evidence for risperidone monotherapy in the acute treatment of children and adolescents with bipolar disorder includes two prospective open-label studies. The first study was an 8-week open-label trial of risperidone in 30 outpatients (ages 6–17 years) with bipolar disorder (manic, hypomanic, or mixed); doses were titrated weekly according to tolerability and response. Maximum daily doses were 2 mg for participants ≤ 12 years old and up to 4 mg daily for older patients. A statistically significant reduction in YMRS scores was observed by the end of the first week. By week 8, 70% of participants showed a positive response, defined by a much or, at times, very much improved score on the CGI-I scale (≤ 2; Biederman, Mick, Wozniak, et al., 2005; Kafantaris, Coletti, et al., 2001). Significant side effects included weight gain and increased prolactin levels. The second trial was an open-label 8-week study of risperidone and olanzapine monotherapy in 31 preschoolers (ages 4–6 years) with bipolar disorder (Biederman, Mick, Hammerness, et al., 2005; Kafantaris, Coletti, et al., 2001). This was the first study to be done assessing any atypical agent for the treatment of bipolar disorder in preschoolers. The mean daily dose of risperidone was 1.4 ± 0.5 mg/day and of that of olanzapine was 6.3 ± 2.3 mg/day. Both medications led to a significant reduction in scores on the YMRS, and there was no difference in rate of response between those treated with risperidone or with olanzapine. However, only the group treated with risperidone showed significant improvement of depressive symptoms as assessed by the Children's Depression Rating Scale (CDRS). Both treatments resulted in significant increases in weight, but only those children treated with risperidone had significant elevations in prolactin (Biederman, Mick, Hammerness, et al., 2005; Kafantaris, Coletti, et al., 2001).

Finally, there are two prospective trials that evaluate longer term (6 months and 12 months) treatment of youths with mania with a combination of risperidone and lithium or risperidone and divalproex sodium (Pavuluri, Henry, Carbray, et al., 2004; Pavuluri et al., 2006). In the first study, 37 participants (ages 5–18 years) with mixed or manic episodes were enrolled (Pavuluri, Henry, Carbray, et al., 2004). Children in both groups showed significant improvement on all efficacy measures (YMRS, Clinical Global Impressions—Bipolar [CGI-BP], and CDRS—Revised). No differences were found between groups in tolerability or safety. The second study assessed the safety and efficacy of risperidone augmentation of lithium in preschool-onset bipolar disorder among youths who were partial responders to lithium monotherapy (Pavuluri et al., 2006). Thirty-eight participants (mean age: 11.37 ± 3.8 years) with onset of bipolar disorder in the preschool years entered a 12-month trial. All participants received lithium monotherapy, and those who failed to respond to lithium after 8 weeks, as well as those who relapsed after initially responding, were given adjunctive risperidone for up to 11 months. The YMRS was the primary outcome measure in this study (response ≥ 50% decrease in YMRS from baseline). A substantial number (21 out of 38) of these youths were either nonresponders or partial responders to lithium monotherapy. Subsequent augmentation of lithium with risperidone was well tolerated and efficacious in 18 out of 21 youths receiving the combined treatment. These two studies are notably the only long-term studies of any atypical antipsychotic used for treating children with a mood disorder. See Table 5.1 for more details on prospective studies of atypical antipsychotics in early-onset bipolar disorder.

Olanzapine

Olanzapine has the most evidence for mood-stabilizing properties of any antipsychotic medication and has been approved by the FDA for the acute treatment of mania. Five double-blind controlled studies have demonstrated the acute antimanic efficacy of olanzapine monotherapy in adults with bipolar disorder (Pavuluri et al., 2006; Yatham, 2003). In two of these studies, olanzapine was shown to be superior to placebo in treating symptoms of manic or mixed states in adults with bipolar disorder independent of the presence of psychotic symptoms (Pavuluri et al., 2006; Tohen et al., 2000; Tohen et al., 1999). In addition, in a double-blind, placebo-controlled trial in adults with bipolar mania, an intramuscular formulation of olanzapine was reported to be more effective than both placebo and intramuscular lorazepam for the reduction of acute agitation (Meehan et al., 2001).

Published data on the use of olanzapine in the treatment of pediatric bipolar disorder are more limited than in adults. There is one retrospective chart review and one open-label study (Frazier et al., 2001; Pavuluri et al., 2006; Soutullo, Sorter, Foster, McElroy, & Keck, 1999). Olanzapine monotherapy was studied in 23 children and adolescents with bipolar disorder in an 8-week open-label treatment trial (Frazier et al., 2001; Pavuluri et al., 2006). Participants were 5–14 years old and met criteria for bipolar I or bipolar II disorder (manic, hypomanic, or mixed states). Based on response criteria of a 30% decrease in the YMRS and a final Clinical Global Impressions—Severity Scale (CGI-S) ≤ 3, the response rate was reported to be 61% in the 22 of 23 participants completing the study. The mean daily dose of olanzapine was 9.6 ± 4.3 mg. The authors also reported statistically

TABLE 5.1. Prospective Studies with Antipsychotic Medications in Early-Onset Bipolar Disorder

Study	Design	Subjects	Drug/dose	Outcome measures	Results
			Acute treatment		
Monotherapy trials					
Frazier et al. (2001)	8-week open trial; outpatient	23 BPD I or II; 5–14 years	olanzapine 9.6 ± 4.3 mg/day (0.21 ± 0.1 mg/kg/day range, 2.5–20 mg/day)	YMRS, CGI-S BPRS,CDRS	61% response ($\downarrow$ YMRS $\geq$ 30% *and* CGI-S $\leq$ 3)
Biederman, McDonnell, et al. (2005)	4.6 months (average) chart review; outpatient	41 BPD 7–15 years	aripiprazole 16.0 ± 7.9 mg/ day	CGI-I	71% response in aripiprazole (CGI-I $\leq$ 2)
Biederman, Mick, Hammerness, et al. (2005)	8-week open trial; outpatient	31 BPD I, II, or NOS; 4–6 years	risperidone 1.4 ± .5 mg/day olanzapine 6.3 ± 2.3 mg/ day	YMRS, CGI-I CDRS, BPRS	69% response in risperidone 53% response in olanzapine ($\downarrow$ YMRS $\geq$ 30% *or* CGI-I $\leq$ 2)
Biederman, Mick, Wozniak, et al. (2005)	8-week open trial; outpatient	30 BPD I, II, or NOS; 6–17 years	risperidone 1.25 ± 1.5 mg/ day (range, 0.25–2.0 mg/ day)	YMRS, CGI-S BPRS,CDRS	70% response ($\downarrow$ YMRS $\geq$ 30% *or* CGI-I $\leq$ 2)
DelBello, Cecil, et al. (2006)	4-week open trial; outpatient	20 BPD I; 10 HC; 12–18 years	olanzapine 10–20 mg/day	YMRS, CGI-BP-I, CGAS, CDRS-R,	74% response ($\downarrow$ YMRS $\geq$ 50%) 59% remitters ($\downarrow$ YMRS $\leq$ 12, CDRS-R $\leq$ 40, CGI-I $\leq$ 2, *and* CGAS $\geq$ 51)

(continued)

78

Study	Design	Sample	Medication/dose	Measures	Results
DelBello, Kowatch, et al. (2006)	4-week double-blind trial; outpatient	50 BPD I 12–18 years	quetiapine 400–600 mg/day divalproex serum level 80–120 µg/ML	YMRS, CGI-BP-I, PANSS-P, CDRS	60% response in quetiapine 28% response in divalproex ($\downarrow$ YMRS $\leq$ 12 *and* CGI-BP-I $\leq$ 2)
Biederman et al. (2006)	6-week multicenter, double-blind, randomized, parallel-arm trial	110 BPD I	risperidone .01– > 1.5mg/day Mean: 1.52mg/d	NCBRF	
Barzman et al. (2006)	4-week open trial; outpatient	33 BP I, manic or mixed mood + comorbid disruptive behavioral disorder; 12–18 years	quetiapine 400–600 mg/day divalproex serum level 80–120 mg/dL	PANSS EC	Significant within-treatment effects seen for quetiapine and divalproex with no significant group differences in PANSS-EC from baseline to end point

Combination therapy with mood stabilizers

Controlled trial

Study	Design	Sample	Medication/dose	Measures	Results
DelBello et al. (2002)	6-week RDBPC, outpatient follow-up	30 BPD I, manic or mixed; 12–18 years	DVP + quetiapine (QUE) vs. DVP + placebo (Mean DVP level 113 ± 20mg/dL ; Mean QUE dose 432mg/d)	YMRS, PANSS-P CDRS, CGAS	Response ($\downarrow$ YMRS $\geq$ 50%) 87% (DVP+ QUE) vs. 53% (placebo + DVP)

(continued)

79

TABLE 5.1. (*continued*)

Study	Design	Subjects	Drug/dose	Outcome measures	Results
Open trials					
Kafantaris, Coletti, et al. (2001)	Open 4-week COMB (antipsychotic + Li) then 4-week Li	35 BPD I, manic with psychosis; 12–18 years	Li + haloperidol (53.6% of patients, 5 mg/day) or risperidone (21.4% of patients, 2.25 mg/day) or other in 6 patients (olanzapine 10 mg/day, quetiapine 300 mg/day, thiothixene 8 mg/day, chlorpromazine, 100 mg/day)	YMRS, CGI-I Ham-D, CGAS	28/35 completed COMB trial; 8 stable on Li maintenance
Kafantaris, Dicker, et al. (2001)	Open 1-week COMB, then 6-week DBPC discontinuation	10 BPD I, manic 5 psychotic, 5 nonpsychotic; 12–18 years	Li + haloperidol (mean 5 mg daily)	YMRS, Ham-D BPRS	Response ($\downarrow$ YMRS $\geq$ 33% and CGI-S $\leq$ 2) 60% in *non*psychotic participants; 0% in psychotic participants
Maintenance treatment					
Pavuluri, Henry, Naylor, et al. (2004)	Open, outpatients 24 weeks	40 BPD I, manic or mixed; 12.1 ± 3.5 years	Li *or* DVP + risperidone (Mean risp dose: li + risp = 0.75 ± 0.75 mg/day DVP + risp= 0.7 ± 0.67 mg/day)	YMRS, CDRS-R CGI-I, CGAS	Response ($\downarrow$ YMRS $\geq$ 50%, CGI $\leq$ 2 and CGAS $\geq$ 51) same (~80%) – li + risp = DVP + risp

Study	Design	Sample	Intervention	Measures	Outcomes
Pavuluri, Henry, Carbray, et al. (2004)	Open, outpatients 24 weeks	64 BPD I, manic or mixed; 11.2 ± 3.4 years	ALG vs. TAU	YMRS, CGI-S CGI-I-BP, CGAS	Response (final CGI-BP ≤ 2) 68% for ALG group vs. 0% for TAU; only 28% stabilized on monotherapy
Pavuluri et al. (2006)	Open, outpatients 12 months	30 BPD I, manic or mixed, preschool onset 11.37 ± 3.8 years	8 weeks of lithium monotherapy; adjunctive risperidone treatment for insufficient responders	YMRS, CGI, CDRS, CGAS	Response rate (≥ 50% drop in YMRS from baseline) to lithium monotherapy 45%; response rate for combined treatment was 85.7%

Note. ALG, algorithm; BPD, bipolar disorder; BPRS, Brief Psychiatric Rating Scale; CDRS, Children's Depression Rating Scale; CDRS-R, Children's Depression Rating Scale, Revised; CGAS, Children's Global Assessment Scale; CGI-BP, Clinical Global Impression for Bipolar Disorder; CGI-I, Clinical Global Impression of Improvement; CGI-I-BP, Clinical Global Impression of Improvement for Bipolar Disorder; CGI-S, Clinical Global Impression of Severity; DBPC, double-blind placebo-controlled; DVP, divalproex sodium; Ham-D, Hamilton Depression Rating Scale; Li, lithium; NCBRF, Nisonger Child Behavior Rating Form; Ox, oxcarbazepine; PANSS-P, Positive and Negative Symptom Scale—Positive subscale; PANSS-EC, Positive and Negative Symptom Scale—Excited Component; QUE, quetiapine; RDBPC, randomized double-blind placebo controlled; TAU, treatment as usual; YMRS, Young Mania Rating Scale.

significant improvement on all other scales (Brief Psychiatric Rating Scale [BPRS], CDRS) compared with baseline. Overall, the medication was well-tolerated and the only significant side effect was increased body weight (5.0 ± 2.3 kg; $p < .001$ from baseline). Interestingly, 35% ($n = 8$) of the participants were maintained on their stimulant medications, and no differences were seen between those on stimulants and those not with respect to clinical response or weight gain (Frazier et al., 2001; Pavuluri et al., 2006). This study was the first to assess olanzapine in a systematic way in youths with bipolar disorder, and it led to a subsequent open-label study in preschool children with bipolar disorder by Biederman and colleagues (Biederman, Mick, Hammerness, et al., 2005; Pavuluri et al., 2006), as well as a study of adolescents with bipolar disorder by DelBello and colleagues (DelBello, Cecil, et al., 2006; Pavuluri et al., 2006).

DelBello and colleagues studied 20 children with bipolar I disorder in mixed or manic states who were hospitalized for the first time. These participants received olanzapine monotherapy in a 4-week open trial. The researchers found that 74% of the adolescents with bipolar disorder were responders, based on a response criteria of a 50% reduction in YMRS score from baseline to end point. The only significant side effect observed was an increase in body weight from baseline to end point (5.3 ± 3.6 kg; $p < .0001$; DelBello, Cecil, et al., 2006; Pavuluri et al., 2006).

Quetiapine

Quetiapine has been studied as a treatment for bipolar mania in adults, both as an adjunctive agent and as monotherapy. Three placebo-controlled, double-blind acute studies assessed quetiapine as monotherapy for mania and found a significant response, defined by a 50% reduction in YMRS score from baseline to end point (McIntyre, Brecher, Paulsson, Huizar, & Mullen, 2005; Bowden et al., 2005; Vieta, Mullen, Brecher, Paulsson, & Jones, 2005). Furthermore, two double-blind, placebo-controlled studies evaluated the efficacy and tolerability of quetiapine as combination therapy with lithium or DVP and observed significant improvement of the YMRS score from baseline to end point (Sachs et al., 2004; Yatham, Paulsson, Mullen, & Vagero, 2004). Two 3-week, open-label studies were completed examining rapid dose administration of quetiapine as an adjunctive medication in the treatment of bipolar mania; both studies found that patients were able to tolerate rapid titration and showed significant improvement in manic symptoms (Hatim et al., 2006; Pae et al., 2005).

Four studies have examined the use of quetiapine as monotherapy or adjunctive medication to treat mixed states in adults with bipolar disorder who were suboptimally responsive to traditional mood stabilizers. Two of the studies were short term (4–12 weeks; Sajatovic et al., 2001; Sokolski & Denson, 2003), whereas the other two studies followed patients for 6 to 12 months (Altamura, Salvadori, Madaro, Santini, & Mundo, 2003; Hardoy, Garofalo, Carpiniello, Calabrese, & Carta, 2005). All studies found that, overall, quetiapine was well tolerated by adult patients, with only mild side effects.

Published data on quetiapine treatment of bipolar mania in youths consist of two controlled trials and a chart review (Catapano-Friedman, 2001; DelBello, Kowatch, et al., 2006; DelBello et al., 2002; Marchand et al., 2004; Schaller & Behar, 1999). Efficacy for quetiapine as an adjunctive treatment for bipolar mania was first demonstrated in adolescents in a double-blind study by DelBello and colleagues (DelBello et al., 2002; Marchand et al., 2004). These investigators studied quetiapine versus placebo in combination with DVP for the short-term treatment of adolescent mania. Following a loading dose of DVP, 30 adolescents with manic or mixed bipolar I disorder (12–18 years of age) were randomized to receive quetiapine or placebo in combination with DVP for 6 weeks. Quetiapine was titrated to a daily dose of 450 mg (mean dose = 432 mg), and an initial dose of DVP was given at 20 mg/kg/day and titrated to therapeutic levels. Using a criterion of $\geq$ 50% reduction in the YMRS, the authors found a response rate of 87% versus 53% for the quetiapine and placebo groups, respectively. Secondary outcome measures, including the Children's Global Assessment Scale (CGAS), CDRS, and Positive and Negative Symptom Scale (PANSS)— Positive subscale, all showed significant change from baseline, although no group differences were observed for these measures. The most common side effect associated with quetiapine was sedation, which was reported by 80% of participants receiving DVP and quetiapine compared with 33% of participants receiving DVP plus placebo.

Regarding quetiapine monotherapy in bipolar youth, a retrospective chart review completed by Marchand and colleagues (2004) found that children and adolescents with bipolar disorder (I, II, or not otherwise specified) or cyclothymia had significant improvement on quetiapine monotherapy (78.6%) or adjunctive therapy (80%) as defined by a CGI-I score of $\leq$ 2 at end point. Fourteen patients received quetiapine alone, whereas 18 patients received quetiapine with DVP, oxcarbazepine, or lithium and DVP. No serious adverse events occurred, and only a few mild side effects were reported (Marchand et al., 2004). DelBello and colleagues completed a study comparing quetiapine monotherapy with DVP monotherapy (DelBello, Kowatch, et al., 2006; Marchand et al., 2004). This study was a 4-week, double-blind trial in adolescents with bipolar I disorder, ages 12–18 years. Fifty adolescents were randomized, and 19 completed each arm of the study. Both treatment groups showed significant improvement in their YMRS scores from baseline to end point, although there was no statistically significant difference between the groups. The rate of remission (YMRS $\leq$ 12) was greater in the quetiapine group (60%) than the DVP group (28%). Furthermore, the quetiapine group showed a greater response rate in terms of the Clinical Global Impression of Improvement for Bipolar Disorder (CGI-I-BP) (72%), compared with the DVP group (40%). The mean quetiapine dose for responders was 422 mg/day, and 96% of patients in the DVP group achieved therapeutic valproic acid levels (> 80 µg/mL). The two groups did not differ significantly in rates of adverse events, the most common of which were sedation, dizziness, and gastrointestinal upset.

Barzman and colleagues did a post hoc analysis on data from a subset of patients who participated in the larger 4-week, double-blind trial in youths (ages 12–18 years) with bipolar disorder published by DelBello and colleagues (DelBello, Kowatch, et al., 2006). The children in this analysis had bipolar I disorder and a disruptive behavioral disorder, as well as a baseline score of ≥ 1 on the Positive and Negative Symptom Scale—Excited Components (PANSS-EC) and ≥ 4 on at least one of the PANSS-EC items (Barzman et al., 2006; DelBello, Kowatch, et al., 2006). Thirty-three of these adolescents were randomized, with 16 receiving DVP monotherapy and 17 receiving quetiapine. Both treatment groups showed significant decreases in PANSS-EC scores, though there was no significant difference between groups. The most common side effects in both groups were sedation, gastrointestinal upset, and headaches.

Quetiapine monotherapy has also been shown to alleviate bipolar depression in adults, as demonstrated in three double-blind, placebo-controlled, 8-week studies (Thase et al., 2006; Hirschfeld, Weisler, Raines, & Macfadden, 2006; Calabrese et al., 2005). There are no published reports on quetiapine in the treatment of bipolar depression in youths. However, combined data from three double-blind placebo-controlled trials of quetiapine (either monotherapy or as an adjunctive agent) in the treatment of depressive symptoms in 65 adolescents with mood disorders were recently presented (Barzman et al., 2005; Calabrese et al., 2005). These investigators assessed the response of depressive symptoms and suicidal ideation in adolescents with bipolar disorder and in those with other mood disorders and a familial risk for developing bipolar disorder. All studies indicate that depressive symptoms, as rated on the CDRS, significantly decreased from baseline. In addition, the mean CDRS suicidality item score decreased significantly in the 65 patients. These data indicate that quetiapine effectively treats depression in adolescents with or at familial risk for BPD and may improve suicidal ideation.

Ziprasidone

There is one retrospective chart review of 13 adolescents (three with bipolar disorder) treated with ziprasidone (Calabrese et al., 2005; Patel, Sierk, Dorson, & Crismon, 2002). Data on the use of this agent in bipolar disorder are otherwise limited to adult studies. Two relatively large multicenter, double-blind, placebo-controlled trials have been conducted for ziprasidone in the acute treatment of bipolar mania in adults (Calabrese et al., 2005; Keck, Versiani, et al., 2003; Potkin, Keck, Segal, Ice, & English, 2005). Both studies lasted only 21 days and used ziprasidone monotherapy in a flexible-dose design (80–160 mg daily). Response was assessed using the Mania Rating Scale (MRS), derived from the Schedule of Affective Disorders and Schizophrenia—Change Version (SADS-C). Ziprasidone treatment led to decreased scores on the MRS over 3 weeks, with reductions of 45% and 42% for the first and second studies, respectively. In the second study, "separation from placebo" was noted to be statistically significant beginning at day 4, and it was sustained over 3 weeks (Calabrese et al., 2005; Potkin et al., 2005). The most common adverse effects reported for ziprasidone were somnolence, EPS (11%), akathisia (9%), and tremor (8%).

Aripiprazole

The most recently approved antipsychotic medication in the United States is aripiprazole. Although classed with the other SGAs, aripiprazole is unique in its pharmacological profile. The point of distinction is in the mechanism of action of this agent: Aripiprazole acts as both an antagonist and a partial agonist at the dopamine D-2 receptor, in contrast to all other neuroleptics, which function only in dopamine receptor blockade. Aripiprazole is also a partial agonist of serotonin 5-HT1A and a serotonin 5-HT2A receptor antagonist (Calabrese et al., 2005; Potkin et al., 2003).

Aripiprazole has been studied in adults with bipolar mania in a double-blind, placebo-controlled fashion, and the response rate seen with the active agent was 40% compared with 19% for placebo (Calabrese et al., 2005; Keck et al., 2003). The experimental data for the use of aripiprazole in the treatment of early-onset bipolar disorder is at present limited to two systematic chart reviews (Barzman et al., 2004; Biederman, McDonnell, et al., 2005).

Barzman and colleagues (2004) conducted a chart review of youths 5–19 years old who had taken aripiprazole (Barzman et al., 2004). Thirty patients were studied; nine (30%) received aripiprazole monotherapy, and 21 (70%) received it adjunctively. All youths had a diagnosis of either bipolar disorder (Types I, II, or NOS) or schizoaffective disorder, bipolar type. Participants were treated for 1 to 9 months. The mean dose at end point was 10 ± 3mg. Sixty-seven percent of patients were responders as defined by an end point CGI-I score ≤ 2. Twenty percent of responders were taking aripiprazole as monotherapy. The most common side effects were sedation (33%), followed by akathisia (23%), gastrointestinal disturbances (7%), blurry vision (3%), speech disturbance (3%), dystonia (3%), and tremor (3%; Barzman et al., 2004).

Biederman, McDonnell, and colleagues (2005) examined 41 youths (mean age 11.4 ± 3.5 years) with a bipolar spectrum disorder who had been treated with aripiprazole in an academic outpatient clinic for an average of 4.6 months. Participants were in manic, mixed, or hypomanic states at the beginning of the treatment period. Symptom severity prior to treatment and the improvement of symptoms during treatment were assessed with the CGI-S and CGI-I scales, respectively, with ratings based on descriptive chart notes. The mean daily dose of aripiprazole was 16.0 ± 7.9 mg, and the average number of concurrent psychotropic medications was 2.4 ± 1.4, including stimulants (34%), mood stabilizers (39%; lithium and anticonvulsants), selective serotonin reuptake inhibitors (SSRIs; 22%), and others. The final response rate, based on CGI-I scores of 1 or 2, was 71%. Interestingly, 39% of participants were treated concurrently with another antipsychotic medication. Few adverse events were reported, including one case of clear EPS and one of tremor. The most common side effects noted were nausea and insomnia (both 7%), along with vomiting and agitation (both 5%). The authors report that there was no documentation of aripiprazole-associated weight gain in the charts that they reviewed. Of the seven subjects who switched to aripiprazole due to weight gain on other SGAs, two lost weight, and none gained additional weight on aripiprazole.

Algorithm-Based Treatment Study

Based on the existing evidence, Pavuluri and colleagues (Pavuluri, Henry, Devineni, et al., 2004) developed a pharmacotherapy algorithm for the systematic stabilization and maintenance of children with bipolar I disorder over 18 months. The authors then applied the algorithm in a specialty clinic for pediatric mood disorders. Outcomes for a subset of the algorithm group were compared with a matched group of participants who received treatment as usual. The algorithm itself consisted of two phases, the first focused on mood stabilization and the second on adequate response, comorbidity, and other complications. The algorithm group showed a clear advantage both in the short and the long term.

The largest group of participants in this study had manic or mixed episodes without psychotic features; these youths were started on monotherapy with a mood stabilizer (MS; lithium or anticonvulsant). Those with severe symptoms or psychosis began combination therapy of an MS + SGA. Atypical antipsychotic monotherapy was included in the first phase as a first-line option for the subset of cases with predominant irritability and aggression. In support of an SGA monotherapy arm, the authors cite case reports, chart reviews, and open trials with olanzapine (Frazier et al., 2001; Pavuluri, Henry, Devineni, et al., 2004) and risperidone (Biederman, Mick, Wozniak, et al., 2005; Pavuluri, Henry, Devineni, et al., 2004).

In this study, response to treatment was assessed at fixed intervals using the CGI-BP-I. Participants who showed improvement of at least one point on the CGI-BP during the 3 weeks after reaching full dose on the MS were continued for 6 more weeks on their initial regimen. If symptoms worsened before 3 weeks, the original agent was replaced with a second MS before augmentation with an SGA. The SGA was introduced in the combination arm if response was inadequate after 6 weeks, before an alternate MS (or an SGA) was considered. Nonresponders to SGA monotherapy were tried on MS monotherapy. The investigators used a specific titration strategy for each medication, which allowed flexible dosing during both phases of treatment. The algorithm also avoided stimulants and antidepressants as a primary strategy. However, stimulants were used in the second phase as an adjuvant agent.

Results of the first phase of mood stabilization showed that few participants could be successfully stabilized on monotherapy of any kind. Fifty percent ($n = 4$) of participants who began SGA monotherapy (most on risperidone) remained on it for 6 months; only 17% of the 40 participants tried on MS monotherapy showed complete response. The response rate for MS + SGA therapy, however, was 62.3%. Psychostimulants were employed in the second phase to address residual symptoms or ADHD, and these agents were required in only 19% of the algorithm group.

Expert Consensus

Recently, Kowatch and colleagues (Kowatch et al., 2005; Pavuluri, Henry, Devineni, et al., 2004) published treatment guidelines for child and adolescent bipolar disorder, based on the consensus of researchers and clinicians, including members of the pharmaceutical industry, who attended a 2-day meeting. The report consisted primarily of pharmacotherapy recommendations for the acute and maintenance phases of treatment, as well as for the treatment of comorbid psychiatric conditions. The section on acute treatment presented two algorithms: one for the treatment of manic or mixed states *with* psychosis and another for manic or mixed states *without* psychosis. Figure 5.1 presents the concepts of these two algorithms in adapted form.

ATYPICAL ANTIPSYCHOTIC DOSING

To date, the dosing regimens of psychotropic medications, especially the new SGAs, are based on pharmacokinetic (PK), safety, and effectiveness data in adults. The lack of age-specific dosing regimens has resulted in numerous tragedies across many classes of medications, most recently the antidepressants (Kearns et al., 2003; Pavuluri, Henry, Devineni, et al., 2004; Ryan, 2005). Safe and effective age-specific dosing regimens must integrate knowledge of developmental physiology with the pharmacological proper-

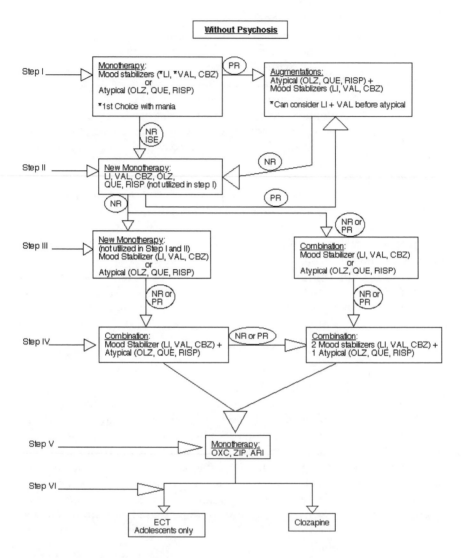

FIGURE 5.1. Treatment decision-making algorithm for early-onset bipolar disorder. Adapted from Pavuluri, Henry, Devineni, et al. (2004) and Kowatch et al. (2005). Copyright 2004, 2005 by the American Academy of Child and Adolescent Psychiatry. Adapted by permission.

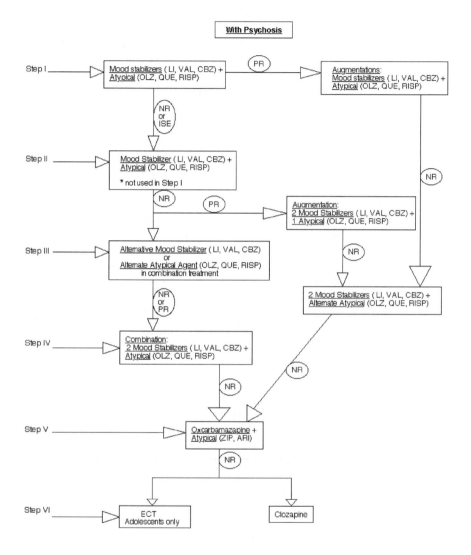

FIGURE 5.1. (*continued*)

ties of each medication. The process of growth and development results in physiological changes in body composition and organ function that may not always follow a linear pattern. For example, renal function and the clearance of renally eliminated drugs increases linearly as a child grows. However, age-dependent changes in both hepatic and extrahepatic metabolic enzymes are not linear. Cytochrome 2D6 (CYP2D6) reaches adult capacity at approximately 6 years of age. CYP1A2 and CYP4A4, other cytochromes that are important to psychotropic metabolism, increase rapidly to exceed the adult levels in children and then decrease slowly after puberty (Evans et al., 1989; Pavuluri, Henry, Devineni, et al., 2004).

Pharmacogenetic differences between individuals at any age additionally increase the complexity of the estimation of drug metabolism. Ultimately, the metabolism of the individual medication in a child depends on the pharmacogenetic profile of the individual, the specific cytochromes required for drug metabolism, and the importance of each cytochrome to the overall process. Growth and development also affect drug distribution. In general, healthy children have a lower proportion of adipose tissue than adults. A greater percentage of the dose of highly lipophilic psychotropics will remain in the child's blood instead of being stored in the adipose tissue; this may increase the risk of adverse effects. PK properties determine drug distribution, metabolism, and elimination. In adults, physiological and PK factors determine the rate and intensity of drug exposure and must be considered when selecting an optimally safe and effective dosing regimen. In children, developmental physiological factors are equally important in drug dosing.

Although Congress and the FDA enacted legislation in the 1990s to improve the availability of pediatric PK and pharmacodynamic data, such data are not available for many older psychotropic medications. For example, dosing recommendations for the typical antipsychotic medications in children are based on small groups of patients and case reports. These studies suggest that children may metabolize typical antipsychotic agents more rapidly than adults (Furlanut et al., 1990; Meyers, Tune, & Coyle, 1980; Morselli, Bianchetti, & Dugas, 1982, 1983; Pavuluri, Henry, Devineni, et al., 2004; Rivera-Calimlim, Griesbach, & Perlmutter, 1979; Sallee et al., 1987). These PK studies should be interpreted with caution because of the limited number of participants and the sometimes conflicting data. The literature underscores the developmental differences and wide patient variability of PK parameters during the first two decades of life.

Recent PK studies of the SGAs are more rigorous, and many take into account aspects of developmental pharmacokinetics. To date, there are five PK studies of SGAs (four publications and one abstract) in children and adolescents (Findling et al., 2004; Frazier et al., 2003; Grothe et al., 2000; McConville et al., 2000; Sallee et al., 2003). Although the majority of these studies were conducted in physically healthy children with schizophrenia, the PK findings can be extrapolated to children with bipolar or psychotic disorders. Clozapine and risperidone are more rapidly metabolized in children than in adults (Casaer, Walleghem, Vandenbussche, Huang, & De Smedt, 1994; Findling et al., 2004; Frazier et al., 2003), which may explain the clinical need for more frequent dosing of these agents during the day in some children. In one PK study, children treated with clozapine had more active metabolite (norclozapine) relative to adult studies. In addition, the clinical response as well as the total number of side effects seen with clozapine in these youths, correlated with the concentrations of the active metabolite of clozapine (norclozapine; Findling et al., 2004; Frazier et al., 2003). Therefore, the authors suggested that both clozapine and norclozapine levels may contribute to the effectiveness, as well as the adverse effects, of this agent in youths. Another report found that olanzapine concentrations in eight youths were similar to those observed in adult patients. The authors recommended a target olanzapine dose of 10 mg/day for most adolescents based on the PK results (Findling et al., 2004; Grothe et al., 2000). Finally, quetiapine, aripiprazole, and ziprasidone appear to be metabolized similarly in children and adults (Findling et al., 2004; McConville et al., 2000; Sallee et al., 2003). Although these studies were more rigorous than those in the past, more pediatric data are necessary to fully describe the pharmacokinetics of the SGAs and the different factors that may alter PK in the individual patient.

Overall, the rate of drug metabolism is variable between patients of the same size, age, and weight. Therefore, it is important for the clinician to exercise caution when initiating and titrating medication doses. Patients with more rapid drug metabolism require larger daily doses of medications. The clinician may divide the medication to be given in two or more doses, thereby avoiding higher peak concentrations and potential adverse effects. Age, weight, and possibly gender of the patient should be considered when choosing an antipsychotic and its dosing strategy. The overall recommended approach to medication treatment, particularly in younger patients, is to start at a low dose and slowly titrate upward in order to minimize the rate and severity of adverse effects.

SIDE EFFECTS OF ATYPICAL ANTIPSYCHOTICS AND MANAGEMENT

Atypical antipsychotics are being prescribed with regularity to youths with bipolar disorder. The rationale for this practice is based largely on data in adults and some emerging data in children that indicate that these agents may have a better side-effect profile, including a lower risk of tardive dyskinesia, than the typical antipsychotics. However, atypicals are not free of side effects, which are dictated by the receptor affinity of each agent. Children appear to be especially vulnerable to EPS, sedation, weight gain, and prolactin elevation (Findling et al., 2004; McConville et al., 2000). Unfortunately, side effects contribute to noncompliance with treatment and, at times, to medication discontinuation, which has been reported in as many as 40% of youths with bipolar disorder and in 64% of youths with bipolar disorder with comorbid externalizing symptoms (Carlson, Lavelle, & Bromet, 1999; Findling et al., 2004). Therefore, it is critical to regularly assess for adverse effects and to intervene appropriately to reduce associated noncompliance and morbidity.

The following discussion about the side effects of atypical agents incorporates information from studies regarding the treatment of youths with these agents regardless of diagnosis. The most common and most serious side effects seen with atypicals are discussed. Common side effects of these agents include EPS, weight gain, sedation, dizziness, hypotension, changes in heart rate, anxiety, hyperprolactinemia, anticholinergic side effects, and glucose dysregulation. Severe side effects include neuroleptic malignant syndrome, serotonin syndrome, agranulocytosis, and myocarditis.

Extrapyramidal Symptoms

EPS include a variety of motor disturbances that usually wax and wane, including acute dystonic reactions, parkinsonian stiffness, akathisia, shuffling, and tremor, as well as withdrawal and tardive dyskinesias. There is evidence that children and adolescents treated with typical and atypical agents may be more susceptible to these side effects than adults (Findling et al., 2004; Keepers, Clappison, & Casey, 1983; Kumra et al., 1996; Mandoki, 1995; Richardson, Haugland, & Craig, 1991). Female patients taking higher doses of typical agents may be more likely to develop the withdrawal symptoms, and the mentally retarded population may be more prone to dyskinetic movements (at baseline and on medication; Findling et al., 2004; Gualtieri, Quade, Hicks, Mayo, & Schroeder, 1984). Atypicals are associated with lower rates of EPS than the typical agents (Findling et al., 2004; Findling, Steiner, & Weller, 2005). Clozapine may have the lowest risk of EPS overall; however, it has other side effects, such as seizures and an increased risk of neutropenia and agranulocytosis, which may be more frequent in the younger age group and may limit its use to the treatment-refractory patient (Findling et al., 2004; Frazier et al., 2003; Kumra et al., 1996; Remschmidt, Schulz, & Martin, 1994).

In the face of EPS, lowering the dose might alleviate the side effects. However, if persistent, intervention with anticholinergic agents may be helpful for dystonias and stiffness, and beta-blockers may help diminish akathisia.

Sedation

The antihistaminergic properties of antipsychotics are associated with sedation. This side effect is more common with the low-potency agents such as clozapine, olanzapine, and quetiapine (Findling et al., 2004; Findling, Kusumakar, et al., 2003). Sedation is of particular concern in youths, as it can diminish capacity to learn in the school setting. This side effect is usually transient, but if persistent, consideration should be given to lowering the dose or to discontinuing the medication and trying an alternative.

Anticholinergic Side Effects

Anticholinergic side effects with antipsychotics are common, particularly on low-potency agents. These adverse effects include dry mouth, constipation, blurry vision, urinary retention, increased heart rate confusion, and decreased learning and memory. Interventions for anticholinergic side effects include lowering the dose, changing agents, and, for constipation specifically, increasing intake of fluids and bulk.

Weight Gain

Almost all antipsychotics have been associated with weight gain (Findling et al., 2004; Kelly, Conley, Love, Horn, & Ushchak, 1998; Sikich et al., 1999; Wirshing, Spellberg, Erhart, Marder, & Wirshing, 1998). Children and adolescents may be more prone than adults toward gaining weight on these agents, but across-the-lifespan studies comparing children with adults have not been done to adequately address this issue (Findling et al., 2004; Frazier et al., 2001). The atypicals have higher risk of weight gain than the typical antipsychotics (Findling et al., 2004; Gothelf et al., 2002; Kelly et al., 1998; Ratzoni et al., 2002; Shaw et al., 2001). The weight gain associated with the SGAs may in part be due to their H_1 and/or $5\text{-}HT_2$ antagonism (Findling et al., 2004; Kelly et al., 1998; Sikich et al., 1999; Wirshing et al., 1998). Weight gain has been reported on clozapine, olanzapine, risperidone, and quetiapine (Findling et al., 2004; Findling, Steiner, & Weller, 2005). Studies of youths on aripiprazole and ziprasidone that fully assess weight parameters are currently in progress.

One child and adolescent 12-week prospective naturalistic study of 25 patients ages 5–18 years recently reported comparative weight gain on three atypical agents. Patients were treated with olanzapine ($n = 11$), risperidone ($n = 8$) or quetiapine ($n = 6$). Height, weight, and fasting glucose and lipid profiles were obtained at baseline and monitored monthly. Those patients on olanzapine and risperidone experienced greater weight gain than those on quetiapine (8.2 ± 3.5 kg and 7.4 ± 4.5 kg vs. 4.1 ± 1.8 kg, respectively). Extreme weight gain (> 7%) was documented in 81% on olanzapine, 75% on risperidone, and 50% on quetiapine (Correll, Saito, Kafantaris, Kumra, & Malhotra, 2002).

Weight gain in youths is of particular concern due to the fact that obesity that begins earlier in life tends to be enduring. Obesity is associated with medical problems such as type II diabetes, hypertension, hyperlipidemia, and orthopedic complications, as well as negative self-esteem, social challenges, and medication noncompliance (Allison & Casey, 2001; Findling et al., 2004).

Monitoring weight at regular intervals and serum glucose and lipids in patients on atypical agents is important. Education about a balanced diet and regular exercise is also important for those who have gained weight on these agents. A recent study has indicated that multimodal weight intervention (nutrition exercise and behavioral intervention) may lead to effective weight loss and improvement in health indicators in adults on atypical agents (Findling et al., 2004; Menza et al., 2004).

Hyperprolactinemia

The hormone prolactin is responsible for breast tissue development and stimulation of lactation. Prolactin elevation is caused by blockade of the D2 receptor in the tuberoinfundibular pathway, and all antipsychotics, including the atypicals, block the D2 receptor. Prolonged elevations in prolactin can be associated with a number of sequelae, such as sexual dysfunction, osteoporosis, and increased cardiovascular risk in premenopausal women (Findling et al., 2004; Wieck & Haddad, 2003; Wudarsky et al., 1999).

Hyperprolactinemia has been reported as occurring in youths treated with clozapine, olanzapine, and risperidone (Findling et al., 2004; Saito et al., 2004; Wudarsky et al., 1999). However, long-term data suggest that the prolactin elevations associated with atypical agents may be transient and asymptomatic (Croonenberghs, Fegert, Findling, De Smedt, & Van Dongen, 2005; Findling et al., 2004; Findling & McNamara, 2004). If prolactin elevation is persistent and associated with side effects, consideration should be given to switching agents.

Diabetes

Individuals with mental illness have double the rate of type II diabetes mellitus reported in the general population. Recent literature indicates that in youths with risk factors for diabetes, treatment with SGAs may hasten the onset of this disorder. Epidemiological data support an association between clozapine, olanzapine, and quetiapine and type II diabetes (Findling et al., 2004; Sernyak, Leslie, Alarcon, Losonczy, & Rosenheck, 2002). There have been a handful of case reports of treatment-emergent diabetes in youths on atypicals, most involving youths on either clozapine or olanzapine (Courvoisie, Cooke, & Riddle, 2004; Findling et al., 2004). Of note, in one retrospective chart review, 5 of 38 (13%) adolescents treated with clozapine had at least one elevated random blood glucose level (Findling et al., 2004). Proposed mechanisms for glucose dysregulation include weight gain from histamine blockade, alterations in the glucose homeostatic system due to 5-HT antagonism, and a prolactin-induced insulin-resistant state. Prudent selection of agent and management includes ongoing consideration of risk factors (family or personal history, central obesity, ethnicity), patient education, weight monitoring, and quick intervention with diet and exercise (Findling et al., 2004; Wirshing et al., 1998).

Cardiovascular Effects

Orthostatic hypotension is the most common cardiovascular side effect of typical and atypical agents and most often is seen with lower-potency medications, including clozapine (Casey, 1997; Findling et al., 2004). This side effect may result from alpha$_1$-adrenergic blockade. Tachycardia may result secondary to hypotension and may be due to the anticholinergic properties of these agents (Findling et al., 2004; Gutgesell et al., 1999).

Prolongation of the QTc interval on electrocardiogram (EKG) has been associated with both typical agents and SGAs. This side effect is of concern, as it increases the risk of arrhythmias. In adult males and females, QTc measurements of > 0.43 and > 0.45, respectively, are considered abnormal; in children the EKG normal range is age-dependent. Of the atypical agents, ziprasidone is most frequently associated with modest QTc prolongation, which seems to be idiosyncratic and not dose-related. In youths, one retrospective chart review revealed that 1 in 10 adolescents treated with ziprasidone had a prolonged QTc, and a prospective study of 20 youths treated with low-dose ziprasidone reported a mean QTc increase of 28 ms, which was unrelated to dose (Findling et al., 2004; McDougle, Kem, & Posey, 2002; Patel et al., 2002). One study reports QTc intervals of approximately 450 ms in 3 of 20 youths treated with low-dose ziprasidone; these investigators recommend close monitoring of EKGs, particularly in children and adolescents on high doses of this agent (Blair, Scahill, State, & Martin, 2005; Findling et al., 2004).

Mania and Anxiety

Treatment-emergent psychiatric symptoms such as mania and anxiety have been reported on atypical agents. Mania or hypomania have been reported on risperidone, olanzapine, quetiapine, and ziprasidone (Findling et al., 2004; Findling, Steiner, & Weller, 2005), although it can be difficult to discern whether symptoms of mania are due to the illness itself or are related to the medication. Treatment-emergent anxiety (school phobias, separation anxiety, and obsessive–compulsive symptomatology) has been reported with typical and atypical antipsychotic treatment in youths (Findling et al., 2004; Hanna, Fluent, & Fischer, 1999; Linet, 1985; Mikkelsen, Detlor, & Cohen, 1981; Rabe-Jablonska, 2001). Data from well-controlled studies are needed to more fully understand the incidence and nature of these side effects. However, if they do occur, discontinuation or a decrease in dose of the atypical may alleviate these treatment-emergent psychiatric symptoms.

OTHER RARE BUT SERIOUS ADVERSE EFFECTS

Neuroleptic Malignant Syndrome

A serious reaction to antipsychotic treatment is neuroleptic malignant syndrome (NMS), a condition associated with muscle rigidity, increased body temperature, delirium, autonomic instability, elevated creatine phosphokinase (CPK) levels and white blood cell (WBC) counts, and rhabdomyolysis. The syndrome may be related to dose increase rather than absolute dose.

Overall, NMS has a similar presentation in children as it does in adults. It can be fatal, and treatment involves discontinuation of the antipsychotic, medical monitoring, and treatment of any sequelae. There have been case reports of NMS in youths treated with olanzapine, risperidone, quetiapine, and aripiprazole (Berry, Pradhan, Sagar, & Gupta, 2003; Chungh, Kim, & Cho, 2005; Findling et al., 2004; Hanft, Eggleston, & Bourgeois, 2004; Mane, Baeza, Morer, Lazaro, & Bernardo, 2005; Spalding, Alessi, & Radwan, 2004; Zalsman et al., 2004). NMS may be prevented by gradual dose titration and by wearing sun-blocking agents and maintaining hydration during the summer (Campbell, Grega, Green, & Bennett, 1983; Connor, Fletcher, & Wood, 2001; Findling et al., 2004; Gualtieri et al., 1984; Kumra et al., 1998; Pearlman, 1986).

Serotonin Syndrome

The serotonin syndrome appears very similar to NMS in terms of symptoms and results from hyperstimulation of both the central and peripheral serotonin receptors. The syndrome most often is associated with treatment with more than one agent that works through the serotonin pathways. Atypical antipsychotics with potent 5-HT blockade, such as clozapine, have been associated with this syndrome, particularly in patients on other serotonergic agents (Findling et al., 2004; Godinho, Thomson, & Bramble,

2002). The intervention is to halt the offending agents, monitor medically, and treat any sequelae.

Agranulocytosis

Generally minor blood dyscrasias can occur on antipsychotic agents, which are often not of clinical significance. However, because neutropenia and agranulocytosis are both side effects of clozapine, weekly blood monitoring is mandated for the first 6 months and every other week thereafter. If a patient's WBC count and absolute neutrophil count remain stable for a year, then patients may move to monthly monitoring. The side effects of neutropenia and agranulocytosis represent significant drops in the type of WBC that fight acute infection (neutrophils). The incidence of these side effects in children and adolescents is not clear; however, there is a suggestion that children may be at least as susceptible and possibly more susceptible to developing moderate neutropenia (< 1500/mm) and agranulocytosis (< 500/mm) on clozapine (Alvir, Lieberman, Safferman, Schwimmer, & Schaaf, 1993; Findling et al., 2004; Frazier et al., 2003; Gerbino-Rosen et al., 2005; Kumra et al., 1996).

If a significant drop in the neutrophil count occurs, clozapine should be discontinued to allow the WBC count to recover. If the patient experienced neutropenia and not agranulocytosis, he or she may be rechallenged upon recovery of WBC and neutrophil counts.

Myocarditis

Although rare and, to date, reported only in adults, myocarditis and cardiomyopathy have been associated with clozapine treatment, and the etiology is not well understood (Findling et al., 2004; Hagg, Spigset, Bate, & Soderstrom, 2001; Wehmeier, Schuler-Springorum, Heiser, & Remschmidt, 2004). These conditions should be considered in patients developing dyspnea, fatigue, chest pain, and/or edema, and medical consultation should be sought.

DRUG–DRUG INTERACTIONS

Many interactions between antipsychotics and other medications are due to a shared metabolism in the cytochrome P450 (CYP) systems. Most psychotropic medications are metabolized by four isozymes: CYP1A2, CYP2C, CYP2D6, and CYP3A3/4; CYP1A2 and CYP2D6 are generally responsible for the metabolism of both typical and atypical antipsychotics. Children and adolescents are more efficient users of these different isozymes, which may lead to developmental differences in the metabolism of antipsychotic agents (Findling et al., 2004; Frazier et al., 2003).

Medications that inhibit isozymes that a particular antipsychotic uses may increase the antipsychotic levels in the blood, leading to increased adverse effects. Because SSRIs can inhibit certain isozymes, coadministration of an SSRI and an antipsychotic that are metabolized through the same isozyme system should be performed cautiously. For example, like risperidone, paroxetine and fluoxetine are metabolized by CYP2D6. The combination of risperidone with either paroxetine or fluoxetine can lead to increased antipsychotic levels. Fluvoxamine is an inhibitor of CYP1A2, which is also responsible for the metabolism of olanzapine and clozapine (Findling et al., 2004; Findling, McNamara, et al., 2003).

MONITORING

Table 5.2 summarizes suggested clinical monitoring during the treatment of children and adolescents with BPD.

CONCLUSION

The extant data suggest that SGAs have a place in the treatment of bipolar disorder in children and adolescents. They may be useful as monotherapy or adjunctive treatment. The use of these agents to treat youths with bipolar disorder is guided predominantly by acute studies, with only one report of long-term therapy that assessed the safety and efficacy of risperidone in youths with bipolar disorder (Pavuluri, Henry, Carbray, et al., 2004). However, data are emerging that suggest that the majority of youths with bipolar disorder would benefit from combined treatment with an atypical and another agent such as lithium or an anticonvulsant (DelBello et al., 2002; Findling et al., 2004; Pavuluri, Henry, Carbray, et al., 2004).

Given the increased prescriptive practice of these medications in youths with bipolar disorder, longitudinal double-blind studies of these agents compared and in combination with mood stabilizers are critically needed in order to determine the long-term safety and efficacy of these medications (Chang & Ketter, 2000; Findling et al., 2004). Long-term maintenance studies would more fully determine whether these agents would be effective as monotherapeutic agents for bipolar disorder in youths and would provide information about dosing, as the use of these agents in acute mania may differ from their use in maintenance treatment.

TABLE 5.2. Suggested Monitoring Procedures and Intervals for Treatment of Children and Adolescents with Atypical Antipsychotic Medications

	Baseline	4 weeks	8 weeks	12 weeks	Quarterly	Annually	Every 5 years
Patient and family medical history	√					√	
Weight (BMI)[a]	√	√	√	√	√		
Waist circumference	√					√	
Vitals: blood pressure, heart rate[b]	√			√		√	
Fasting glucose	√			√		√	
Fasting lipid profile[c]	√			√		√	√
CBC[d] with diff* (for clozapine specifically see text under side effects for monitoring guidelines)	*						
Serum prolactin[e]*	*						
Pregnancy test[f],* toxic screen*	*						
Electrocardiogram (EKG)[g] (for ziprasidone specifically)	*						
Abnormal Involuntary Movement Scale/Barnes	√	√	√	√	√	√	
Clinical Global Impressions Scale—Severity and Improvement (if available)	√	√	√	√	√	√	
Physical exam (done by primary care provider)	√					√	

Note. Data in **bold** are from American Diabetes Association et al. (2004). Tests marked with an asterisk (*), when applicable, should be done and repeated on an as-needed basis according to clinical indication.

[a]BMI, Body mass index.

[b]Consider orthostatic vital signs in case of dizziness.

[c]Total cholesterol, LDL, HDL, and serum triglycerides.

[d]CBC, complete blood count.

[e]Routine serum prolactin measurements have not been supported; measurements should be made in the case of clinical signs of hyperprolactinemia.

[f]Pregnancy tests are indicated for females of child-bearing age and should be accompanied by education regarding the potential adverse effects and necessity of contraceptive measures.

[g]Baseline EKG for any medication, particularly if there is a family history of congenital heart disease. In case of ziprasidone therapy, repeat EKG is recommended with dose increases to monitor for QT_c interval prolongation.

REFERENCES

Allison, D. B., & Casey, D. E. (2001). Antipsychotic-induced weight gain: A review of the literature. *Journal of Clinical Psychiatry, 62*, 22–31.

Altamura, A. C., Salvadori, D., Madaro, D., Santini, A., & Mundo, E. (2003). Efficacy and tolerability of quetiapine in the treatment of bipolar disorder: Preliminary evidence from a 12-month open-label study. *Journal of Affective Disorders, 76*, 267–271.

Alvir, J. M., Lieberman, J. A., Safferman, A. Z., Schwimmer, J. L., & Schaaf, J. A. (1993). Clozapine-induced agranulocytosis: Incidence and risk factors in the United States. *New England Journal of Medicine, 329*, 162–167.

American Diabetes Association, American Psychiatric Association, American Association of Clinical Endocrinologists, & North American Association for the Study of Obesity. (2004). Consensus Development Conference on Antipsychotic Drugs and Obesity and Diabetes. *Diabetes Care, 27*, 596–601.

Barbini, B., Scherillo, P., Benedetti, F., Crespi, G., Colombo, C., & Smeraldi, E. (1997). Response to clozapine in acute mania is more rapid than that of chlorpromazine. *International Clinical Psychopharmacology, 12*, 109–112.

Barzman, D., Adler, C., DelBello, M. P., Stanford, K., Kowatch, R., & Strakowski, S. M. (2005). Quetiapine efficacy in bipolar adolescents with depressive symptoms [Abstract No. 44]. Presented at the annual meeting of the American College of Neuropsychopharmacology, Waikoloa Village, Kona, HI.

Barzman, D. H., DelBello, M. P., Adler, C. M., Stanford, K. E., & Strakowski, S. M. (2006). The efficacy and tolerability of quetiapine versus divalproex for the treatment of impulsivity and reactive aggression in adolescents with co-occurring bipolar disorder and disruptive behavior disorder(s). *Journal of Child and Adolescent Psychopharmacology, 16*, 665–670.

Barzman, D. H., DelBello, M. P., Kowatch, R. A., Gernert, B., Fleck, D. E., Pathak, S., et al. (2004). The effectiveness and tolerability of aripiprazole for pediatric bipolar disorders: A retrospective chart review. *Journal of Child and Adolescent Psychopharmacology, 14*, 593–600.

Berry, N., Pradhan, S., Sagar, R., & Gupta, S. K. (2003). Neuroleptic malignant syndrome in an adolescent receiving olanzapine–lithium combination therapy. *Pharmacotherapy, 23*, 255–259.

Biederman, J., McDonnell, M. A., Wozniak, J., Spencer, T., Aleardi, M., Falzone, R., et al. (2005). Aripiprazole in the treatment of pediatric bipolar disorder: A systematic chart review. *CNS Spectrums, 10*, 141–148.

Biederman, J., Mick, E., Bostic, J. Q., Prince, J., Daly, J., Wilens, T. E., et al. (1998). The naturalistic course of pharmacologic treatment of children with maniclike symptoms: A systematic chart review. *Journal of Clinical Psychiatry, 59*, 628–637.

Biederman, J., Mick, E., Faraone, S. V., Wozniak, J., Spencer, T., & Pandina, G. (2006). Risperidone for the treatment of affective symptoms in children with disruptive behavior disorder: A post hoc analysis of data from a 6-week, multicenter, randomized, double-blind, parallel-arm study. *Clinical Therapeutics, 28*, 794–800.

Biederman, J., Mick, E., Hammerness, P., Harpold, T., Aleardi, M., Dougherty, M., et al. (2005). Open-label, 8-week trial of olanzapine and risperidone for the treatment of bipolar disorder in preschool-age children. *Biological Psychiatry, 58*, 589–594.

Biederman, J., Mick, E., Prince, J., Bostic, J. Q., Wilens, T. E., Spencer, T., et al. (1999). Systematic chart review of the pharmacologic treatment of comorbid attention deficit hyperactivity disorder in youth with bipolar disorder. *Journal of Child and Adolescent Psychopharmacology, 9*, 247–256.

Biederman, J., Mick, E., Wozniak, J., Aleardi, M., Spencer, T., & Faraone, S. V. (2005). An open-label trial of risperidone in children and adolescents with bipolar disorder. *Journal of Child and Adolescent Psychopharmacology, 15*, 311–317.

Blair, J., Scahill, L., State, M., & Martin, A. (2005). Electrocardiographic changes in children and adolescents treated with ziprasidone: A prospective study. *Journal of the American Academy of Child and Adolescent Psychiatry, 44,* 73–79.

Bowden, C. L., Grunze, H., Mullen, J., Brecher, M., Paulsson, B., Jones, M., et al. (2005). A randomized, double-blind, placebo-controlled efficacy and safety study of quetiapine or lithium as monotherapy for mania in bipolar disorder. *Journal of Clinical Psychiatry, 66,* 111–121.

Bowles, T. M., & Levin, G. M. (2003). Aripiprazole: A new atypical antipsychotic drug. *Annals of Pharmacotherapy, 37,* 687–694.

Brambilla, P., Barale, F., & Soares, J. C. (2003). Atypical antipsychotics and mood stabilization in bipolar disorder. *Psychopharmacology (Berl), 166,* 315–332.

Calabrese, J. R., Keck, P. E., Jr., Macfadden, W., Minkwitz, M., Ketter, T. A., Weisler, R. H., et al. (2005). A randomized, double-blind, placebo-controlled trial of quetiapine in the treatment of bipolar I or II depression. *American Journal of Psychiatry, 162,* 1351–1360.

Calabrese, J. R., Meltzer, H. Y., & Markovitz, P. J. (1991). Clozapine prophylaxis in rapid cycling bipolar disorder. *Journal of Clinical Psychopharmacology, 11,* 396–397.

Campbell, M., Grega, D. M., Green, W. H., & Bennett, W. G. (1983). Neuroleptic-induced dyskinesias in children. *Clinical Neuropharmacology, 6,* 207–222.

Carlson, G. A., Lavelle, J., & Bromet, E. J. (1999). Medication treatment in adolescents vs. adults with psychotic mania. *Journal of Child and Adolescent Psychopharmacology, 9,* 221–231.

Carlson, G. A., Loney, J., Salisbury, H., Kramer, J. R., & Arthur, C. (2000). Stimulant treatment in young boys with symptoms suggesting childhood mania: A report from a longitudinal study. *Journal of Child and Adolescent Psychopharmacology, 10,* 175–184.

Casaer, P., Walleghem, D., Vandenbussche, I., Huang, M. L., & De Smedt, G. (1994). Pharmacokinetics and safety of risperidone in autistic children. *Pediatric Neurology, 11,* 89.

Casey, D. E. (1997). Will the new antipsychotics bring hope of reducing the risk of developing extrapyramidal syndromes and tardive dyskinesia? *International Clinical Psychopharmacology, 12,* S19–S27.

Catapano-Friedman, L. (2001). Effectiveness of quetiapine in the management of psychotic depression in an adolescent boy with bipolar disorder, mixed, with psychosis. *Journal of Child and Adolescent Psychopharmacology, 11,* 205–206.

Chang, K. D., & Ketter, T. A. (2000). Mood stabilizer augmentation with olanzapine in acutely manic children. *Journal of Child and Adolescent Psychopharmacology, 10,* 45–49.

Cheng-Shannon, J., McGough, J. J., Pataki, C., & McCracken, J. T. (2004). Second-generation antipsychotic medications in children and adolescents. *Journal of Child and Adolescent Psychopharmacology, 14,* 372–394.

Chungh, D. S., Kim, B. N., & Cho, S. C. (2005). Neuroleptic malignant syndrome due to three atypical antipsychotics in a child. *Journal of Psychopharmacology, 19,* 422–425.

Connor, D. F., Fletcher, K. E., & Wood, J. S. (2001). Neuroleptic-related dyskinesias in children and adolescents. *Journal of Clinical Psychiatry, 62,* 967–974.

Correll, C. U., Saito, E., Kafantaris, V., Kumra, S., & Malhotra, A. K. (2002). *Atypical antipsychotics: Nutritional and metabolic effects on children and adolescents.* Abstract presented at the annual meeting of the American Academy of Child and Adolescent Psychiatry, Miami, FL.

Courvoisie, H. E., Cooke, D. W., & Riddle, M. A. (2004). Olanzapine-induced diabetes in a seven-year-old boy. *Journal of Child and Adolescent Psychopharmacology, 14,* 612–616.

Croonenberghs, J., Fegert, J. M., Findling, R. L., De Smedt, G., & Van Dongen, S. (2005). Risperidone in children with disruptive behavior disorders and subaverage intelligence: A 1-year, open-label study of 504 patients. *Journal of the American Academy of Child and Adolescent Psychiatry, 44,* 64–72.

Delay, J., Deniker, P., & Harl, J. M. (1952). Utilisation en thérapeutique psychiatrique d'une phénothiazine d'action centrale élective (4560 RP) [Therapeutic use in psychiatry of phenothiazine of central elective action]. *Annales Médico Psychologiques (Paris)*, *110*, 112–117.

DelBello, M. P., Cecil, K. M., Adler, C. M., Daniels, J. P., & Strakowski, S. M. (2006). Neurochemical effects of olanzapine in first-hospitalization manic adolescents: A proton magnetic resonance spectroscopy study. *Neuropsychopharmacology*, *31*, 1264–1273.

DelBello, M. P., Findling, R. L., Kushner, S., Wang, D., Olson, W. H., Capece, J. A., et al. (2005). A pilot controlled trial of topiramate for mania in children and adolescents with bipolar disorder. *Journal of the American Academy of Child and Adolescent Psychiatry*, *44*, 539–547.

DelBello, M. P., Kowatch, R. A., Adler, C. M., Stanford, K. E., Welge, J. A., Barzman, D. H., et al. (2006). A double-blind randomized pilot study comparing quetiapine and divalproex for adolescent mania. *Journal of the American Academy of Child and Adolescent Psychiatry*, *45*, 305–313.

DelBello, M. P., Schwiers, M. S., Rosenberg, H. L., & Strakowski, S. (2002). A double-blind, randomized, placebo-controlled study of quetiapine as adjunctive treatment for adolescent mania. *Journal of the American Academy of Child and Adolescent Psychiatry*, *41*, 1216–1223.

Evans, W. E., Relling, M. V., Petros, W. P., Meyer, W. H., Mirro, J., Jr., & Crom, W. R. (1989). Dextromethorphan and caffeine as probes for simultaneous determination of debrisoquin-oxidation and N-acetylation phenotypes in children. *Clinical Pharmacology and Therapeutics*, *45*, 568–573.

Findling, R. L., Blumer, J. L., Kauffman, R., Batterson, J., Gilbert, D., Bramer, S. L., et al. (2004, June). *Pharmacokinetic effects of aripiprazole in children and adolescents with conduct disorder.* Presented at the 24th Collegium Internationale Neuro-Psychopharmacologicum Congress, Paris, France.

Findling, R. L., Kusumakar, V., Daneman, D., Moshang, T., De Smedt, G., & Binder, C. (2003). Prolactin levels during long-term risperidone treatment in children and adolescents. *Journal of Clinical Psychiatry*, *64*, 1362–1369.

Findling, R. L., & McNamara, N. K. (2004). Atypical antipsychotics in the treatment of children and adolescents: Clinical applications. *Journal of Clinical Psychiatry*, *65*, S30–S44.

Findling, R. L., McNamara, N. K., Youngstrom, E. A., Branicky, L. A., Demeter, C. A., & Schulz, S. C. (2003). A prospective, open-label trial of olanzapine in adolescents with schizophrenia. *Journal of the American Academy of Child and Adolescent Psychiatry*, *42*, 170–175.

Findling, R. L., McNamara, N. K., Youngstrom, E. A., Stansbrey, R., Gracious, B. L., Reed, M. D., et al. (2005). Double-blind 18-month trial of lithium versus divalproex maintenance treatment in pediatric bipolar disorder. *Journal of the American Academy of Child and Adolescent Psychiatry*, *44*, 409–417.

Findling, R. L., Steiner, H., & Weller, E. B. (2005). Use of antipsychotics in children and adolescents. *Journal of Clinical Psychiatry*, *66*, S29–S40.

Fleischhacker, W. W. (2002). Second generation antipsychotics. *Psychopharmacology (Berl)*, *162*, 90–91.

Frazier, J. A., Biederman, J., Tohen, M., Feldman, P. D., Jacobs, T. G., Toma, V., et al. (2001). A prospective open-label treatment trial of olanzapine monotherapy in children and adolescents with bipolar disorder. *Journal of Child and Adolescent Psychopharmacology*, *11*, 239–250.

Frazier, J. A., Cohen, L. G., Jacobsen, L. J., Grother, D., Flood, J., Baldessarini, R. J., et al. (2003). Clozapine pharmacokinetics in children and adolescents with childhood-onset schizophrenia. *Journal of Clinical Psychopharmacology*, *23*, 87–91.

Frazier, J. A., Gordon, C. T., McKenna, K., Lenane, M. C., Jih, D., & Rapoport, J. L. (1994). An open trial of clozapine in 11 adolescents with childhood-onset schizophrenia. *Journal of the American Academy of Child and Adolescent Psychiatry*, *33*, 658–663.

Frazier, J. A., Meyer, M. C., Biederman, J., Wozniak, J., Wilens, T. E., Spencer, T. J., et al. (1999). Risperidone treatment for juvenile bipolar disorder: A retrospective chart review. *Journal of the American Academy of Child and Adolescent Psychiatry*, *38*, 960–965.

Fuchs, D. C. (1994). Clozapine treatment of bipolar disorder in a young adolescent. *Journal of the American Academy of Child and Adolescent Psychiatry, 33*, 1299–1302.

Furlanut, M., Benetello, P., Baraldo, M., Zara, G., Montanari, G., & Donzelli, F. (1990). Chlorpromazine disposition in relation to age in children. *Clinical Pharmacokinetics, 18*, 329–331.

Geller, B., Cooper, T. B., Sun, K., Zimerman, B., Frazier, J., Williams, M., et al. (1998). Double-blind and placebo-controlled study of lithium for adolescent bipolar disorders with secondary substance dependency. *Journal of the American Academy of Child and Adolescent Psychiatry, 37*, 171–178.

Gerbino-Rosen, G., Roofeh, D., Tompkins, D. A., Feryo, D., Nusser, L., Kranzler, H., et al. (2005). Hematological adverse events in clozapine-treated children and adolescents. *Journal of the American Academy of Child and Adolescent Psychiatry, 44*, 1024–1031.

Godinho, E. M., Thomson, A. E., & Bramble, D. J. (2002). Neuroleptic withdrawal versus serotonergic syndrome in an 8-year-old child. *Journal of Child and Adolescent Psychopharmacology, 12*, 265–270.

Gothelf, D., Falk, B., Singer, P., Kairi, M. M., Phillip, M., Zigel, L., et al. (2002). Weight gain associated with increased food intake and low habitual activity levels in male adolescent schizophrenic inpatients treated with olanzapine. *American Journal of Psychiatry, 159*, 1055–1057.

Gracious, B. L., Youngstrom, E. A., Findling, R. L., & Calabrese, J. R. (2002). Discriminative validity of a parent version of the Young Mania Rating Scale. *Journal of the American Academy of Child and Adolescent Psychiatry, 41*, 1350–1359.

Green, A. I., Tohen, M., Patel, J. K., Banov, M., DuRand, C., Berman, I., et al. (2000). Clozapine in the treatment of refractory psychotic mania. *American Journal of Psychiatry, 157*, 982–986.

Grothe, D. R., Calis, K. A., Jacobsen, L., Kumra, S., DeVane, C. L., Rapoport, J. L., et al. (2000). Olanzapine pharmacokinetics in pediatric and adolescent inpatients with childhood-onset schizophrenia. *Journal of Clinical Psychopharmacology, 20*, 220–225.

Gualtieri, C. T., Quade, D., Hicks, R. E., Mayo, J. P., & Schroeder, S. R. (1984). Tardive dyskinesia and other clinical consequences of neuroleptic treatment in children and adolescents. *American Journal of Psychiatry, 141*, 20–23.

Gutgesell, H., Atkins, D., Barst, R., Buck, M., Franklin, W., Humes, R., et al. (1999). AHA Scientific Statement: Cardiovascular monitoring of children and adolescents receiving psychotropic drugs. *Journal of the American Academy of Child and Adolescent Psychiatry, 38*, 1047–1050.

Hagg, S., Spigset, O., Bate, A., & Soderstrom, T. G. (2001). Myocarditis related to clozapine treatment. *Journal of Clinical Psychopharmacology, 21*, 382–388.

Hanft, A., Eggleston, C. F., & Bourgeois, J. A. (2004). Neuroleptic malignant syndrome in an adolescent after brief exposure to olanzapine. *Journal of Child and Adolescent Psychopharmacology, 14*, 481–487.

Hanna, G. L., Fluent, T. E., & Fischer, D. J. (1999). Separation anxiety in children and adolescents treated with risperidone. *Journal of Child and Adolescent Psychopharmacology, 9*, 277–283.

Hardoy, M. C., Garofalo, A., Carpiniello, B., Calabrese, J. R., & Carta, M. G. (2005). Combination quetiapine therapy in the long-term treatment of patients with bipolar I disorder. *Clinical Practice and Epidemiology in Mental Health, 1*, 7.

Hatim, A., Habil, H., Jesjeet, S. G., Low, C. C., Joseph, J., Jambunathan, S. T., et al. (2006). Safety and efficacy of rapid dose administration of quetiapine in bipolar mania. *Human Psychopharmacology, 21*, 313–318.

Hirschfeld, R. M., Baker, J. D., Wozniak, P., Tracy, K., & Sommerville, K. W. (2003). The safety and early efficacy of oral-loaded divalproex versus standard-titration divalproex, lithium, olanzapine, and placebo in the treatment of acute mania associated with bipolar disorder. *Journal of Clinical Psychiatry, 64*, 841–846.

Hirschfeld, R. M., Weisler, R. H., Raines, S. R., & Macfadden, W. (2006). Quetiapine in the treatment of anxiety in patients with bipolar I or II depression: A secondary analysis from a randomized, double-blind, placebo-controlled study. *Journal of Clinical Psychiatry, 67,* 355–362.

Hunt, N., & Silverstone, T. (1991). Tardive dyskinesia in bipolar affective disorder: A catchment area study. *International Clinical Psychopharmacology, 6,* 45–50.

Janicak, P. G., Newman, R. H., & Davis, J. M. (1992). Advances in the treatment of mania and related disorders: A reappraisal. *Psychiatric Annals, 22,* 92–103.

Kafantaris, V., Coletti, D. J., Dicker, R., Padula, G., & Kane, J. M. (2001). Adjunctive antipsychotic treatment of adolescents with bipolar psychosis. *Journal of the American Academy of Child and Adolescent Psychiatry, 40,* 1448–1456.

Kafantaris, V., Dicker, R., Coletti, D. J., & Kane, J. M. (2001). Adjunctive antipsychotic treatment is necessary for adolescents with psychotic mania. *Journal of Child and Adolescent Psychopharmacology, 11,* 409–413.

Kapur, S., & Seeman, P. (2000). Antipsychotic agents differ in how fast they come off the dopamine D2 receptors: Implications for atypical antipsychotic action. *Journal of Psychiatry and Neuroscience, 25,* 161–166.

Kearns, G. J., Abdel-Rahman, S. M., Alander, S. W., Blowey, D. L., Leeder, J. S., & Kauffman, R. E. (2003). Developmental pharmacology: Drug disposition, action, and therapy in infants and children. *New England Journal of Medicine, 349,* 1157–1167.

Keck, P. E., Jr., Marcus, R., Tourkodimitris, S., Ali, M., Liebeskind, A., Saha, A., et al. (2003). A placebo-controlled, double-blind study of the efficacy and safety of aripiprazole in patients with acute bipolar mania. *American Journal of Psychiatry, 160,* 1651–1658.

Keck, P. E., Jr., Versiani, M., Potkin, S., West, S. A., Giller, E., & Ice, K. (2003). Ziprasidone in the treatment of acute bipolar mania: A three-week, placebo-controlled, double-blind, randomized trial. *American Journal of Psychiatry, 160,* 741–748.

Keepers, G. A., Clappison, V. J., & Casey, D. E. (1983). Initial anticholinergic prophylaxis for neuroleptic-induced extrapyramidal syndromes. *Archives of General Psychiatry, 40,* 1113–1117.

Kelly, D. L., Conley, R. R., Love, R. C., Horn, D. S., & Ushchak, C. M. (1998). Weight gain in adolescents treated with risperidone and conventional antipsychotics over six months. *Journal of Child and Adolescent Psychopharmacology, 8,* 151–159.

Kowatch, R. A., Fristad, M., Birmaher, B., Dineen Wagner, K., Findling, R. L., & Hellander, M. (2005). Treatment guidelines for children and adolescents with bipolar disorders. *Journal of the American Academy of Child and Adolescent Psychiatry, 44,* 213–235.

Kowatch, R. A., Suppes, T., Carmody, T. J., Bucci, J. P., Hume, J. H., Kromelis, M. R., et al. (2000). Effect size of lithium, divalproex sodium, and carbamazepine in children and adolescents with bipolar disorder. *Journal of the American Academy of Child and Adolescent Psychiatry, 39,* 713–720.

Kowatch, R. A., Suppes, T., Gilfillan, S. K., Fuentes, R. M., Grannemann, B. D., & Emslie, G. J. (1995). Clozapine treatment of children and adolescents with bipolar disorder and schizophrenia: A clinical case series. *Journal of Child and Adolescent Psychopharmacology, 5,* 241–253.

Krakowski, M., Czobor, P., & Volavka, J. (1997). Effect of neuroleptic treatment on depressive symptoms in acute schizophrenic episodes. *Psychiatry Research, 71,* 19–26.

Kumra, S., Frazier, J. A., Jacobsen, L. K., McKenna, K., Gordon, C. T., Lenane, M. C., et al. (1996). Childhood-onset schizophrenia. A double-blind clozapine–haloperidol comparison. *Archives of General Psychiatry, 53,* 1090–1097.

Kumra, S., Jacobsen, L. K., Lenane, M., Smith, A., Lee, P., Malanga, C. J., et al. (1998). Case series: Spectrum of neuroleptic-induced movement disorders and extrapyramidal side effects in childhood-onset schizophrenia. *Journal of the American Academy of Child and Adolescent Psychiatry, 37,* 221–227.

Linet, L. S. (1985). Tourette syndrome, pimozide, and school phobia: The neuroleptic separation anxiety syndrome. *American Journal of Psychiatry, 142*, 613–615.

Mandoki, M. W. (1995). Risperidone treatment of children and adolescents: Increased risk of extrapyramidal side effects? *Journal of Child and Adolescent Psychopharmacology, 5*, 49–67.

Mane, A., Baeza, I., Morer, A., Lazaro, M. L., & Bernardo, M. (2005). Neuroleptic malignant syndrome associated with risperidone in a male with early-onset schizophrenia. *Journal of Child and Adolescent Psychopharmacology, 15*, 844–845.

Marchand, W. R., Wirth, L., & Simon, C. (2004). Quetiapine adjunctive and monotherapy for pediatric bipolar disorder: A retrospective chart review. *Journal of Child and Adolescent Psychopharmacology, 14*, 405–411.

Martin, B. C., Miller, L. S., & Kotzan, J. A. (2001). Antipsychotic prescription use and costs for persons with schizophrenia in the 1990s: Current trends and five year time series forecasts. *Schizophrenia Research, 47*, 281–292.

Masi, G., & Milone, A. (1998). Clozapine treatment in an adolescent with bipolar disorder. *Panminerva Medica, 40*, 254–257.

Masi, G., Mucci, M., & Millepiedi, S. (2002). Clozapine in adolescent inpatients with acute mania. *Journal of Child and Adolescent Psychopharmacology, 12*, 93–99.

McConville, B. J., Arvanitis, L. A., Thyrum, P. T., Yeh, C., Wilkinson, L. A., Chaney, R. O., et al. (2000). Pharmacokinetics, tolerability, and clinical effectiveness of quetiapine fumarate: An open-label trial in adolescents with psychotic disorders. *Journal of Clinical Psychiatry, 61*, 252–260.

McDougle, C. J., Kem, D. L., & Posey, D. J. (2002). Case series: Use of ziprasidone for maladaptive symptoms in youths with autism. *Journal of the American Academy of Child and Adolescent Psychiatry, 41*, 921–927.

McIntyre, R. S., Brecher, M., Paulsson, B., Huizar, K., & Mullen, J. (2005). Quetiapine or haloperidol as monotherapy for bipolar mania—a 12-week, double-blind, randomised, parallel-group, placebo-controlled trial. *European Neuropsychopharmacology, 15*, 573–585.

Meehan, K., Zhang, F., David, S., Tohen, M., Janicak, P., Small, J., et al. (2001). A double-blind, randomized comparison of the efficacy and safety of intramuscular injections of olanzapine, lorazepam, or placebo in treating acutely agitated patients diagnosed with bipolar mania. *Journal of Clinical Psychopharmacology, 21*, 389–397.

Meltzer, H. Y. (1999). The role of serotonin in antipsychotic drug action. *Neuropsychopharmacology, 21*, 106S–115S.

Menza, M., Vreeland, B., Minsky, S., Gara, M., Radler, D. R., & Sakowitz, M. (2004). Managing atypical antipsychotic-associated weight gain: 12-month data on a multimodal weight control program. *Journal of Clinical Psychiatry, 65*, 471–477.

Meyers, B., Tune, L. E., & Coyle, J. T. (1980). Clinical response and serum neuroleptic levels in childhood schizophrenia. *American Journal of Psychiatry, 137*, 483–484.

Mikkelsen, E. J., Detlor, J., & Cohen, D. J. (1981). School avoidance and social phobia triggered by haloperidol in patients with Tourette's disorder. *American Journal of Psychiatry, 138*, 1572–1576.

Miller, C. H., Mohr, F., Umbricht, D., Woerner, M., Fleischhacker, W. W., & Lieberman, J. A. (1998). The prevalence of acute extrapyramidal signs and symptoms in patients treated with clozapine, risperidone, and conventional antipsychotics. *Journal of Clinical Psychiatry, 59*, 69–75.

Morselli, P. L., Bianchetti, G., & Dugas, M. (1982). Haloperidol plasma level monitoring in neuropsychiatric patients. *Therapeutic Drug Monitoring, 4*, 51–58.

Morselli, P. L., Bianchetti, G., & Dugas, M. (1983). Therapeutic drug monitoring of psychotropic drugs in children. *Pediatric Pharmacology, 3*, 149–156.

Naber, D., Holzbach, R., Perro, C., & Hippius, H. (1992). Clinical management of clozapine patients in relation to efficacy and side-effects. *British Journal of Psychiatry. Supplement*, 54–59.

Pae, C. U., Nassir Ghaemi, S., Kim, T. S., Kim, J. J., Lee, S. J., Lee, C. U., et al. (2005). Rapid titration versus conventional titration of quetiapine in the treatment of bipolar mania: A preliminary trial. *International Clinical Psychopharmacology, 20*, 327–330.

Patel, N. C., Sierk, P., Dorson, P. G., & Crismon, L. (2002). Experience with ziprasidone. *Journal of the American Academy of Child and Adolescent Psychiatry, 41*, 495.

Pavuluri, M. N., Henry, D. B., Carbray, J. A., Naylor, M. W., & Janicak, P. G. (2005). Divalproex sodium for pediatric mixed mania: A 6-month prospective trial. *Bipolar Disorders, 7*, 266–273.

Pavuluri, M. N., Henry, D. B., Carbray, J. A., Sampson, G., Naylor, M. W., & Janicak, P. G. (2004). Open-label prospective trial of risperidone in combination with lithium or divalproex sodium in pediatric mania. *Journal of Affective Disorders, 82*, S103–S111.

Pavuluri, M. N., Henry, D. B., Carbray, J. A., Sampson, G. A., Naylor, M. W., & Janicak, P. G. (2006). A one-year open-label trial of risperidone augmentation in lithium nonresponder youth with preschool-onset bipolar disorder. *Journal of Child and Adolescent Psychopharmacology, 16*, 336–350.

Pavuluri, M. N., Henry, D. B., Devineni, B., Carbray, J. A., Naylor, M. W., & Janicak, P. G. (2004). A pharmacotherapy algorithm for stabilization and maintenance of pediatric bipolar disorder. *Journal of the American Academy of Child and Adolescent Psychiatry, 43*, 859–867.

Pavuluri, M. N., Henry, D., Naylor, M., Sampson, G., Carbray, J., & Janicak, P. G. (2004). A prospective trial of combination therapy of risperidone with lithium or divalproex sodium in pediatric mania. *Journal of Affective Disorders, 82*, 103–111.

Pearlman, C. A. (1986). Neuroleptic malignant syndrome: A review of the literature. *Journal of Clinical Psychopharmacology, 6*, 257–273.

Potkin, S. G., Keck, P. E., Jr., Segal, S., Ice, K., & English, P. (2005). Ziprasidone in acute bipolar mania: A 21-day randomized, double-blind, placebo-controlled replication trial. *Journal of Clinical Psychopharmacology, 25*, 301–310.

Potkin, S. G., Saha, A. R., Kujawa, M. J., Carson, W. H., Ali, M., Stock, E., et al. (2003). Aripiprazole, an antipsychotic with a novel mechanism of action, and risperidone vs. placebo in patients with schizophrenia and schizoaffective disorder. *Archives of General Psychiatry, 60*, 681–690.

Rabe-Jablonska, J. (2001). Obsessive-compulsive disorders in adolescents with diagnosed schizophrenia. *Psychiatria Polska, 35*, 47–57.

Ranjan, R., & Meltzer, H. Y. (1996). Acute and long-term effectiveness of clozapine in treatment-resistant psychotic depression. *Biological Psychiatry, 40*, 253–258.

Ratzoni, G., Gothelf, D., Brand-Gothelf, A., Reidman, J., Kikinzon, L., Gal, G., et al. (2002). Weight gain associated with olanzapine and risperidone in adolescent patients: A comparative prospective study. *Journal of the American Academy of Child and Adolescent Psychiatry, 41*, 337–343.

Remschmidt, H., Schulz, E., & Martin, C. L. (1994). An open trial of clozapine in thirty-six adolescents with schizophrenia. *Journal of Child and Adolescent Psychopharmacology, 4*, 31–41.

Richardson, M. A., Haugland, G., & Craig, T. J. (1991). Neuroleptic use, parkinsonian symptoms, tardive dyskinesia, and associated factors in child and adolescent psychiatric patients. *American Journal of Psychiatry, 148*, 1322–1328.

Richelson, E. (1999). Receptor pharmacology of neuroleptics: Relation to clinical effects. *Journal of Clinical Psychiatry, 60*, 5–14.

Rivera-Calimlim, L., Griesbach, P. H., & Perlmutter, R. (1979). Plasma chlorpromazine concentrations in children with behavioral disorders and mental illness. *Clinical Pharmacology and Therapeutics, 26*, 114–121.

Ryan, N. D. (2005). Treatment of depression in children and adolescents. *Lancet, 366*, 933–940.

Sachs, G., Chengappa, K. N., Suppes, T., Mullen, J. A., Brecher, M., Devine, N. A., et al. (2004).

Quetiapine with lithium or divalproex for the treatment of bipolar mania: A randomized, double-blind, placebo-controlled study. *Bipolar Disorders, 6,* 213–223.

Sachs, G. S., Grossman, F., Ghaemi, S. N., Okamoto, A., & Bowden, C. L. (2002). Combination of a mood stabilizer with risperidone or haloperidol for treatment of acute mania: A double-blind, placebo-controlled comparison of efficacy and safety. *American Journal of Psychiatry, 159,* 1146–1154.

Saito, E., Correll, C. U., Gallelli, K., McMeniman, M., Parikh, U. H., Malhotra, A. K., et al. (2004). A prospective study of hyperprolactinemia in children and adolescents treated with atypical antipsychotic agents. *Journal of Child and Adolescent Psychopharmacology, 14,* 350–358.

Sajatovic, M., Brescan, D. W., Perez, D. E., DiGiovanni, S. K., Hattab, H., Ray, J. B., et al. (2001). Quetiapine alone and added to a mood stabilizer for serious mood disorders. *Journal of Clinical Psychiatry, 62,* 728–732.

Sallee, F. R., Gilbert, D. L., Vinks, A. A., Miceli, J. J., Robarge, L., & Wilner, K. (2003). Pharmacodynamics of ziprasidone in children and adolescents: Impact on dopamine transmission. *Journal of the American Academy of Child and Adolescent Psychiatry, 42,* 902–907.

Sallee, F. R., Pollock, B. G., Stiller, R. L., Stull, S., Everett, G., & Perel, J. M. (1987). Pharmacokinetics of pimozide in adults and children with Tourette's syndrome. *Journal of Clinical Pharmacology, 27,* 776–781.

Schaller, J. L., & Behar, D. (1999). Quetiapine for refractory mania in a child [Letter to the editor]. *Journal of the American Academy of Child and Adolescent Psychiatry, 38,* 498–499.

Segal, J., Berk, M., & Brook, S. (1998). Risperidone compared with both lithium and haloperidol in mania: A double-blind randomized controlled trial. *Clinical Neuropharmacology, 21,* 176–180.

Sernyak, M. J., Leslie, D. L., Alarcon, R. D., Losonczy, M. F., & Rosenheck, R. (2002). Association of diabetes mellitus with use of atypical neuroleptics in the treatment of schizophrenia. *American Journal of Psychiatry, 159,* 561–566.

Shaw, J. A., Lewis, J. E., Pascal, S., Sharma, R. K., Rodriguez, R. A., Guillen, R., et al. (2001). A study of quetiapine: Efficacy and tolerability in psychotic adolescents. *Journal of Child and Adolescent Psychopharmacology, 11,* 415–424.

Shen, W. W. (1999). A history of antipsychotic drug development. *Comprehensive Psychiatry, 40,* 407–414.

Sikich, L., Williamson, K., Malekpour, A., Bashford, R., Hooper, S., Sheitman, B., et al. (1999, December). *Double-blind comparison of haloperidol, risperidone and olanzapine in psychotic youth.* Abstract presented at the annual meeting of the American College of Neuropsychopharmacology. Acapulco, Mexico.

Sokolski, K. N., & Denson, T. F. (2003). Adjunctive quetiapine in bipolar patients partially responsive to lithium or valproate. *Progress in Neuropsychopharmacology and Biological Psychiatry, 27,* 863–866.

Soutullo, C. A., Sorter, M. T., Foster, K. D., McElroy, S. L., & Keck, P. E. (1999). Olanzapine in the treatment of adolescent acute mania: A report of seven cases. *Journal of Affective Disorders, 53,* 279–283.

Spalding, S., Alessi, N. E., & Radwan, K. (2004). Aripiprazole and atypical neuroleptic malignant syndrome. *Journal of the American Academy of Child and Adolescent Psychiatry, 43,* 1457–1458.

Stahl, S. M. (1999). *Psychopharmacology of antipsychotics.* London: Dunitz.

Suppes, T., Phillips, K. A., & Judd, C. R. (1994). Clozapine treatment of nonpsychotic rapid cycling bipolar disorder: A report of three cases. *Biological Psychiatry, 36,* 338–340.

Thase, M. E., Macfadden, W., Weisler, R. H., Chang, W., Paulsson, B., Khan, A., et al. (2006). Efficacy of quetiapine monotherapy in bipolar I and II depression: A double-blind, placebo-controlled study (the BOLDER II study). *Journal of Clinical Psychopharmacology, 26,* 600–609.

Tohen, M., Jacobs, T. G., Grundy, S. L., McElroy, S. L., Banov, M. C., Janicak, P. G., et al. (2000). Efficacy of olanzapine in acute bipolar mania: A double-blind, placebo-controlled study. *Archives of General Psychiatry, 57,* 841–849.

Tohen, M., Sanger, T. M., McElroy, S. L., Tollefson, G. D., Chengappa, R., Daniel, D. G., et al. (1999). Olanzapine versus placebo in the treatment of acute mania. *American Journal of Psychiatry, 156,* 702–709.

Vieta, E., Mullen, J., Brecher, M., Paulsson, B., & Jones, M. (2005). Quetiapine monotherapy for mania associated with bipolar disorder: Combined analysis of two international, double-blind, randomised, placebo-controlled studies. *Current Medical Research and Opinion, 21,* 923–934.

Voruganti, L. P., & Awad, A. G. (2004). Is neuroleptic dysphoria a variant of drug-induced extrapyramidal side effects? *Canadian Journal of Psychiatry, 49,* 285–289.

Wagner, K. D., Weller, E. B., Carlson, G. A., Sachs, G., Biederman, J., Frazier, J. A., et al. (2002). An open-label trial of divalproex in children and adolescents with bipolar disorder. *Journal of the American Academy of Child and Adolescent Psychiatry, 41,* 1224–1230.

Wehmeier, P. M., Schuler-Springorum, M., Heiser, P., & Remschmidt, H. (2004). Chart review for potential features of myocarditis, pericarditis, and cardiomyopathy in children and adolescents treated with clozapine. *Journal of Child and Adolescent Psychopharmacology, 14,* 267–271.

Wieck, A., & Haddad, P. M. (2003). Antipsychotic-induced hyperprolactinaemia in women: Pathophysiology, severity and consequences. Selective literature review. *British Journal of Psychiatry, 182,* 199–204.

Wirshing, D. A., Spellberg, B. J., Erhart, S. M., Marder, S. R., & Wirshing, W. C. (1998). Novel antipsychotics and new onset diabetes. *Biological Psychiatry, 44,* 778–783.

Wudarsky, M., Nicolson, R., Hamburger, S. D., Spechler, L., Gochman, P., Bedwell, J., et al. (1999). Elevated prolactin in pediatric patients on typical and atypical antipsychotics. *Journal of Child and Adolescent Psychopharmacology, 9,* 239–245.

Yatham, L. N. (2002). The role of novel antipsychotics in bipolar disorders. *Journal of Clinical Psychiatry, 63,* 10–14.

Yatham, L. N. (2003). Acute and maintenance treatment of bipolar mania: The role of atypical antipsychotics. *Bipolar Disorders, 5,* 7–19.

Yatham, L. N., Paulsson, B., Mullen, J., & Vagero, A. M. (2004). Quetiapine versus placebo in combination with lithium or divalproex for the treatment of bipolar mania. *Journal of Clinical Psychopharmacology, 24,* 599–606.

Young, R. C., Biggs, J. T., Ziegler, V. E., & Meyer, D. A. (1978). A rating scale for mania: Reliability, validity and sensitivity. *British Journal of Psychiatry, 133,* 429–435.

Zalsman, G., Lewis, R., Konas, S., Loebstein, O., Goldberg, P., Burguillo, F., et al. (2004). Atypical neuroleptic malignant syndrome associated with risperidone treatment in two adolescents. *International Journal of Adolescent Medicine and Health, 16,* 179–182.

CHAPTER 6

Mood Stabilizers

ROBERT A. KOWATCH

Mood stabilizers can be categorized into the "traditional" mood stabilizers—lithium, valproate, and carbamazepine—and the newer antiepileptic agents that are also sometimes used as mood stabilizers, for example, oxcarbazepine, lamotrigine, and topiramate (Weisler, Cutler, Ballenger, Post, & Ketter, 2006). Several well-controlled studies have demonstrated the efficacy of lithium, valproate, and carbamazepine for the treatment of mania in adults (Ketter, Nasrallah, & Fagiolini, 2006). There is also emerging evidence about the effectiveness of the newer antiepileptic agents in treating mania and bipolar depression in adults with bipolar disorder (Weisler et al., 2006). Lithium and valproate are often used to treat bipolar disorder in children and adolescents, and the evidence base for the safety and efficacy of these two mood stabilizers and the newer antiepileptic agents in children and adolescents is steadily increasing (Kowatch & DelBello, 2006; Pavuluri, Birmaher, & Naylor, 2005). Both the traditional and newer mood-stabilizing agents are often used to treat children and adolescents with bipolar disorder; the purpose of this chapter is to present and review this information.

VALPROATE

Valproate (divalproex sodium; 2-propylpentanoate) is a simple branched-chain carboxylic acid that was first introduced in the United States in 1978 as an antiseizure agent. It is currently approved by the Food and Drug Administration (FDA) for the treatment of partial-complex seizures, migraines, and manic episodes of manic–depressive illness in adults.

Research Studies

A review of the five controlled studies of valproate for the acute treatment of mania in adults showed an average response rate of 54%, demonstrating efficacy for valproate versus placebo (McElroy & Keck, 2000). In many of these studies, positive results were obtained even though patients were selected from a population previously refractory to lithium treatment and those characterized by rapid cycling, mixed affective states, and irritability. There have been several case reports and open-prospective trials suggesting the effectiveness of valproate for the treatment of children and adolescents with bipolar disorders (Deltito, Levitan, Damore, Hajal, & Zambenedetti, 1998; Kastner & Friedman, 1992; Kastner, Friedman, Plummer, Ruiz, & Henning, 1990; Papatheodorou & Kutcher, 1993; Papatheodorou, Kutcher, Katic, & Szalai, 1995; West & McElroy, 1995; West et al., 1994; Whittier, West, Galli, & Raute, 1995). In a 6-week prospective study, Kowatch and colleagues (2000) directly compared the effectiveness of lithium, valproate, and carbamazepine for manic, hypomanic, or mixed episodes associated with bipolar disorder, types I or II. Using a $\geq$ 50% change from baseline to end point in the Young Mania Rating Scale (YMRS) scores to define response, the response rates were 38%, 38%, and 53% for carbamazepine, lithium, and divalproex, respectively ($\chi^2 = 0.85$, $p = .60$). Wagner and colleagues (2006) published the results of an open-label study of valproate in 40 children and adolescents (ages 7–19 years) with bipolar disorder. In the initial open-label phase of this study, participants were given a starting dosage of divalproex of 15 mg/kg/day. The mean final dosage was 17 mg/kg/day. Twenty-two participants (55%) scored $\geq$ 50% on the YMRS during the open phase of treatment, suggesting that approximately half of children and adolescents with mania will respond to divalproex.

Recently, the results of a large, randomized, placebo-controlled, double-blind, multicenter study designed to evaluate the safety and efficacy of Depakote ER in the treatment of bipolar I disorder, manic or mixed episode, in children and adolescents ages 10–17 years were released (Abbott, 2006). During this trial 150 participants with current clinical diagnoses of bipolar I disorder, manic or mixed episode, were enrolled at 20 study sites. Participants were outpatients with manic or mixed episodes and with YMRS scores of greater than or equal to 20 at screening and baseline. Participants were randomized in a 1:1 ratio to receive active study medication (250 mg and/or 500 mg tablets of Depakote ER) or matching placebo tablets. The duration of the study was 6 weeks, including a screening period lasting 3–14 days, a 4-week treatment period, and an optional 1-week taper period. The primary efficacy variable, the change from baseline to the final evaluation for YMRS, did not demonstrate a statistically significant treatment difference. Likewise, Depakote ER therapy did not result in statistically significant clinical benefits in psychopathology, as measured by any of the secondary end points. Also, a higher increase in ammonia levels was observed in the Depakote ER group (18.63 ± 25.72 mcmol/L) than in the placebo group (2.12 ± 22.21 mcmol/L). This trial may have been negative because the active treatment period of 4 weeks was not long enough or because the serum levels of divalproex were not high enough. It is important to recognize that in adult trials of marketed antidepressants, antidepressant drugs were superior to placebo in only 45 out of 93 (48%) randomized controlled trials (Yang, Cusin, & Fava, 2005), which means that more than half of these trials were negative. The result of one, possibly negative trial, of valproate in children and adolescents with bipolar disorder must be interpreted with caution, and child psychiatrists should not stop using valproate to treat child and adolescent bipolar disorder until there is a more indepth examination of this trial and subsequent replications.

Clinical Use

Dosing

Valproate is readily absorbed from the gastrointestinal system, with peak levels occurring 2–4 hours after each dose. But if valproate is given with meals to decrease nausea, peak levels may be reached in 5–6 hours. Valproate is highly protein bound, metabolized in the liver, and has a serum half-life between 8 and 16 hours in children and young adolescents (Cloyd, Fischer, Kriel, & Kraus, 1993). A starting dose of divalproex sodium of 15 mg/kg/day in 2–3 divided doses in children and adolescents will produce serum valproate levels in the range of 50–60 mg/ml. Once this low serum level has been obtained, the dose is usually titrated upward depending on the participant's tolerance and response, and it is optimal to measure serum valproate levels 12 hours after the last dose. Optimum serum levels for treating mania among adults are between 85 and 110 mg/ml, and the same is thought to be true in children and adolescents (Bowden et al., 1996).

Laboratory Studies

Baseline studies prior to initiating treatment with valproate should include general medical history and physical examination, liver function tests, complete blood count (CBC) with differential and platelets, and a pregnancy test for sexually active females. A complete blood count with differential, platelet count, and liver functions should be checked every 6 months or when clinically indicated.

Adverse Effects

Common side effects of valproate in children and adolescents include nausea, increased appetite, weight gain, sedation, thrombocytopenia, transient hair loss, tremor, and vomiting. Rarely, pancreatitis (Sinclair, Berg, & Breault, 2004; Werlin & Fish, 2006) and liver failure (Ee et al., 2003; Konig et al., 1994; Treem, 1994) can also occur in children treated with valproate. Fetal exposure to valproate is associated with an increased rate of neural tube defects (Ketter et al., 2006).

There have been recent concerns about the possible association between valproate and polycystic ovarian syndrome (PCOS). COS is an endocrine disorder characterized by ovulatory dysfunction and hyperandrogenism that affects between 3 and 5% of women who are not taking psychotropic medications (Rasgon, 2004). Common symptoms of PCOS include irregular or absent menstruation, lack of ovulation, weight gain, hirsutism, and/or acne. The initial reports of the association between PCOS and divalproex exposure were in women with epilepsy. The association was particularly strong if their exposure had occurred during adolescence (Isojarvi, Laatikainen, Pakarinen, Juntunen, & Myllyla, 1993). In a recent report, an increased (7.5 times) risk of new-onset oligoamenorrhea with hyperandrogenism was also found in bipolar women who were exposed to valproate (Joffe et al., 2006). Females who are treated with valproate should have a baseline assessment of menstrual cycle patterns and be continually monitored for menstrual irregularities, weight gain, hirsutism, and/or acne that may develop during valproate treatment. If symptoms of PCOS develop, referral to an endocrinologist should be considered.

Drug Interactions

Valproate is metabolized in the liver by cytochrome P450 enzymes and has interactions with several medications that also are metabolized by this system. Medications that will increase valproate levels include erythromycin, SSRIs, cimetidine, and salicylates. Valproate may increase the levels of phenobarbital, primidone, carbamazepine, phenytoin, tricyclics, and lamotrigine.

Contraindications

Valproate should be administered cautiously and serum levels and liver functions monitored carefully in patients with significant liver dysfunction

(Asconape, 2002) or in patients with inborn errors of ammonia metabolism (Konig et al., 1994; Treem, 1994).

CARBAMAZEPINE

Carbamazepine is an anticonvulsant agent structurally similar to imipramine that was first introduced in the United States in 1968 for the treatment of seizures. Two recent controlled studies of a long-acting preparation of carbamazepine in adults with bipolar disorder demonstrated efficacy for carbamazepine as monotherapy for mania in adults (Weisler et al., 2006). There have been no controlled studies of carbamazepine for the treatment of children and adolescents with bipolar disorder and the majority of reports in the literature concern its use in children and adolescents with attention-deficit/hyperactivity disorder (ADHD) or conduct disorder (Cueva et al., 1996; Evans, Clay, & Gualtieri, 1987; Kafantaris et al., 1992; Puente, 1975). Pleak, Birmaher, Gavrilescu, Abichandani, and Williams (1988) reported the worsening of behavior in 6 of 20 child and adolescent patients treated with carbamazepine for ADHD and conduct disorder. Thus there is not good evidence to support the use of carbamazepine as a first-line agent for children and adolescents with bipolar disorder, and this drug's numerous P450 drug interactions make its clinical use difficult.

Dosing

In patients 6–12 years of age, a reasonable starting dose of carbamazepine is 100 mg twice daily and, in patients age 12 and older, 100 mg three times daily. Carbamazepine serum levels between 8 and 11 mg/ml are necessary for seizure control; however, the level for therapeutic effects in youths with bipolar disorder are unknown. The maximum daily dose of carbamazepine should not exceed 1000 mg/day in children ages 6–12 years and 1200 mg/day in patients age 13 and older.

Laboratory Studies

Carbamazepine is metabolized by the P450 hepatic system to an active metabolite, carbamazepine-10,11-epoxide. Carbamazepine induces its own metabolism, and this "autoinduction" is complete 3–5 weeks after achieving a fixed dose. Initial carbamazepine serum half-lives range from 25 to 65 hours and then decrease to 9–15 hours after autoinduction of the P450 enzymes (Wilder, 1992). Complete pretreatment blood counts, including platelets, should be obtained as a baseline. If a patient in the course of treatment exhibits low or decreased white blood cell or platelet counts, the patient should be monitored closely.

Adverse Events

Common side effects of carbamazepine in children and adolescents include sedation, ataxia, dizziness, blurred vision, nausea, and vomiting. Uncommon side effects of carbamazepine include aplastic anemia, hyponatremia, and Stevens–Johnson syndrome (Devi, George, Criton, Suja, & Sridevi, 2005; Keating & Blahunka, 1995).

Drug Interactions

Carbamazepine has many clinically significant drug interactions in children and adolescents because of its stimulation of the hepatic P450 isoenzyme system. Carbamazepine may decrease levels of such medications as oral contraceptives and lamotrigine (Ciraulo, Shader, Greenblatt, & Creelman, 1995).

Contraindications

Carbamazepine can cause fetal harm when administered to a pregnant woman.

Table 6.1 summarizes clinical information about lithium, valproate, and carbamazepine.

NOVEL ANTIEPILEPTIC AGENTS

Several newer antiepileptic agents developed for the treatment of epilepsy are sometimes used as mood stabilizers in adults, children, and adolescents. These agents include gabapentin, topiramate, oxcarbazepine, lamotrigine, levetiracetam, tiagabine, and zonisamide. The data are presently limited regarding the efficacy and tolerability of these agents for the treatment of pediatric bipolar disorder. There have been several recent controlled trials of these agents in adults with mania or mixed moods (Bowden & Karren, 2006). There are two controlled studies of these newer agents, one with oxcarbazepine and one with topiramate, in children and adolescents with bipolar disorder (DelBello et al., 2005; Wagner et al., 2006).

Lamotrigine

Lamotrigine (Lamictal) has a novel mechanism of action by blocking voltage-sensitive sodium channels and secondarily inhibiting the release of excit-

TABLE 6.1. Mood Stabilizer Dosing/Monitoring in Children and Adolescents with Bipolar Disorder

Generic name	U.S. trade name	How supplied (mg)	Starting dose	Target dose	Therapeutic serum level	Cautions
Carbamazepine Carbamazepine XR	Tegretol Tegretol XR Equetro	100, 200 100, 200, 400	Outpatients: 7 mg/kg/day 2–3 daily doses	Based on response and serum levels	8–11 mg/L	Monitor for P450 drug interactions
Gabapentin	Neurontin	100, 300, 400	100 mg two or three times per day	Based on response	N/A	Watch for behavioral disinhibition
Lamotrigine	Lamictal	25, 100, 200	12.5 mg daily	Increase weekly based on response	N/A	Monitor carefully for rashes, serum sickness
Li⁺carbonate Li⁺carbonate Li⁺citrate	Lithobid Eskalith Cibalith-S	300 (& 150 generic) 300 or 450 CR Li-citrate 5 cc = 300 mg	Outpatients: 25 mg/kg/day 2–3 daily doses	30 mg/kg/day 2–3 daily doses	0.8–1.2 mEq/L	Monitor for hypothyroidism Avoid in pregnancy
Oxcarbazepine	Trileptal	150, 300, 600	150 mg two times per day	20–29 kg 900 mg/day 30–39 kg 1200 mg/day >39 kg 1800 mg/day	N/A	Monitor for hyponatremia
Topiramate	Topamax	25, 100	25 mg daily	100–400 mg/day	N/A	Monitor for memory problems, kidney stones
Valproic acid Divalproex sodium	Depakene Depakote	125, 250, 500	20 mg/kg/day 2 daily doses	20 mg/kg/day 2–3 daily doses	90–120 mg/L	Monitor liver functions, for pancreatitis & PCOS in females Avoid in pregnancy

Note. N/A, not applicable.

115

atory neurotransmitters, particularly glutamate and aspartate (Ketter, Wang, Becker, Nowakowska, & Yang, 2003). Lamotrigine also inhibits serotonin reuptake, suggesting that it might possess antidepressant properties. In 2003 the FDA approved lamotrigine for the maintenance treatment of bipolar I disorder in adults to delay the time to occurrence of mood episodes (depression, mania, hypomania, mixed episodes) in patients treated for acute mood episodes with standard therapy. Several prospective studies in adults with bipolar disorder suggest that lamotrigine may be beneficial for the treatment of mood (especially depressive) symptoms in bipolar disorder (Bowden et al., 2003; Calabrese et al., 1999).

Chang, Saxena, and Howe (2006) published an 8-week, open-label trial of lamotrigine alone or as adjunctive therapy for the treatment of 20 adolescents ages 12–17 years (mean age = 15.8 years) with bipolar disorders who were experiencing a depressive or mixed episode. The mean final dose was 131.6 mg/day, and 84% of these participants were rated as much or very much improved on the Clinical Global Improvement (CGI) scale. Larger, placebo-controlled studies of lamotrigine in bipolar children and adolescents are needed.

Dosing

It is critical to follow the revised dosing guidelines for lamotrigine to avoid serious rashes. These guidelines can be found at *http://www.lamictal.com/epilepsy/hcp/dosing/pediatric_dosing.html*. The starting dose of lamotrigine for an adolescent not on valproate is 25 mg/day for 2 weeks, with a gradual titration to 200–400 mg/day.

Laboratory Studies

Prior to starting lamotrigine, a patient's CBC, differential, platelet count, and liver function tests should be checked.

Adverse Events

The most common side effects of lamotrigine are dizziness, tremor, somnolence, nausea, and headache. Rashes develop in 12% of patients and typically within the first 8 weeks of lamotrigine therapy. Rarely, severe cutaneous reactions such as Stevens–Johnson syndrome and toxic epidermal necrolysis have been described. The risk of developing a serious rash is greater in children and adolescents less than 16 years old compared with adults, in whom the incidence is approximately 0.1% (Goodwin et al., 2004; Ketter et al., 2005). The frequency of serious rash associated with lamotrigine (defined as rashes requiring hospitalization and discontinuation of treatment), including Stevens–Johnson syndrome, is approximately 1 in 100 (1%) in children age less than 16 years and 3 in 1,000 (0.3%) in adults (Glaxo, 2001).

Drug Interactions

Lamotrigine is primarily eliminated by hepatic metabolism through glucuronidation processes (Sabers & Gram, 2000). The glucuronidation of lamotrigine is inhibited by valproic acid and is induced by carbamazepine. Concomitant treatment with valproate increases lamotrigine blood levels, and therefore, it is advisable to use lower lamotrigine doses and to proceed very cautiously when coadministering these medications. Additionally, when coadministered with oral contraceptives, increased lamotrigine doses may be required as estrogen induces the metabolism of lamotrigine. However, postpartum or following discontinuation of oral contraceptives doses should be decreased, because lamotrigine levels may double for a given dose (Reimers, Helde, & Brodtkorb, 2005).

Contraindications

Lamotrigine is contraindicated in patients who have demonstrated hypersensitivity to it.

Gabapentin

Gabapentin (Neurontin) is structurally similar to gamma-aminobutyric acid (GABA). It increases GABA release from glia and may modulate sodium channels. Adult double-blind controlled studies of gabapentin as adjunctive therapy to lithium or valproate and as monotherapy suggest that it is no more effective than placebo for the treatment of mania (Pande, Crockatt, Janney, Werth, & Tsaroucha, 2000); however, gabapentin may be useful in combination with other mood-stabilizing agents for the treatment of anxiety disorders in individuals with bipolar disorder (Keck, Strawn, & McElroy, 2006).

Dosing

The effective dose of gabapentin is 600 to 1800 mg/day given in divided doses (three times a day), with a starting dose of 50–100 mg three times a day. Gabapentin has a saturable absorption, and, therefore, patients may benefit from administering it in divided doses. However, the bioavailability of gabapentin is decreased by 20% with concomitant use of aluminum/magnesium hydroxide antacids.

Adverse Effects

Gabapentin has a relatively benign side-effect profile. The most common side effects in studies involving patients with bipolar disorder are sedation, dizziness, tremor, headache, ataxia, fatigue, and weight gain. Gabapentin has rarely been associated with rashes, thyroiditis, sexual dysfunction, or renal impairment.

Interactions

Gabapentin is not metabolized or protein bound and does not alter hepatic enzymes or interact with other anticonvulsants.

Topiramate

Topiramate (Topamax) is a sulfamate-substitued monosaccharide with several potential mechanisms of action, including blockade of voltage-gated sodium channels, antagonism of the kainate/AMPA subtype of glutamate receptor, enhancement of GABA activity, and carbonic anhydrase inhibition. Topiramate is a weak inducer of cytochrome P450 enzymes and, therefore, is potentially associated with a risk of oral contraceptive failure (particularly with low-dose estrogen oral contraceptives).

Preliminary data from case reports and open studies suggest that topiramate has antimanic properties when used as adjunctive treatment and as monotherapy in children and adolescents with bipolar disorder (DelBello, Schwiers, Rosenberg, & Strakowski, 2002; Barzman et al., 2005). DelBello et al. (2005) published the results of a double-blind, placebo-controlled study of topiramate monotherapy for acute mania in children and adolescents with bipolar disorder. This trial was unfortunately discontinued early by the pharmaceutical company after several trials with topiramate failed to show efficacy in adults with mania. During the pediatric trial, 56 children and adolescents (6–17 years) with a diagnosis of bipolar disorder type I were randomized in a double-blind study to topiramate (52%) or placebo (48%). Topiramate was started at 25 mg twice daily and titrated to 400 mg over 5 days, after which it was allowed to be decreased. The mean final dose was 278 ± 121 mg/day. Decreased appetite and nausea were the most frequent side effects that were significantly greater in the topiramate than the placebo group. The reduction on the primary outcome variable, the mean YMRS score from baseline to final visit using the last observation carried forward (LOCF), was not statistically different between the topiramate group and the placebo group. The only statistically significant differences in efficacy measures between treatment groups were the difference between slopes of the linear mean profiles of the YMRS using a post hoc repeated-measures regression and the change in Brief Psychiatric

Rating Scale (BPRS) for Children at day 28 using observed data. This is considered a negative trial, with the caveat that the results are inconclusive because of premature termination resulting in a limited sample size.

Side effects of topiramate include sedation, fatigue, paresthesias, impaired concentration, and psychomotor slowing. In patients with epilepsy, there is a 1–2% rate of nepholithiasis because of carbonic anhydrase inhibition. In contrast to other antiepileptic drugs (AEDs) and antipsychotics used to treat bipolar disorder, topiramate is associated with anorexia and weight loss. Body weight reduction seems to be dose-related and is more common in patients with larger body mass indices. Word-finding difficulties have been reported in up to one-third of adult patients treated with topiramate and have also been reported to occur in children. Cognitive disturbances might be worse in patients treated with concomitant divalproex. Additionally, topiramate is associated with limb agenesis in rodents and therefore should be used with caution in females of childbearing potential.

Oxcarbazepine

Oxcarbazepine (Trileptal), the 10-keto analogue of carbamazepine, is biotransformed by hydroxylation to its active metabolite 10,11-dihydro-10-hydroxy carbamazepine (MHD). MHD is the primary active metabolite and accounts for its antiseizure properties.

Recently, Wagner and colleagues reported the results of a multicentered, randomized double-blind placebo-controlled study (Wagner et al., 2006). In this study, 116 youths with bipolar disorder (mean age = 11.1 ± 2.9 years) were randomized to receive either oxcarbazepine or placebo. The difference in the primary outcome variable, change in YMRS mean scores, between the treatment groups was not statistically or clinically significant. This is a negative trial that does not support the use of oxcarbazepine as monotherapy in the treatment of mania in children and adolescents. Whether this medication may be useful for the treatment of hypomania, bipolar disorder not otherwise specified, or cyclothymia is unknown.

Zonisamide

Zonisamide (Zonegran) is a sulfonamide derivative antiepileptic that has several potential mechanisms of action, including blockade of voltage-sensitive sodium channels and calcium currents, modulation of GABAergic and dopaminergic systems, carbonic anhydrase inhibition, and free-radical scavenging. Zonisamide is protein-bound (40–60%) but does not appear to affect the protein binding of other drugs. Concurrent administration with enzyme-inducing anticonvulsants such as carbamazepine stimulate zonisamide metabolism and decrease serum zonisamide levels at steady state.

Open-label studies suggest that zonisamide may be useful for the treatment of adults with bipolar disorder (McElroy et al., 2005); however, there have been no studies examining zonisamide for the treatment of children and adolescents with bipolar disorder. Common side effects of zonisamide in patients with epilepsy include nepholithiasis, drowsiness, ataxia, and loss of appetite. Rare but serious side effects include severe rashes (i.e., Stevens–Johnson syndrome and toxic epidermal necrolysis), as well as hematological and immunological abnormalities, such as aplastic anemia or agranulocytosis, IgA and IgG2 deficiency, and oligohydrosis and hyperthermia in pediatric patients. Zonisamide should be used with caution in patients with sulfa allergy.

Miscellaneous Antiepileptic/Mood-Stabilizing Agents

Other new AEDs include vigabatrin (Sabril), and levetiracetam (Keppra). Vigabatrin, which inhibits GABA catabolism, is of limited use in patients with bipolar disorder because it appears to induce depression and is associated with visual field constriction. Levetiracetam is a novel AED, whose mechanism of action remains unclear. Levetiracetam rapidly achieves steady-state concentrations, is primarily eliminated unchanged in the urine, and is minimally protein-bound. Risk for drug interactions is minimal with levetiracetam because it does not induce or get metabolized by cytochrome P450 enzymes. Common side effects of levetiracetam include sedation, dizziness, and asthenia. Although the efficacy of levetiracetam in the treatment of bipolar disorder remains to be evaluated, based on its pharmacodynamic properties and side-effect profile, it may prove to be a promising new agent for the treatment of bipolar disorder.

Table 6.2 summarizes clinical information about the antiepileptic agents.

SUMMARY

It is clear from the studies reviewed herein that lithium is efficacious in the treatment of bipolar disorder in children and adolescents. But lithium is difficult for many children and adolescents to tolerate in the long term because of side effects, such as exacerbation of acne and enuresis. Lithium treatment by itself is rarely effective in children and adolescents with bipolar disorder over the long term (Findling et al., 2005). It is less clear whether valproate is efficacious for the treatment of mania because of the one large negative controlled trial that was discussed earlier. The efficacy data on the newer mood stabilizers are less clear, and clinicians should use these agents cautiously in children and adults until further positive results emerge.

TABLE 6.2. Mood Stabilizer Dosing/Monitoring in Children and Adolescents with Bipolar Disorder

Generic name	U.S. trade name	How supplied (mg)	Starting dose	Target dose	Cautions
Gabapentin	Neurontin	100, 300, 400	100 mg two or three times per day	Based on response	Watch for behavioral disinhibition
Lamotrigine	Lamictal	25, 100, 200	12.5 mg daily	Increase per titration guidelines and response	Monitor carefully for rashes, serum sickness
Oxcarbazepine	Trileptal	150, 300, 600	150 mg two times per day	20–29 kg 900 mg/day 39–39 kg 1200 mg/day >39 kg 1800 mg/day	Monitor for hyponatremia
Tiagabine	Gabitril				
Topiramate	Topamax	25, 100	25 mg daily	100–400 mg/day	Monitor for memory problems, kidney stones

The pharmacotherapy of pediatric bipolar disorder is often complex, and mood stability is sometimes achieved only with several medications, including mood stabilizers and antipsychotics. DelBello et al. (2002) published the results of a double-blind and placebo-controlled study that examined the efficacy, safety, and tolerability of quetiapine as an adjunct to valproate for acute mania in adolescents with bipolar disorder versus valproate alone. In this study, 30 adolescent inpatients with mania or mixed bipolar I disorder, ages 12–18 years, received an initial divalproex dose of 20 mg/kg and were randomized in a double-blind study to 6 weeks of quetiapine, which was titrated to 450 mg/day ($n = 15$), or placebo ($n = 15$). The divalproex (valproate) plus quetiapine group demonstrated a statistically significant greater reduction in YMRS scores from baseline to end point than did the valproate-plus-placebo group, $F(1, 27) = 5.04$, $p = .03$. Moreover, YMRS response rate was significantly greater in the valproate-plus-quetiapine group than in the valproate-plus-placebo group (87% vs. 53%). The findings of this study indicate that quetiapine in combination with divalproex was more effective for the treatment of adolescent bipolar mania than divalproex alone.

There is also emerging evidence that the traditional mood stabilizers, lithium and valproate, may be "neuroprotective" in the central nervous system (Chuang, 2004; Rowe & Chuang, 2004). The mechanisms of these possible neuroprotective effects are complex, but they mediate changes at the level of the genome (Zhou et al., 2005). Ultimately, the best treatment for children and adolescents with bipolar disorder may involve the use of a traditional mood stabilizer, in concert with an atypical antipsychotic. Future studies hopefully will determine this.

REFERENCES

Abbott, L. (2006). A double-blind, placebo-controlled trial to evaluate the safety and efficacy of depakote ER for the treatment of mania associated with bipolar disorder in children and adolescents (Protocol No. M01-342). Retrieved February 2008, from *www.clinicalstudy results.org*.

Asconape, J. J. (2002). Some common issues in the use of antiepileptic drugs. *Seminars in Neurology*, 22(1), 27–39.

Barzman, D. H., DelBello, M. P., Kowatch, R. A., Warner, J., Rofey, D., Stanford, K., et al. (2005). Adjunctive topiramate in hospitalized children and adolescents with bipolar disorders. *Journal of Child and Adolescent Psychopharmacology*, 15(6), 931–937.

Bowden, C. L., Calabrese, J. R., Sachs, G., Yatham, L. N., Asghar, S. A., Hompland, M., et al. (2003). A placebo-controlled 18-month trial of lamotrigine and lithium maintenance treatment in recently manic or hypomanic patients with bipolar I disorder. *Archives of General Psychiatry*, 60(4), 392–400.

Bowden, C. L., Janicak, P. G., Orsulak, P., Swann, A. C., Davis, J. M., Calabrese, J. R., et al. (1996). Relation of serum valproate concentration to response in mania. *American Journal of Psychiatry*, 153(6), 765–770.

Bowden, C. L., & Karren, N. U. (2006). Anticonvulsants in bipolar disorder. *Australian New Zealand Journal of Psychiatry*, 40(5), 386–393.

Calabrese, J., Bowden, C., Sachs, G., Ascher, J., Monaghan, E., & Rudd, G. (1999, February). A double-blind placebo-controlled study of lamotrigine monotherapy in outpatients with bipolar I depression. *Journal of Clinical Psychiatry*, 60, 79–88.

Chang, K., Saxena, K., & Howe, M. (2006). An open-label study of lamotrigine adjunct or monotherapy for the treatment of adolescents with bipolar depression. *Journal of the American Academy of Child and Adolescent Psychiatry*, 45(3), 298–304.

Chuang, D. M. (2004). Neuroprotective and neurotrophic actions of the mood stabilizer lithium: Can it be used to treat neurodegenerative diseases? *Critical Reviews in Neurobiology*, 16(1–2), 83–90.

Ciraulo, D. A., Shader, R. J., Greenblatt, D. J., & Creelman, W. L. (Eds.). (1995). *Drug interactions in psychiatry*. Baltimore: Williams & Wilkins.

Cloyd, J. C., Fischer, J. H., Kriel, R. L., & Kraus, D. M. (1993). Valproic acid pharmacokinetics in children: IV. Effects of age and antiepileptic drugs on protein binding and intrinsic clearance. *Clinical Pharmacology and Therapeutics*, 53(1), 22–29.

Cueva, J. E., Overall, J. E., Small, A. M., Armenteros, J. L., Perry, R., & Campbell, M. (1996). Carbamazepine in aggressive children with conduct disorder: A double-blind and placebo-controlled study. *Journal of the American Academy of Child and Adolescent Psychiatry*, 35(4), 480–490.

DelBello, M. P., Findling, R. L., Kushner, S., Wang, D., Olson, W. H., Capece, J. A., et al. (2005). A pilot controlled trial of topiramate for mania in children and adolescents with bipolar disorder. *Journal of the American Academy of Child and Adolescent Psychiatry*, 44(6), 539–547.

DelBello, M., Schwiers, M., Rosenberg, H., & Strakowski, S. (2002). Quetiapine as adjunctive treatment for adolescent mania associated with bipolar disorder. *Journal of the American Academy of Child and Adolescent Psychiatry, 41*(10), 1216–1223.

Deltito, J. A., Levitan, J., Damore, J., Hajal, F., & Zambenedetti, M. (1998). Naturalistic experience with the use of divalproex sodium on an in-patient unit for adolescent psychiatric patients. *Acta Psychiatrica Scandinavica, 97*(3), 236–240.

Devi, K., George, S., Criton, S., Suja, V., & Sridevi, P. K. (2005). Carbamazepine—the commonest cause of toxic epidermal necrolysis and Stevens–Johnson syndrome: A study of 7 years. *Indian Journal of Dermatology, Venereology, and Leprology, 71*(5), 325–328.

Ee, L. C., Shepherd, R. W., Cleghorn, G. J., Lewindon, P. J., Fawcett, J., Strong, R. W., et al. (2003). Acute liver failure in children: A regional experience. *Journal of Paediatrics and Child Health, 39*(2), 107–110.

Evans, R. W., Clay, T. H., & Gualtieri, C. T. (1987). Carbamazepine in pediatric psychiatry. *Journal of the American Academy of Child and Adolescent Psychiatry, 26*(1), 2–8.

Findling, R. L., McNamara, N. K., Youngstrom, E. A., Stansbrey, R., Gracious, B. L., Reed, M. D., et al. (2005). Double-blind 18-month trial of lithium versus divalproex maintenance treatment in pediatric bipolar disorder. *Journal of the American Academy of Child and Adolescent Psychiatry, 44*(5), 409–417.

Glaxo, W. I. (2001). Lamictal (lamotrigine) product information. In *Physicians desk reference*. Research Triangle Park, NC: Thomson Healthcare.

Goodwin, G. M., Bowden, C. L., Calabrese, J. R., Grunze, H., Kasper, S., White, R., et al. (2004). A pooled analysis of 2 placebo-controlled 18-month trials of lamotrigine and lithium maintenance in bipolar I disorder. *Journal of Clinical Psychiatry, 65*(3), 432–441.

Isojarvi, J. I., Laatikainen, T. J., Pakarinen, A. J., Juntunen, K. T., & Myllyla, V. V. (1993). Polycystic ovaries and hyperandrogenism in women taking valproate for epilepsy. *New England Journal of Medicine, 329*(19), 1383–1388.

Joffe, H., Cohen, L. S., Suppes, T., McLaughlin, W. L., Lavori, P., Adams, J. M., et al. (2006). Valproate is associated with new-onset oligoamenorrhea with hyperandrogenism in women with bipolar disorder. *Biological Psychiatry, 59*(11), 1078–1086.

Kafantaris, V., Campbell, M., Padron-Gayol, M. V., Small, A. M., Locascio, J. J., & Rosenberg, C. R. (1992). Carbamazepine in hospitalized aggressive conduct disorder children: An open pilot study. *Psychopharmacology Bulletin, 28*(2), 193–199.

Kastner, T., & Friedman, D. L. (1992). Verapamil and valproic acid treatment of prolonged mania. *Journal of the American Academy of Child and Adolescent Psychiatry, 31*(2), 271–275.

Kastner, T., Friedman, D. L., Plummer, A. T., Ruiz, M. Q., & Henning, D. (1990). Valproic acid for the treatment of children with mental retardation and mood symptomatology. *Pediatrics, 86*(3), 467–472.

Keating, A., & Blahunka, P. (1995). Carbamazepine-induced Stevens–Johnson syndrome in a child. *Annals of Pharmacotherapy, 29*(5), 538–539.

Keck, P. E., Jr., Strawn, J. R., & McElroy, S. L. (2006). Pharmacologic treatment considerations in co-occurring bipolar and anxiety disorders. *Journal of Clinical Psychiatry, 67*(Suppl. 1), 8–15.

Ketter, T. A., Nasrallah, H. A., & Fagiolini, A. (2006). Mood stabilizers and atypical antipsychotics: Bimodal treatments for bipolar disorder. *Psychopharmacology Bulletin, 39*(1), 120–146.

Ketter, T. A., Wang, P. W., Becker, O. V., Nowakowska, C., & Yang, Y. S. (2003). The diverse roles of anticonvulsants in bipolar disorders. *Annals of Clinical Psychiatry, 15*(2), 95–108.

Ketter, T. A., Wang, P. W., Chandler, R. A., Alarcon, A. M., Becker, O. V., Nowakowska, C., et al. (2005). Dermatology precautions and slower titration yield low incidence of lamotrigine treatment-emergent rash. *Journal of Clinical Psychiatry, 66*(5), 642–645.

Konig, S. A., Siemes, H., Blaker, F., Boenigk, E., Gross-Selbeck, G., Hanefeld, F., et al. (1994). Severe hepatotoxicity during valproate therapy: An update and report of eight new fatalities. *Epilepsia, 35*(5), 1005–1015.

Kowatch, R. A., & DelBello, M. P. (2006). Pediatric bipolar disorder: Emerging diagnostic and treatment approaches. *Child and Adolescent Psychiatric Clinics of North America, 15*(1), 73–108.

Kowatch, R. A., Suppes, T., Carmody, T. J., Bucci, J. P., Hume, J. H., Kromelis, M., et al. (2000). Effect size of lithium, divalproex sodium and carbamazepine in children and adolescents with bipolar disorder. *Journal of the American Academy of Child and Adolescent Psychiatry, 39*(6), 713–720.

McElroy, S., & Keck, P. J. (2000). Pharmacologic agents for the treatment of acute bipolar mania. *Biological Psychiatry, 48*, 539–557.

McElroy, S. L., Suppes, T., Keck, P. E., Jr., Black, D., Frye, M. A., Altshuler, L. L., et al. (2005). Open-label adjunctive zonisamide in the treatment of bipolar disorders: A prospective trial. *Journal of Clinical Psychiatry, 66*(5), 617–624.

Pande, A. C., Crockatt, J. G., Janney, C. A., Werth, J. L., & Tsaroucha, G. (2000, September). Gabapentin in bipolar disorder: A placebo-controlled trial of adjunctive therapy. *Bipolar Disorders, 2*, 249–255.

Papatheodorou, G., & Kutcher, S. P. (1993). Divalproex sodium treatment in late adolescent and young adult acute mania. *Psychopharmacology Bulletin, 29*(2), 213–219.

Papatheodorou, G., Kutcher, S. P., Katic, M., & Szalai, J. P. (1995). The efficacy and safety of divalproex sodium in the treatment of acute mania in adolescents and young adults: An open clinical trial. *Journal of Clinical Psychopharmacology, 15*(2), 110–116.

Pavuluri, M. N., Birmaher, B., & Naylor, M. W. (2005). Pediatric bipolar disorder: A review of the past 10 years. *Journal of the American Academy of Child and Adolescent Psychiatry, 44*(9), 846–871.

Pleak, R. R., Birmaher, B., Gavrilescu, A., Abichandani, C., & Williams, D. T. (1988). Mania and neuropsychiatric excitation following carbamazepine. *Journal of the American Academy of Child and Adolescent Psychiatry, 27*(4), 500–503.

Puente, R. M. (1975). The use of carbamazepine in the treatment of behavioural disorders in children. In W. Birkmayer (Ed.), *Epileptic seizures—behaviour—pain* (pp. 243–252). Baltimore: University Park Press.

Rasgon, N. (2004). The relationship between polycystic ovary syndrome and antiepileptic drugs: A review of the evidence. *Journal of Clinical Psychopharmacology, 24*(3), 322–334.

Reimers, A., Helde, G., & Brodtkorb, E. (2005). Ethinyl estradiol, not progestogens, reduces lamotrigine serum concentrations. *Epilepsia, 46*(9), 1414–1417.

Rowe, M. K., & Chuang, D. M. (2004). Lithium neuroprotection: Molecular mechanisms and clinical implications. *Expert Reviews in Molecular Medicine, 6*(21), 1–18.

Sabers, A., & Gram, L. (2000). Newer anticonvulsants: Comparative review of drug interactions and adverse effects. *Drugs, 60*(1), 23–33.

Sinclair, D. B., Berg, M., & Breault, R. (2004). Valproic acid-induced pancreatitis in childhood epilepsy: Case series and review. *Journal of Child Neurology, 19*(7), 498–502.

Treem, W. R. (1994). Inherited and acquired syndromes of hyperammonemia and encephalopathy in children. *Seminars in Liver Disease, 14*(3), 236–258.

Wagner, K. D., Kowatch, R. A., Emslie, G. J., Findling, R. L., Wilens, T. E., McCague, K., et al. (2006). A double-blind, randomized, placebo-controlled trial of oxcarbazepine in the treatment of bipolar disorder in children and adolescents. *American Journal of Psychiatry, 163*(7), 1179–1186.

Weisler, R. H., Cutler, A. J., Ballenger, J. C., Post, R. M., & Ketter, T. A. (2006). The use of antiepileptic drugs in bipolar disorders: A review based on evidence from controlled trials. *CNS Spectrums, 11*(10), 788–799.

Werlin, S. L., & Fish, D. L. (2006). The spectrum of valproic acid-associated pancreatitis. *Pediatrics*, *118*(4), 1660–1663.

West, K., & McElroy, S. L. (1995). Oral loading doses in the valproate treatment of adolescents with mixed bipolar disorder. *Journal of Child and Adolescent Psychopharmacology*, *5*, 225–231.

West, S. A., Keck, P. E. J., McElroy, S. L., Strakowski, S. M., Minnery, K. L., McConville, B. J., et al. (1994). Open trial of valproate in the treatment of adolescent mania. *Journal of Child and Adolescent Psychopharmacology*, *4*, 263–267.

Whittier, M. C., West, S. A., Galli, V. B., & Raute, N. J. (1995). Valproic acid for dysphoric mania in a mentally retarded adolescent. *Journal of Clinical Psychiatry*, *56*(12), 590–591.

Wilder, B. J. (1992). Pharmacokinetics of valproate and carbamazepine. *Journal of Clinical Psychopharmacology*, *12*(Suppl. 1), 64S–68S.

Yang, H., Cusin, C., & Fava, M. (2005). Is there a placebo problem in antidepressant trials? *Current Topics in Medicinal Chemistry*, *5*(11), 1077–1086.

Zhou, R., Gray, N. A., Yuan, P., Li, X., Chen, J., Chen, G., et al. (2005). The anti-apoptotic, glucocorticoid receptor cochaperone protein bag-1 is a long-term target for the actions of mood stabilizers. *Journal of Neuroscience*, *25*(18), 4493–4502.

CHAPTER 7

Newer Drugs

ADELAIDE S. ROBB *and* PARAMJIT T. JOSHI

Bipolar disorder in children and adolescents, as with adults, is treated pharmacologically with the more traditional mood stabilizers, considered to be first-line agents. These mood stabilizers include lithium carbonate and divalproex sodium. Two drugs are approved by the Food and Drug Administration (FDA) for the treatment of pediatric bipolar disorder: lithium in children 12 and older and risperidone in children 10 and older. While divalproex sodium is FDA-approved for the treatment of epilepsy in children over the age of 2 years, it is approved for bipolar disorder only in adults with bipolar mixed or manic episodes. Other agents that are FDA-approved for the treatment of bipolar disorder in adults include aripiprazole, lamotrigine, olanzapine, quetiapine, risperdal, and ziprasidone. In addition to these medications, other antipsychotic and antiepileptic agents are also used for mood stabilization. All of these mood-stabilizing medications are described in other chapters in this volume.

Despite this wide range of treatment options, many patients are treatment resistant and/or require polypharmacy (Denicoff, Smith-Jackson, Bryan, Ali, & Post, 1997). In a review of the National Institute of Mental Health (NIMH) intramural bipolar clinic records, Post and colleagues found that more patients have become treatment resistant to monotherapy over the three decades that the clinic has been seeing patients with bipolar disorder (Post et al., 2000). These authors also noted a shift, both in the number of medications used and in the number of patients who were considered rapid cyclers over the three decades. In the 1970s the percentage of patients with bipolar disorder requiring polypharmacy was 25%, with 29% being rapid cyclers. By the 1990s the number requiring polypharmacy was 67%, and the ones considered rapid cyclers had increased markedly to 70% of cases. These findings of mixed, rapid cycling and hard-to-treat patients have also been shown in patients with pediatric bipolar disorder by a number of investigators (Geller et al., 1995; Geller & Luby, 1997; Strober et al., 1988).

Several pediatric investigators have examined the response rates of pediatric bipolar disorder to monotherapy and combination therapy with the standard mood-stabilizing agents. This subject is covered extensively in other chapters in this volume and is highlighted here as Table 7.1. In the Findling et al. (2003) study remission was defined prior to study onset as 4 consecutive weeks with Young Mania Rating Scale (YMRS) < 12.5, Child Depression Rating Scale (CDRS-R) < 40, and Children's Global Assessment scale (CGAS) > 51. In the study by Kowatch, Sethuraman, Home, Kromelis, and Weinberg (2003) patients from the earlier study by Kowatch and colleagues (2000) received open-label treatment, including two mood stabilizers, stimulants, antidepressants, and antipsychotics. Fifty-eight percent of patients were on combination treatment, and 80% of them improved.

When patients do not respond to the conventional mood stabilizers and antipsychotics, clinicians look beyond to other treatment options. Other treatments for pediatric bipolar disorder include electroconvulsive therapy (ECT), dietary supplements such as omega-3 fatty acids, and various psychotherapies, including individual, group and family modalities, which are discussed elsewhere (see Chapters 9 and 10, this volume). This chapter focuses on newer medications and drug regimens that have been studied, recommended, and used for the treatment of bipolar disorder. Most of these newer agents have been studied in adults with bipolar disorder and are discussed in the text and summarized in Table 7.2. Pediatric

TABLE 7.1. Pediatric Studies in Bipolar Disorder

Study	Kowatch et al. (2000)	Findling et al. (2003)	Kowatch et al. (2003)
Number	42	90	35
Length	6–8 weeks	20 weeks	16 weeks
Design	Double blind	Open 2 drug	Open 2 drug
Response	50% ↓ YMRS		
% Response/effect size lithium	38%/1.06		
% Response/effect size valproic acid	58%/1.63		
% Response/effect size carbamazepine	38%/1.00		
% Remission on lithium and valproic acid		47%	
% on 2 drugs/% response on 2 drugs			58%/80%

TABLE 7.2. New Adult Medications

Study	Population	Type	Number	First drug	New drug	Response
Giannini et al. (1984), Hoschl & Kozeny (1989), Garza-Trevino et al. (1992)	BP	OL, CR	86, 20	Multiple	Verapamil	Positive
Prien & Gelenberg (1989), Dubovsky (1993)	BP	OL, CS	Multiple studies	Multiple	Verapamil	Positive
Janicak et al. (1998)	BP	DB, PBO	32	PBO	Verapamil 480mg	MRS, HAM-D, BPRS, no change either group
Walton et al. (1996)	BP, acute mania	DB	40	Lithium	Verapamil	Li > verapamil on all measures—BPRS, MRS, GAF, CGI
Lenzi et al. (1995)	BP mixed, manic	OL	15	Chlorpromazine	Verapamil	BPRS, CGI, 14/15 needed both meds, verapamil monotherapy did not work
Giannini et al. (2000)	BP maintenance	DB	20	PBO or magnesium	Verapamil	Magnesium add-on decreased BPRS scores
Wisner et al. (2002)	BP pregnant	OL	37		Verapamil	HAM-D, BPRS, 9/11 manic mixed better, safe in pregnant patients with BP
Goodnick (1996)	BP manic	OL	12		Verapamil	YMRS improved by 32%, improvement predicted by ↑ calcium levels, magnesium did not predict response

(continued)

Reference	Diagnosis	Design	N	Comparator	Drug	Results
Brunet et al. (1990)	BP	OL, CS	6		Nimodipine	MRS, BPRS improved
Manna (1991)	BPRC	OL	12	Lithium	Nimodipine	↓ length and number cycles
Pazzaglia et al. (1993)	TR mood disorder	OL	12	Carbamazepine add on	Nimodipine	5/9 respond to nimodipine, 2/3 respond to add-on carbamazepine
Pazzaglia et al. (1998)	TR mood disorder	OL	30	Verapamil	Nimodipine	10/30 better on nimodipine, relapse on verapamil
Goodnick et al. (1995)	TR, BPRC, CS	OL	2	Multiple	Nimodipine	Both better with nimodipine monotherapy
Grunze et al. (1996)	CR	OL	1	Lithium	Nimodipine	Did better on combination, relapse on stopping nimodipine
Yingling et al. (2002)	pregnant BP, CR	OL	1	Lithium, carbamazepine	Nimodipine	Did fine on monotherapy through pregnancy
De Beaurepaire (1992)	TR, BP, SA	OL	7	Neuroleptic	Nifedipine	5/7 responded to combination, withdrawal from nifedipine caused relapse
Caillard (1985)	BP mania	OL	6		Diltiazem	Worked in short-term treatment
Silverstone & Birkett (2000)	TR BP	OL	8	MS, AP, AD, thyroid, clonazepam	Diltiazem	On combination ↓ frequency and severity of manic symptoms
Davanzo et al. (1999)	**BPRC teen**	**OL**	**1**	**Multiple drugs**	**Nimodipine**	**Stable for 3 years**
Bebchuk et al. (2000)	BP manic	DB	7		Tamoxifen	YMRS ↓ 10.29 points, 5/7 50% ↓ YMRS
Cohen et al. (1982)	BP manic	OL	8	Lithium	Lecithin	Combination 4/8 marked improvement

(continued)

TABLE 7.2. (*continued*)

Study	Population	Type	Number	First drug	New drug	Response
Stoll et al. (1996)	TR BPRC	OL	6	Lithium	Choline	5/6 rapid improvement in manic symptoms on both drugs, less effect on depressive symptoms
Schreier (1982)	**BP manic teen**	**OL**	**1**	**Lithium and haldol**	**Lecithin**	**Lecithin plus lithium remission**
Burt et al. (1999)	TR mood	OL	11	Multiple	Donepezil	6/11 responded, 54.5% markedly improved
Schaffer et al. (2000)	BPRC	OL	20	Failed Li, VPA, CBZ	Mexiletine	53% full or partial response

Note. Pediatric cases are in **bold**. YMRS, Young Mania Rating Scale; HAM-D, Hamilton Depression Rating Scale; BPRS, Brief Psychiatric Rating Scale; MRS, Mania Rating Scale; OL, open label; CR, case report; CS, case series; DB, double blind; CGI, Clinical Global Impression; GAF, Global Assessment of Functioning; BPRC, bipolar rapid cycling; BP, bipolar; TR, treatment resistant; SA, schizoaffective; AP, antipsychotics; AD, antidepressants; MS, mood stabilizers; Li, lithium; VPA, valproic acid; CBZ, carbamazepine; PBO, placebo.

studies for these newer agents, when available, are noted in this chapter. These medications fall into three categories:

1. Medications that affect the hypothalamic–pituitary–adrenal (HPA) axis.
2. Medications that affect second-messenger systems.
3. Other medications.

MEDICATIONS THAT AFFECT THE HYPOTHALAMIC–PITUITARY–ADRENAL AXIS

Endocrinologists and psychiatrists have noted that patients with disturbances in the thyroid, parathyroid, and adrenal glands can present with a variety of psychiatric symptoms. The following three sections explore the affective symptoms associated with disturbances in these endocrine symptoms and how clinicians and researchers have used modification of these major endocrine systems to treat the treatment-resistant patient with bipolar disorder.

Thyroid Dysfunction

Patients with thyroid dysfunction can have hypothyroidism or hyperthyroidism. In general, women and older people are more likely to have thyroid dysfunction (Hollowell et al., 2002).

Hypothyroidism is classified from grades I to III.

- Grade I is considered overt hypothyroidism characterized by low T3 (triiodothyronine) and T4 (thyroxine) levels and elevated TSH (thyroid-stimulating hormone).
- Grade II, or subclinical, hypothyroidism has normal T3 and T4 levels with elevated TSH.
- Grade III shows normal T3, T4, and TSH levels with exaggerated TSH response to TRH (thyrotropin-releasing hormone; Ladenson et al., 2000).

In patients with clinical and subclinical hypothyroidism, affective symptoms are a common presentation (Geffken, Ward, Staab, Carmichael, & Evans, 1998). *Hyperthyroidism* can occur from overproduction of thyroid hormone in the thyroid or another site in the body and from taking too much exogenous thyroid hormone. The most common cause of hyperthyroidism in up to 80% of patients is Graves' disease. Clinical hyperthyroidism includes elevated T3 and T4 with low TSH. Subclinical hyperthyroidism is characterized by a normal level of T3 and T4 with low

TSH. Patients with hyperthyroidism present with psychiatric symptoms that more closely resemble those of bipolar disorder and may also present with anxiety symptoms similar to those of panic disorder. These psychiatric presentations are summarized in Table 7.3. Pediatric symptoms of hypothyroidism are similar to those in adults, while symptoms of pediatric hyperthyroidism include irritability and weight loss (Birrell & Cheetham, 2004). Lazar et al. (2000) broke down presentations by pubertal status and noted that prepubertal patients frequently showed weight loss and loose stools, while pubertal patients showed irritability, palpitations, and tremor.

Thyroid Dysfunction in Major Depression and Bipolar Disorder

While patients with primary endocrine disorders of the thyroid can present with psychiatric symptoms, patients with primary affective disorder are known to have alterations in their thyroid hormone levels and elevations of antithyroid antibodies. Table 7.4 summarizes these findings of thyroid dysfunction in mood disorder. Zarate and colleagues studied thyroid indices in patients over the age of 18 presenting with first episode of bipolar mixed or manic episode (Zarate, Tohen, & Zarate, 1997). Seventy-two patients were assessed for TSH, T4, and T3RU (reverse uptake). Patients with mixed episodes of bipolar disorder tend to have higher TSH levels than patients with pure manic episodes. Up to 92% of people with rapid-cycling bipolar disorder have thyroid dysfunction, while only 32% of non-rapid-cycling bipolar patients have thyroid dysfunction (Cowdry, Wehr, Zis, & Goodwin, 1983). Patients with rapid-cycling bipolar disorder are also more likely to have antithyroid antibodies, which correlate with severity of illness (Oomen, Schipperijin, & Drexhage, 1996). Frye and colleagues noted that patients with low or below normal thyroid function had poorer outcome (Frye et al., 1999). Cole and colleagues noted that patients with low free thyroid index (FTI) and elevated TSH had poorer treatment response (Cole et al., 2002). Ramasubbu (2003) postulated in a letter to the editor that T4 was best for bipolar disorder and T3 for unipolar depression. Gyulai et al. (2003) decided to determine the interaction between lithium treatment and the development of thyroid hypofunction seen in patients with rapid-cycling bipolar disorder. They completed a trial of 20 medication-free patients with rapid-cycling bipolar disorder and 20 age- and sex-matched controls. Both groups were treated for 4 weeks with lithium and achieved serum levels of 0.7–1.2 mEq/L. At baseline both groups were comparable in thyroid function tests and in response to TRH challenge. Both groups had decreases in T4 and increases in TSH with lithium treatment; however, more patients developed grade III hypothyroidism. No people in either group developed antimicrosomal or antithyroglobulin antibodies, and thyroid status did not correlate with scores on depression or mania rating scales. The authors

TABLE 7.3. Endocrine Disorders and Psychiatric Symptoms

	Hypothyroid	Hyperthyroid	Hyperparathyroid	Hypoparathyroid	Hypercortisol	Hypocortisol
Labs	↑ TSH ↓ T3/T4	↓ TSH, ↑ T3/T4	↑ Calcium	↓ Calcium	↑ Glucocorticoids	↓ Glucocorticoids
Acute adult	Depressed mood; low energy; hypersomnia; weight gain; short-term memory; cognitive impairment; fatigue	Bipolar/panic, irritability, mood lability, fatigue, weight loss, insomnia	Apathy, fatigue, mood symptoms, poor concentration, 4–57% psychiatric symptoms	Intellectual impairment, neurosis, psychosis	Cushing's, 85%; anxiety; mood changes; crying; fatigue; memory, concentration deficits; insomnia; social withdrawal	Addison's, fatigue, anorexia, apathy, negativism, depression, irritability, anhedonia, impaired thinking, social withdrawal
Chronic adult	Irritable mood, delirium, dementia, restlessness, hypersexuality, delusions, hallucinations					
Toxic		Delirium, manic mood, psychotic symptoms	Somnolence, coma		Suicidal, psychotic	Coma, delirium
Pediatric	Similar to adult	Prepubertal—weight loss, loose stools; Pubertal—irritability, palpitations, tremor				

TABLE 7.4. Thyroid Dysfunction and Affective Disorder

Study	Population	Thyroid labs	Findings	Treatment
Zarate et al. (1997)	Adult BP	TSH, T4, T3RU	Mixed TSH > manic TSH	
Cowdry et al. (1983)	Adult BP, RC, NRC	TSH	↑ TSH 92% RC, 32% NRC; Hypothyroid 50.7% RC, 0% NRC	
Oomen et al. (1996)	Adult BP	Antithyroid antibodies	Correlate with severity	
Frye et al. (1999)	Adult BP		Low or below normal TFTs poorer outcome	
Cole et al. (2002)	Adult BPD	FTI, TSH	Low FTI, ↑ TSH poorer outcome	
Gyulai et al. (2003)	Adult BPRC vs. Control	TSH, T4	BPRC more grade III hypothyroid	Lithium
Sokolov et al. (1994)	Adolescent BPD, MDD vs. Control	T4, T3	↑ T4 mania & depression ↑ RT3 ↓ T3 mania	
West et al. (1996)	Adolescent BP+ADHD	TSH, T3,T4	↓ T4 BP+ADHD	

Note. BP, bipolar; BPD, bipolar depressed; MDD, major depressive disorder; RT3, reverse T3; FTI, free thyroid index; RC, rapid cycling; NRC, nonrapid cycling; TSH, thyroid-stimulating hormone; TFT, thyroid function tests; ADHD, attention-deficit/hyperactivity disorder.

concluded that lithium challenge unmasked thyroid hypofunction and precipitated rapid-cycling phenotype. Sokolov, Kutcher, and Joffe (1994) examined adolescents on their first admission to a psychiatric unit for their thyroid function tests, including T4, free T4, T3, reverse T3, FTI, and T3 resin uptake. All patients were free of history of thyroid illness and medications that cause thyroid dysfunction, including lithium. The authors noted that T4 was elevated in patients with depression and mania compared with controls. Patients with mania also had decreased T3 and increased reverse T3. These results mirrored the findings of adult studies of thyroid dysfunction in mood disorder.

Thyroid Supplementation

Thyroid supplementation (see Table 7.5 for a summary of all the studies using thyroid supplementation for mood disorder) for the treatment of resistant unipolar and bipolar depression was reported by Joffe and colleagues (Joffe, Singer, Levitt, & MacDonald, 1993), who compared lithium and triiodothyronine in patients who were resistant to treatment with tricyclic

antidepressants. In this 2-week trial 50 outpatients were given either placebo (n = 16), 37.5 micrograms of T3 (n = 17) or lithium up to 1200 mg
daily with a mean serum level of 0.55 nmol/L (n = 17). Ten patients on T3
responded, 9 responded to lithium, and 3 to placebo. Bauer and colleagues
studied a group of patients with bipolar depression and treated them with
levothyroxine augmentation (Bauer, Hellweg, Graf, & Baumgartner, 1998).
Bauer et al. (1998) treated 17 patients (12 with bipolar and 5 with unipolar
disorder) with resistance to two or more antidepressants given in adequate
trials. At mean doses of 482 micrograms of levothyroxine, patients showed
reductions on the Hamilton Rating Scale for Depression (HAM-D) from
26.6 to 11.6, with 8 patients achieving full remission at 8 weeks and 10 in
remission at 12 weeks. The remitted patients stayed on levothyroxine for
27 months, with 7 of the 10 maintaining remission, 2 with partial remission, and 1 relapsing. A second open-label study with 320 micrograms
daily of levothyroxine in women with refractory bipolar depression showed
7 out of 10 patients to be full responders (Bauer et al., 2005).

Suparaphysiological doses of thyroid hormone for rapid-cycling bipolar
disorder were used by Gjessing (1938). Desiccated thyroid at doses high
enough to cause tachycardia was administered to treat patients who would
be classified as rapid cycling today (Gjessing, 1938). Bauer and Whybrow
(1990) did an early study of 11 patients with rapid-cycling bipolar disorder
treated with thyroxine at 150–400 micrograms daily. They were treated
with thyroxine as an add-on to their primary mood stabilizer (the majority
of the participants were on lithium). Improvement was noted in both manic
and depressive symptoms. Baumgartner, Bauer, and Hellweg (1994) treated
6 patients with non-rapid-cycling bipolar disorder with open-label levothyroxine, 250–500 micrograms daily. Relapses dropped by 80% and hospitalizations by 90%. Bauer and colleagues studied the use of supraphysiological doses of thyroxine in patients with depressive disorders and in
normal controls (Bauer et al., 2002). Thirteen patients with refractory unipolar and bipolar depression and 13 controls were given 50 micrograms of
thyroxine that was titrated up to 500 micrograms by day 28 and maintained for a second 4 weeks. Both groups were followed for 8 weeks for
discontinuation due to side effects. Patients with mood disorder remained
on a constant dose of their other psychotropic drugs, including mood stabilizers, antipsychotics, and antidepressants. Individuals in both groups
showed elevations in heart rate and decreased blood pressure. Patients with
depression tolerated the thyroxine better and showed smaller increments in
their serum thyroid indices than controls. None of the patients discontinued because of side effects, and 38% of the controls discontinued due to
adverse effects that mimicked hyperthyroidism.

The use of supplemental thyroid hormone as a combination/add-on
strategy was studied by Tremont and Stern (2000) as a way to minimize the
cognitive side effects of lithium treatment and electroconvulsive therapy.

TABLE 7.5. Thyroid Supplementation for Mood Disorder

Study	Population	Resistant	First drug	Thyroid	Second drug	Response
Joffe et al. (1993)	Adult MDD, BPD	Yes	TCA	T3 37.5 µg	Lithium 1200 mg	10/17 T3, 9/17 Li
Bauer et al. (1998)	Adult MDD, BPD	Yes 2+AD		T4 482 µg		8@8weeks 10@12 weeks
Bauer et al. (2001)	Women BPD			T4 320 µg		7/10 full respond
Bauer & Whybrow (1990)	Adult BPRC		MS—lithium	T4 150–400 µg		Manic and depressive symptoms better
Baumgartner et al. (1994)	Adult BP NRC			T4 250–500 µg		↓ relapse by 80% ↓ hospitalization by 90%
Bauer et al. (2002)	Adult MDD BPD vs. Control	Yes	MS, AD, AP	T4 250–500 µg		↑ pulse ↓ blood pressure 38% control quit hyperthyroid
Tremont & Stern (2000)	Adult BP		Li, ECT	T3 50 µg		↓ memory problem ↓ # ECTs
Prohaska et al. (1995)	Adult BP euthyroid, subclinical hypothyroid		Li	T3 0, 25, 50 µg		Both groups better processing speed and motor speed on thyroid
Weeston & Constantino (1996)	Adolescent BPRC	Yes; multi-drug		T4 125 µg		Stable for 9 months

Note. BP, bipolar; BPD, bipolar depressed; MDD, major depressive disorder; RC, rapid cycling; NRC, nonrapid cycling; AD, antidepressant; AP, antipsychotic; ECT, electroconvulsive therapy; MS, mood stabilizer; TCA, tricyclic antidepressant; Li, lithium.

136

Up to 50% of patients on lithium reported neuropsychological side effects, such as memory and concentration difficulties (Gitlin, Cochran, & Jamison, 1989). Dubovsky noted that in patients treated with ECT up to 75% reported memory problems (Dubovsky, 1995). In the augmentation of ECT with 50 micrograms of T3 versus placebo condition, patients in the thyroid group needed fewer ECT treatments and had less memory impairment (Stern et al., 1991; Stern et al., 2000).

Prohaska and colleagues conducted a double-blind crossover trial of 8 euthyroid and 8 subclinical hypothyroid patients on lithium maintenance treatment. Patients were on placebo for 4 weeks and T3 at 25 micrograms for 2 weeks and at 50 micrograms for 2 weeks. Patients of normal and subclinical status both did better in information processing speed and motor speed on thyroid hormone given in combination with lithium (Prohaska, Stern, Mason, Nevels, & Prange, 1995).

Although thyroid supplementation has been reasonably well tolerated in adults, the risk for osteoporosis remains a concern. Gyulai et al. (2001) examined the effects on bone mineral density (BMD) in pre- and postmenopausal patients treated with long-term T4 therapy at suppressive doses. Twenty-six patients were treated for at least 12 months with T4 and had pre- and posttreatment BMD assessments. They found no changes after 12 months, and there was also no difference reported in the BMD of patients before and after menopause when compared with sex-matched population standards.

There is a paucity of literature on the study of thyroid supplementation in patients with pediatric bipolar disorder. A study by West and colleagues (West et al., 1996) examined the difference in thyroid indices of adolescents with acute mania with and without comorbid attention-deficit/ hyperactivity disorder (ADHD). They examined thyroid indices on admission to the hospital in 30 adolescents with mania, 20 of whom had comorbid ADHD. The two groups did not differ in TSH and T3 levels, but the patients with comorbid ADHD and mania had significantly lower serum T4 concentrations. It was postulated that perhaps patients with comorbid ADHD and bipolar mania might be a group that might respond to thyroid supplementation. Weeston and Constantino (1996) reported on the use of high-dose T4 for an adolescent with rapid-cycling bipolar disorder. They treated an adolescent boy who had been hospitalized for more than 111 days for bipolar disorder, shifting rapidly between mania and depression. A number of interventions had failed, including ECT, lithium, carbamazepine, valproate, multiple neuroleptics, calcium-channel blockers, clonidine, and antidepressants. The patient was started on a combination of clonazepam, haloperidol, and valproate, causing sedation but no improvement in the mania symptoms. Levothyroxine was then added to this regimen as an add-on strategy. The starting dose of 25 micrograms was titrated up to 125 micrograms, with resolution of his symptoms over the next 2 weeks. He remained stable on valproate and levothyroxine 9 months later.

Parathyroid Dysfunction

The parathyroid gland uses the secretion of parathyroid hormone (PTH) to regulate serum calcium levels through a negative feedback loop. Low calcium leads to increased PTH levels, which then promotes bone resorption, increases abdominal absorption of dietary calcium, and promotes retention of calcium through the kidneys (Geffken et al., 1998). Patients with alterations of calcium metabolism and parathyroid dysfunction may present with psychiatric symptoms.

Hyperparathyroidism presents with hypercalcemia and can result from an adenoma that secretes excess PTH or secondary to renal failure, due to malignancy, granulomatous disease, hyperthyroidism, and hypocortisolism (Geffken et al., 1998). Calcium levels range from normal (8.9–10.1 mg/dl), to mildly elevated (12–16 mg/dl), moderate elevation (16–19 mg/dl), and severe elevation (> 19 mg/dl). Psychiatric symptoms change as the calcium level increases, as shown in Table 7.3 (Hall & Stickney, 1986; Hasket & Rose, 1981; Leigh & Kramer, 1984). Rates of psychiatric symptoms in patients with hyperparathyroidism can range from 4 to 57% of patients (Alarcon & Franceschini, 1984).

Hypoparathyroidism is characterized by low serum calcium levels and may be due to undersecretion of PTH, lack of vitamin D, or unresponsiveness to PTH or vitamin D. Although some cases of hypoparathyroidism are autoimmune or familial, most cases are due to local trauma to the neck. Patients can also have pseudohypoparathyroidism characterized by unresponsiveness to high-circulating PTH with low calcium and elevated phosphate levels. Psychiatric symptoms appear in Table 7.3 (Denko & Kaelbling, 1962).

Cortisol Dysfunction

Cortisol is regulated through the HPA. Adrenocorticotropic hormone (ACTH) is a pituitary hormone responsible for the release of cortisol and other glucocorticoids from the adrenal cortex. Corticotropin-releasing hormone (CRH) regulates the levels of ACTH. ACTH levels inhibit further ACTH release through a negative feedback loop on the anterior pituitary and at the hypothalamus by decreasing CRH secretion from the hypothalamus (Geffken et al., 1998).

Hypercortisolism is due to excess of glucocorticoids levels. Psychiatric symptoms include weight gain, decreased libido, emotional lability, irritability, anxiety, and depression. Up to 85% of patients with Cushing's syndrome have psychiatric and mental changes, described in Table 7.3 (Hasket,

1985; Kelly, Kelly, & Faragher, 1996). Mood symptoms are more likely to be fluctuating, may correlate with ACTH levels, and may precede the medical symptoms. Treatment of Cushing's syndrome leads to resolution of depressive symptoms. Antidepressants may be helpful while waiting for cortisol levels to normalize (Sonino, Fava, Belluardo, Girelli, & Boscaro, 1993).

Hypocortisolism is usually due to Addison's disease with diminished cortisol secretion. Patients may also have lowered cortisol secretion due to impaired or lowered levels of ACTH or CRH. Psychiatric symptoms are listed in Table 7.3 (Engel & Margolin, 1975).

MEDICATIONS THAT AFFECT SECOND-MESSENGER SYSTEMS

Calcium and Second-Messenger Systems

Free intracellular calcium ion concentrations are elevated in lymphocytes and platelets of patients with bipolar mania and depression but not in unipolar or control individuals (Dubovsky, 1998). Patients with bipolar disorder are thought to have "hyperactivity of intracellular calcium release" (Dubovsky, Murphy, Thomas, & Rademacher, 1992). Calcium influx is also important for presynaptic release of neurotransmitters (Stanley, 1997).

Mood stabilizers have been shown to have an effect on calcium and the second-messenger systems. Lithium inhibits inositol monophosphatase and calcium entry into the cell (Lenox & Manji, 1998). Carbamazepine interferes with phosphorylation stimulated by the calcium calmodulin (Meyer et al., 1995). Patients given combinations of lithium and calcium-channel blockers may experience neurotoxicity or cardiac toxicity (Wright & Jarrett, 1991; Dubovsky, Franks, & Allen, 1987). Carbamazepine in combination with calcium-channel blockers may cause elevated levels of carbamazepine and neurotoxicity (Gadde & Calabrese, 1990; MacPhee, McInnes, Thompson, & Brodie, 1986).

Calcium-channel blockers (CCBs) include a variety of medications that alter voltage- or ligand-gated channels. The four main types of voltage-gated channels are L, T, N, and P. CCBs are primarily the L subtype of voltage-gated channels through the alpha-1 subunit (Triggle, 1992). Nifedipine antagonizes voltage-dependent interactions, and verapamil and diltiazem antagonize frequency-dependent interactions. The second-generation agents differ in selectivity for site, with felodipine selective for vascular L channels and nimodipine for cerebral vascular and neuronal L channels (Triggle, 1992). One study compared patients with hypertension on beta-blockers with those on CCBs and noted 1.60 relative risk for patients to have a myocardial infarction during 4 years of treatment (Jespersen, Hansen, & Mortensen, 1994). A naturalistic study of elderly individuals that controlled for cancer risk factors noted a 1.72-fold increased relative risk for the development of cancer in patients treated with CCBs (Pahor et al., 1996). Hollister and Garza-Trevino (1999) reviewed all the results from 61 trials of calcium-channel blockers: 37 anecdotal, 7 partially controlled, and 17 controlled trials. The authors noted that the anecdotal reports were favorable, while controlled trials were less likely to be positive. Patients who responded to trials of CCBs were more likely to have bipolar disorder with rapid-cycling courses than to have major depression, schizophrenia, or dementia (the other types of illnesses examined in at least one study [Hollister & Garza-Trevino, 1999] with the use of a CCB). The following calcium-channel blockers have been studied and used for the treatment of bipolar disorder.

Verapamil has been the most studied of the calcium-channel blockers in the treatment of bipolar disorder. It is a phenylalkamine-type CCB that interferes with the sodium–calcium counterexchange, inhibits TSH release, inhibits antidiuretic hormone (ADH), and blocks adenyl cyclase activity (Giannini, Houser, Loiselle, Giannini, & Price, 1984; Hoschl & Kozeny, 1989). Verapamil may also function as an anticonvulsant and act as an antidopaminergic agent (Sachs, 1989). Early case reports and open-label studies showed a positive treatment response for bipolar disorder (Giannini et al., 1984; Hoschl & Kozeny, 1989; Garza-Trevino, Overall, & Hollister, 1992). These early trials were case series with use of concomitant medications and less-ill patients with bipolar disorder (Prien & Gelenberg, 1989; Dubovsky, 1993). Janicak and colleagues examined verapamil versus placebo for acute mania in 32 patients (17 on verapamil and 15 on placebo; Janicak, Sharma, Panday, & Davis, 1998). Verapamil doses were up to 480 mg daily and there was no difference reported in the improvement on the Mania Rating Scale (MRS), HAM-D, or Brief Psychiatric Rating Scale (BPRS) in either group. Walton and colleagues conducted a double-blind trial of verapamil versus lithium for bipolar mania (Walton, Berk, & Brook, 1996). Forty patients who were consecutively admitted to an acute inpatient psychiatric unit presenting with DSM-IV acute mania were studied. Twenty-one patients were assigned to verapamil and 19 to lithium. Eighteen patients in each group completed the trial. Patients on verapamil were started on 40 mg three times a day and increased to 80 to 120 mg three times a day. Four patients were maintained on 80 mg three times a day and 14 on 120 mg three times a day. Patients assigned to lithium started on 250 mg three times a day and were adjusted to a mean dose of 832 mg with a mean lithium level of 0.51 mmol/L. Patients were rated on the BPRS, MRS, Global Assessment of Function (GAF) scale, and Clinical Global Impression (CGI) scale. Lorazepam was used on an as-needed basis for agitation. At the end of 28 days, the patients assigned to lithium showed significant improvement on BPRS, MRS, GAF, and CGI compared with the verapamil group. The only side effect noted on lithium was tremor, and no side effects were reported on verapamil. Both groups needed lorazepam at similar doses.

Lenzi and colleagues conducted a trial of verapamil and chlorpromazine in patients with severe manic or mixed episodes (Lenzi, Marazziti, Raffaelli, & Cassano, 1995). Fifteen inpatient women with mixed or manic episodes were treated with verapamil from 240 mg daily to a maximum dose of 400 mg daily. Chlorpromazine from 50 to 400 mg was used as needed. The BPRS and CGI were used to measure outcomes. Statistically significant decreases in symptoms occurred from day 10 onward. Fourteen patients needed both verapamil and chlorpromazine, and the authors concluded that monotherapy with verapamil was ineffective in this population.

Another combination approach with the use of verapamil and magnesium was conducted by Giannini and colleagues (Giannini, Nakoneczie, Melemis, Ventresco, & Condon, 2000). Magnesium inhibits calcium activity through calmodulin and calcium channels and was thought to potentiate the antimanic effects of verapamil. Twenty men with bipolar disorder were on maintenance verapamil for 6 to 24 months. They were randomized to verapamil 320 mg daily plus placebo or verapamil plus 375 mg magnesium oxide. All the patients were on a low-magnesium diet (chocolate, freeze-dried coffee, and peanuts). They were followed for 120 days with BPRS scores. Patients who had been randomized to the placebo add-on did not demonstrate a decrease in the BPRS scores, while those on magnesium showed a significant decrease in their BPRS scores.

A case report of a patient on lithium, lisinopril, aspirin, and verapamil shows severe lithium toxicity and confusion (Chandragiri, Pasol, & Gallagher, 1998). The lithium dose had remained constant after lisinopril, verapamil, and aspirin were instituted after a stroke. The patient presented with an altered mental status and had a lithium level of 4.9 mEq/L and serum creatinine of 2.3 mg/dL. She was dialyzed, and lithium and verapamil were discontinued. Lithium in combination with verapamil has been reported to cause ataxia, dysarthria, tremor, and nausea (Dubovsky et al., 1987; Price & Giannini, 1986).

Wisner and colleagues describe the use of verapamil for women with bipolar disorder (Wisner et al., 2002). Thirty-seven women with bipolar disorder seen in a clinic were selected to use verapamil as their mood stabilizer; some of the patients were pregnant. The women were titrated up to a maximum dose of 480 mg daily. Scores for the HAM-D and MRS were used to evaluate response. Nine of 11 patients with mania or mixed state responded. The investigators concluded that verapamil was safe to use during pregnancy and lactation and may offer an alternative for the treatment of bipolar disorder in pregnant women.

Goodnick (1996) treated 12 patients who were manic with verapamil in doses up to 360 mg daily and followed the YMS scores, as well as the calcium and magnesium levels. Mean improvement in the YMRS score was

32%. Improvement in manic symptoms was predicted by increases in plasma calcium. Decreasing plasma magnesium did not predict resolution of manic symptoms or changes in calcium levels.

Nimodipine is a second-generation 1,4-dihydropyridine-derivative CCB with selective binding to vascular sites, increased lipophilic, and minimal inotropic effects (Langley & Sorkin, 1989). It is used to treat subarachnoid hemorrhage (SH; Barker & Ogilvy, 1996; Freedman & Waters, 1987). It is more lipid soluble than the other CCBs and has some antidopaminergic and anticonvulsant properties (de Falco, Bartiromo, Majello, DiGeronimo, & Mundo, 1992). Nimodipine has been shown to increase cerebrospinal fluid (CSF) levels of somatotropin release-inhibiting factor (SRIF; Pazzaglia, George, Post, Rubinow, & Davis, 1995). Multiple studies of nimodipine have been positive in the treatment of bipolar disorder, including treatment-resistant and rapid-cycling bipolar disorder.

An early case series of 6 female inpatients with bipolar disorder showed improvement on mania and brief psychiatric rating scales (Brunet et al., 1990). Patients were rapidly titrated up to 360 mg daily of nimodipine and had marked improvement in rating scale scores within 7 days.

Manna (1991) conducted another open trial in 12 patients with rapid-cycling bipolar disorder at 90 mg daily dose). Patients on lithium plus nimodipine had the best outcome compared with monotherapy on lithium or nimodipine. The authors also noted a decrease in the length and number of ill cycles.

The NIMH group studied 12 patients with treatment-resistant mood disorder using nimodipine 120 to 480 mg daily (Pazzaglia, Post, Ketter, George, & Marangell, 1993). Five of the 9 who completed the study responded to nimodipine. In patients who were followed over a longer period of time, two of the three rapid cyclers relapsed and responded to the addition of carbamazepine. While nimodipine blocks calcium influx into the cell through voltage-dependent channels, carbamazepine blocks calcium influx through a blockade of the N-methyl-D-aspartate (NMDA) receptors with effects on kinases and transcriptional regulation. The same authors had a second, larger case series of 30 patients who were treatment unresponsive to at least two conventional mood stabilizers (Pazzaglia et al., 1998). Ten patients showed moderate or marked improvement on CGI—Improvement (CGI-I) scales with nimodipine treatment. Substitution with verapamil led to recurrence of affective symptoms. In their earlier work on nimodipine, Pazzaglia and colleagues noted that nimodipine led to increases in CSF levels of SRIF in patients with mood disorders (Pazzaglia et al., 1995). CSF samples were collected from 14 affectively ill patients who were medication free (for at least 2 weeks) and then after nimodipine was administered up to 720 mg daily dose for a mean length of 26 days. Eleven of 14 patients had significant increases in CSF SRIF, which did not correlate with mood ratings or other mental or cognitive symptoms.

A case report series in 1995 by Goodnick examined a 53-year-old woman with rapid-cycling bipolar disorder who had failed trials of lithium, valproate, thyroid supplementation, and verapamil, all as monotherapies and in combination (Goodnick, 1995). She was hospitalized and washed out of all prior medications and started on nimodipine at 30 mg three times a day for 1 week, with mood shifts decreasing to one to two episodes daily. She was then titrated up to 60 mg three times a day by the end of the second week. Her mood improved dramatically, and her mood swings stopped. Her mood remained stable for 12 months of follow-up. The second patient in this case series was a 58-year-old man with a 37-year history of bipolar disorder. His illness course had deteriorated, and he was having four cycles per year with frequent hospitalizations. He had failed lithium in combination with carbamazepine and with antidepressants. He was hospitalized and washed out of all medications for 2 weeks. He was started on nimodipine as monotherapy, and his mood stabilized. He resumed his previous medications and discontinued nimodipine, with recurrence of depressive symptoms. He was hospitalized a second time and started on nimodipine 30 mg three times a day and titrated up to 60 mg three times a day with a tapering of his other psychotropic medications. He remained on nimodipine monotherapy with good symptom control at 5-month follow-up.

Grunze and colleagues did a case report of a patient on lithium and nimodipine (Grunze, Walden, Wolf, & Berger, 1996). The patient experienced good relief of symptoms on an unchanged dose of lithium and nimodipine up to 270 mg daily. After discharge, symptoms returned 2 months after discontinuation of nimodipine.

Yingling and colleagues report the use of nimodipine in the treatment of a pregnant patient with bipolar disorder (Yingling, Utter, Vengail, & Mason, 2002). She was being treated for hypothyroidism and hypertension with levothyroxine, methyldopa, and lithium carbonate. She developed nephrogenic diabetes insipidus on lithium, and a trial of carbamazepine failed. She was started on a nimodipine dose of 180 mg that was increased to 360 mg daily, with improvement in her bipolar symptoms and hypertension. Her mood remained stable through the pregnancy and delivery and at 1 year postpartum.

Nifedipine is a first-generation 1,4-dihydropyridine-derivative CCB. One open-label series studied 7 treatment-resistant patients with bipolar and schizoaffective disorder. They were being treated with neuroleptics, and nifedipine was added as augmentation up to 120 mg daily (De Beaurepaire, 1992). Five patients showed some response: 2 responded rapidly, and 3 improved more slowly. Withdrawal of the nifedipine led to relapse of symptoms.

Diltiazem is a benzothiazepine-type CCB. It acts on a different site on the L-type calcium channels than do verapamil and nimodipine (Silverstone & Grahame-Smith, 1992). One open study showed that diltiazem was effective in the short-term treatment of 6 patients with mania (Caillard, 1985).

Silverstone and Birkett (2000) conducted a longer term study in Canada of 8 female patients in an outpatient mood disorders clinic who had histories of treatment-resistant bipolar disorder. All patients were treated with long-acting diltiazem up to 240 mg daily in combination with mood stabilizers (lithium, carbamazepine, or sodium valproate), antipsychotics (moclobemide, chlorpromazine), thyroid hormone, clonazepam, and antidepressants (imipramine and paroxetine). They were followed over 6 months on the combination of diltiazem and other agents. They reported a decrease in both the frequency and severity of manic and depressive symptoms. Side effects were minimal; 2 patients had nausea and 1 had headaches.

A paucity of studies have been conducted in children with bipolar disorder and the use of CCBs. An adolescent was successfully treated for ultradian-cycling bipolar disorder with nimodipine by Davanzo, Krah, Kleiner, and McCracken (1999). This 13-year-old boy had failed trials of lithium, clonidine, fluoxetine, and levothyroxine. Trials of carbamazepine and divalproex sodium were also unsuccessful. He was started on nimodipine at 30 mg daily and titrated up to 180 mg daily. Concomitant medications included lithium, chlorpromazine, and levothyroxine. Lithium was then tapered and discontinued. He has remained stable on nimodipine for 3 years.

Protein Kinase C

Lithium and valproate both cause specific reductions in protein kinase C (PKC) alpha and epsilon isozymes (Manji, Etchenberrigaray, Chen, & Olds, 1993; Manji, Potter, & Lenox, 1995; Chen, Manji, Hawver, Wright, & Potter, 1994). PKC regulates neuronal excitability, neurotransmitter release, and long-term synaptic events (Nishizuka, 1992; Conn & Sweatt, 1994). Tamoxifen citrate is the only selective PKC inhibitor available for human use and is a synthetic nonsteroidal antiestrogen that is used for breast cancer. It acts through the estrogen receptor antagonism and the PKC inhibition. Tamoxifen crosses the blood–brain barrier. Patients on long-term tamoxifen have experienced mild to moderate depression (Cathcart et al., 1993). Bebchuk and colleagues conducted a trial of adults with DSM-IV mania and a YMRS score > 14 (Bebchuk et al., 2000). They were started on blinded tamoxifen 10 mg twice a day and titrated up to a maximum dose of 80 mg daily. For the 7 patients in the study, the mean decrease in the YMRS was 10.29, with 5 out of 7 patients having greater than a

50% reduction in the YMRS score. Only one patient had side effects of flushing at the maximum dose, and that patient was able to tolerate 60 mg daily.

Choline and Lecithin

Lithium affects several second-messenger systems, including the phosphatidylinositol-associated second-messenger system (Manji et al., 1995). Phosphatidylcholine is an important precursor for the second messenger diacylglycerol (Besterman, Duronio, & Cuatrecasa, 1986). Phosphatidylinositol and phosphatidylcholine affect different points in the same cell-signaling cascade. Use of both lithium and an agent that affects choline can target the cascade in two places, converting patients who are unresponsive or partially responsive to lithium into complete responders.

A second hypothesis, "adrenergic-cholinergic balance," postulates that mania arises from an excess of adrenergic activity and a low level of cholinergic activity. Because choline is converted into acetylcholine, the administration of choline may reduce manic symptoms by correcting the underactive levels of central choline (Janowsky, el-Yousef, Davis, & Sekerke, 1972).

Choline and its precursor lecithin (phosphatidylcholine) play a role in mood disorder. Cholinomimetic drugs, including pilocarpine, have been used to treat manic symptoms (Willoughby, 1889). Cholinergic antagonists, including scopolamine, can precipitate manic symptoms (Safer & Allen, 1971). Lithium is known to inhibit choline transport, and erythrocyte choline levels were elevated in some of the patients with bipolar disorder with manic episodes (Stoll, Cohen, Snyder, & Hanin, 1991). In their study of inpatients with bipolar disorder and controls, patients had higher erythrocyte choline concentrations than controls. Of the patients with bipolar disorder, a subgroup had extremely elevated choline levels, and they were less likely to be lithium responders, needed more neuroleptics, and had more severe illness at admission. Patients low in choline had a 4:1 ratio of manic to depressive episodes, while patients high in choline had equal numbers of depressive and manic episodes. A choline precursor, lecithin, has been effective in some patients with bipolar mania (Cohen, Lipinski, & Altesman, 1982; Schreier, 1982; Leiva, 1990). In the Schreier (1982) case report, lecithin was found to be helpful in an adolescent girl with mania. She had multiple episodes of mania, lasting several days to weeks, that were unresponsive to lithium and haloperidol. A trial of 15 grams of 90% pure lecithin, in combination with lithium, led to symptom remission. When a psychosocial stressor precipitated minor manic symptoms, increasing her lecithin to 23 grams led to a long-term stable mood. Cohen and colleagues reviewed the literature to determine whether lecithin might be helpful in treating bipolar disorder (Cohen et al., 1982). They treated 8 bipolar patients in the manic phase with 15 to 30 grams a day of lecithin. Four of the patients showed marked improvement. As this coadministration of a choline precursor and lithium proved moderately successful for some patients, researchers developed a "choline trapping" hypothesis (Stoll, Sachs, et al., 1996), postulating that coadministration of these two agents would be more effective than monotherapy with either lithium or the choline precursor alone. Stoll and colleagues decided to augment the choline levels in the brain by coadministering lithium and choline to treatment-refractory patients with rapid-cycling bipolar disorder (Stoll, Sachs et al., 1996). Six patients with rapid-cycling bipolar disorder were maintained on lithium and other medications. Choline bitartrate capsules were added, starting at 2–4 grams of free choline daily and increasing to 3–8 grams as maintenance. Five of 6 patients had two or more proton magnetic resonance spectroscopy (H-MRS) scans that showed an increase in brain choline signal (choline trapping). Five of the six patients experienced clinically significant antimanic response to combination lithium and choline therapy. Effects on mania were more pronounced and rapid than effects on depressive symptoms.

OTHER MEDICATIONS FOR THE TREATMENT OF BIPOLAR DISORDER

Donepezil is a reversible acetylcholinesterase inhibitor (AChE) that is used primarily in the treatment of Alzheimer-type mild to moderate dementia. It binds selectively to the central AChEs rather than the (BuChE), which cause more peripheral side effects such as nausea, diarrhea, and lassitude (Burt, Sachs, & Demopulos, 1999). It has been thought to increase depressive symptoms and have antimanic properties. Burt and colleagues (1999) conducted a prospective open-label study on 11 patients with treatment-resistant affective disorder in which donepezil was added to current medication regimens. Four patients had mania; 5, mixed moods; 1, hypomania; and 1, depression. Patients were resistant to or intolerant of at least two other mood-stabilizing medications. Patients remained on lithium or other mood stabilizers, and donepezil was added. Patients were started on 5 mg/day for 4 weeks and then increased to 10 mg/day of donepezil. Six of the 11 patients responded; 54.5% were markedly improved by 6 weeks. Three other patients did not respond, even at a dose of 10 mg. Five patients had side effects, including nausea, insomnia, diarrhea, and mild sedation. One patient ended the study due to nausea and diarrhea.

Mexiletine is a medication with antiarrhythmic, anticonvulsant, and analgesic properties. Schaffer and colleagues conducted a trial on 20 patients with rapid-cycling bipolar disorder who had failed trials of lithium, valproic acid, and carbamazepine (Schaffer, Levitt, & Joffe, 2000). They were dosed from 200 to 1,200 mg daily and monitored for response with mood rating scales. Fifty-three percent of the patients had a full or partial response to mexiletine. Postulated mechanisms include gamma-aminobutyric acid (GABA), blockade of fast sodium channels, prevention of sodium leakage and calcium overload, and activation of delta$_1$-opioid receptors.

CONCLUSIONS

For many patients with bipolar disorder, therapy and successful mood stabilization requires treatment beyond monotherapy with a classic mood stabilizer. As patients have rapid-cycling symptoms or cannot tolerate one of the conventional agents, clinicians must turn to other options. Thyroid augmentation has the best evidence for both a role in causation of rapid-cycling bipolar disorder and as an effective treatment for these patients, especially when given in combination with another mood stabilizer. CCBs have mixed evidence for efficacy in bipolar disorder, although nimodipine has more positive evidence than the other agents in that group. Other agents that have been shown to be helpful in case reports and small open-label trials include tamoxifen, lecithin, choline, donepezil, and mexiletine. These agents should be used with caution and after more conventional mood stabilizers have been unsuccessful in patients.

REFERENCES

Alarcon, R., & Franceschini, J. (1984). Hyperparathyroidism and paranoid psychosis: Case report and review of the literature. *British Journal of Psychiatry, 145*, 477–486.

Barker, F. N., & Ogilvy, C. (1996). Efficacy of prophylactic nimodipine for delayed ischemic deficit after subarachnoid hemorrhage: A meta-analysis. *Journal of Neurosurgery, 84*, 405–414.

Bauer, M., Baur, H., Berghofer, A., Strohle, A., Hellweg, R., Muller-Oerlinghausen, B., et al. (2002). Effects of supraphysiological thyroxine administration in healthy controls and patients with depressive disorders. *Journal of Affective Disorders, 68*, 285–294.

Bauer, M., Hellweg, R., Graf, K., & Baumgartner, A. (1998). Treatment of refractory depression with high dose thyroxine. *Neuropsychopharmacology, 18*, 444–455.

Bauer, M., London, E. D., Rasgon, N., Berman, S. M., Frye, M. S., Altshuler, L. L., et al. (2005, May). Supraphysiological doses of levothyroxine alter regional cerebral metabolism and improve mood in bipolar depression. *Molecular Psychiatry, 10*(5), 456–469.

Bauer, M., & Whybrow, P. (1990). Rapid cycling bipolar affective disorder: II. Treatment of refractory rapid cycling with high-dose thyroxine: A preliminary study. *Archives of General Psychiatry, 47*, 435–440.

Baumgartner, A., Bauer, M., & Hellweg, R. (1994). Treatment of intractable nonrapid cycling bipolar affective disorder with high-dose thyroxine: An open clinical trial. *Neuropsychopharmacology, 10*, 183–189.

Bebchuk, J., Arfken, C., Dolan-Manjis, S., Murph, J., Hasanat, K., Manji, H. K. (2000). A preliminary investigation of a protein kinase C inhibitor in the treatment of acute mania. *Archives of General Psychiatry, 57,* 95–97.

Besterman, J., Duronio, V., & Cuatrecasa, P. (1986). Rapid formation of diacylglycerol from phosphatidylcholine: A pathway for generation of a second messenger. *Proceedings of the National Academy of Sciences of the USA, 83,* 6785–6789.

Birrell, G., & Cheetham, T. (2004). Juvenile thyrotoxicosis: Can we do better? *Archives of Diseases in Children, 89,* 745–750.

Brunet, G., Gerlich, B., Robert, P., Dumas, S., Souetre, E., & Darcourt, G. (1990). Open trial of calcium antagonist nimodipine in acute mania. *Clinical Neuropharmacology, 13,* 224–228.

Burt, T., Sachs, G., & Demopulos, C. (1999). Donepezil in treatment-resistant bipolar disorder. *Biological Psychiatry, 45,* 959–964.

Caillard, V. (1985). Treatment of mania using a calcium antagonist: Preliminary trial. *Neuropsychobiology, 14,* 23–26.

Cathcart, C., Jones, S., Pumroy, C. S., Peters, G. N., Knox, S. M., & Cheek, J. H. (1993). Clinical recognition and management of depression in node negative breast cancer patients treated with tamoxifen. *Breast Cancer Research and Treatment, 27,* 277–281.

Chandragiri, S. S., Pasol, E., & Gallagher, R. M. (1998). Lithium, ACE inhibitors, NSAIDs, and verapamil. *Psychosomatics, 39*(3), 281–282.

Chen, G., Manji, H., Hawver, D. B., Wright, C. B., & Potter, W. Z. (1994). Chronic sodium valproate selectively decreases protein kinase C α and ε in vitro. *Journal of Neurochemistry, 63,* 2361–2364.

Cohen, B., Lipinski, J., & Altesman, R. I. (1982). Lecithin in the treatment of mania: Double-blind placebo-controlled trials. *American Journal of Psychiatry, 139,* 1162–1164.

Cole, D., Thase, M., Mallinger, A. G., Soares, J. C., Luther, J. F., Kupfer, D. J., et al. (2002). Slower treatment response in bipolar depression predicted by lower pretreatment thyroid function. *American Journal of Psychiatry, 159,* 116–121.

Conn, P., & Sweatt, J. (1994). *Protein kinase C in the nervous system.* New York: Oxford University Press.

Cowdry, R., Wehr, T., Zis, A. P., & Goodwin, F. K. (1983). Thyroid abnormalities associated with rapid-cycling bipolar illness. *Archives of General Psychiatry, 40*(4), 414–420.

Davanzo, P. A., Krah, N., Kleiner, J., & McCracken, J. (1999). Nimodipine treatment of an adolescent with ultradian cycling bipolar affective illness. *Journal of Child and Adolescent Psychopharmacology, 9*(1), 51–61.

De Beaurepaire, R. (1992). Treatment of neuroleptic-resistant mania and schizoaffective disorders. *American Journal of Psychiatry, 149,* 1614–1615.

de Falco, F., Bartiromo, U., Majello, L., DiGeronimo, G., & Mundo, P. (1992). Calcium antagonist nimodipine in intractable epilepsy. *Epilepsia, 33,* 343–345.

Denicoff, K., Smith-Jackson, E., Bryan, A. L., Ali, S. O., & Post, R. M. (1997). Valproate prophylaxis in a prospective clinical trial of refractory bipolar disorder. *American Journal of Psychiatry, 154,* 1456–1458.

Denko, I., & Kaelbling, R. (1962). The psychiatric aspects of hypoparathyroidism: Review of the literature and case report. *Acta Psychiatria Scandanavica, 164*(Suppl.), 5–38.

Dubovsky, S. (1993). Calcium antagonists in manic depressive illness. *Neuropsychobiology, 27,* 184–192.

Dubovsky, S. (1995). Electroconvulsive therapy. In H. I. Kaplan & B. J. Sadock (Eds.), *Comprehensive textbook of psychiatry* (6th ed., pp. 2129–2140). Baltimore: Williams & Wilkins.

Dubovsky, S. (1998). *Calcium channel antagonists as novel agents for the treatment of bipolar disorder.* Washington, DC: American Psychiatric Press.

Dubovsky, S., Franks, R., & Allen, S. (1987). Verapamil: A new antimanic drug with potential interactions with lithium. *Journal of Clinical Psychiatry, 48,* 371–372.

Dubovsky, S., Murphy, J., Thomas, M., & Rademacher, J. (1992). Abnormal intracellular calcium ion concentration in platelets and lymphocytes of bipolar patients. *American Journal of Psychiatry, 149*, 118–120.

Engel, G., & Margolin, S. (1975). Neuropsychiatric disturbances in Addison's disease and the role of impaired carbohydrate metabolism in the production of abnormal cerebral function. *Archives of Neurology and Psychiatry, 45*, 881–884.

Findling, R., McNamara, N., Gracious, B. L., Youngstrom, E. A., Stransbrey, R. J., Reed, M. D., et al. (2003). Combination lithium and divalproex sodium in pediatric bipolarity. *Journal of the American Academy of Child and Adolescent Psychiatry, 42*(8), 895–901.

Freedman, D., & Waters, D. (1987). Second generation dihydropyridine calcium antagonists. Greater vascular selectivity and some unique applications. *Drugs, 34*, 578–598.

Frye, M., Denicoff, K., Bryan, A. L., Smith-Jackson, E. E., Ali, S. O., Luckenbaugh, D., et al. (1999). Association between lower serum free T4 and greater mood instability and depression in lithium-maintained bipolar patients. *American Journal of Psychiatry, 156*, 1909–1914.

Gadde, K., & Calabrese, J. (1990). Diltiazem effect of carbamazepine levels in manic depression. *Journal of Clinical Psychopharmacology, 10*, 378–379.

Garza-Trevino, E., Overall, J., & Hollister, L. (1992). Verapamil versus lithium in acute mania. *American Journal of Psychiatry, 149*, 121–122.

Geffken, G., Ward, H., Staab, J., Carmichael, S., & Evan, D. (1998). Psychiatric morbidity in endocrine disorders. *Psychiatric Clinics of North America, 21*(2), 473–489.

Geller, B., & Luby, J. (1997). Child and adolescent bipolar disorder: A review of the past 10 years. *Journal of the American Academy of Child and Adolescent Psychiatry, 36*(9), 1168–1176.

Geller, B., Sun, K., Zimerman, B., Luby, J., Frazier, J., & Williams, M. (1995). Complex and rapid cycling in bipolar children and adolescents: A preliminary study. *Journal of Affective Disorders, 34*, 259–268.

Giannini, A., Houser, W. J., Loiselle, R., Giannini, M., & Price, W. (1984). Antimanic effects of verapamil. *American Journal of Psychiatry, 141*, 1602–1603.

Giannini, A., Nakoneczie, A., Melemis, A., Ventresco, J., & Condon, M. (2000). Magnesium oxide augmentation of verapamil maintenance therapy in mania. *Psychiatry Research, 93*, 83–87.

Gitlin, M., Cochran, S., & Jamison, R. (1989). Maintenance lithium treatment: Side effects and compliance. *Journal of Clinical Psychiatry, 50*, 127–131.

Gjessing, L. (1938). Disturbances of somatic function in catatonia with a periodic course and their compensation. *Journal of Mental Science, 84*, 608–621.

Goodnick, P. (1995). Nimodipine treatment of rapid cycling bipolar disorder. *Journal of Clinical Psychiatry, 56*(7), 330.

Goodnick, P. (1996). Treatment of mania: Relationship between response to verapamil and changes in plasma calcium and magnesium levels. *Southern Medical Journal, 89*(2), 225–226.

Grunze, H., Walden, J., Wolf, R., & Berger, M. (1996). Combined treatment with lithium and nimodipine in a bipolar I manic syndrome. *Progress in Neuro-Psychopharmacology and Biological Psychiatry, 20*, 419–426.

Gyulai, L., Bauer, M., Garcia-Espana, F., Cnaan, A., Whybrow, P. C., & Bauer, M. S. (2003). Thyroid hypofunction in patients with rapid-cycling bipolar disorder after lithium challenge. *Biological Psychiatry, 53*, 899–905.

Gyulai, L., Bauer, M., Garcia-Espana, F., Hierholzer, J., Baumgartner, A., Berghofer, A., et al. (2001). Bone mineral density in pre-and postmenopausal women with affective disorder treated with long-term L-thyroxine augmentation. *Journal of Affective Disorders, 66*, 185–191.

Hall, R., & Stickney, S. (1986). Endocrine disease and behavior. *Integrative Psychiatry, 4*, 122–135.

Hasket, R. (1985). Diagnostic categorization of psychiatric disturbance in Cushing's syndrome. *American Journal of Psychiatry, 142*, 911–916.

Hasket, R., & Rose, R. (1981). Neuroendocrine disorders and psychopathology. *Psychiatric Clinics of North America, 4*, 239–252.

Hollister, L., & Garza-Trevino, E. (1999). Calcium channel blockers in psychiatric disorders: A review of the literature. *Canadian Journal of Psychiatry, 44*, 658–664.

Hollowell, J. G., Staehling, N., Flanders, W., Hannon, W., Gunter, E., Spencer, C., et al. (2002). Serum TSH, T₄,and thyroid antibodies in the United States population (1988 to 1994): National Health and Nutrition Examination Survey (NHANES III). *Journal of Clinical Endocrinology and Metabolism, 87*(2), 489–499.

Hoschl, C., & Kozeny, J. (1989). Verapamil in affective disorders: A controlled double-blind study. *Biological Psychiatry, 25*, 128–140.

Janicak, P. G., Sharma, R. P., Panday, G., & Davis, J. (1998). Verapamil for the treatment of acute mania: A double-blind, placebo-controlled trial. *American Journal of Psychiatry, 155*(7), 972–973.

Janowsky, D., el-Yousef, M., Davis, J., & Sekerke, H. (1972). A cholinergic-adrenergic hypothesis in mania and depression. *Lancet, 2*, 632–635.

Jespersen, C., Hansen, J., & Mortensen, L. (1994). The prognostic significance of post-infarction angina pectoris and the effect of verapamil on the incidence of angina pectoris and prognosis. *European Heart Journal, 15*, 270–276.

Joffe, R. T., Singer, W., Levitt, A., & MacDonald, C. (1993). A placebo-controlled comparison of lithium and triiodothyronine augmentation of tricyclic antidepressants in unipolar refractory depression. *Archives of General Psychiatry, 50*(5), 387–393.

Kelly, W., Kelly, M., & Faragher, B. (1996). A prospective study of psychiatric and psychological aspects of Cushing's disease. *Clinical Endocrinology, 45*, 715–720.

Kowatch, R., Sethuraman, G., Home, J., Kromelis, M., & Weinberg, W. (2003). Combination pharmacotherapy in children and adolescents with bipolar disorder. *Biological Psychiatry, 53*(11), 978–984.

Kowatch, R., Suppes, T., Carmody, T., Bucci, J., Home, J., Kromelis, M., et al. (2000). Effect size of lithium, divalproex sodium, and carbamazepine in children and adolescents with bipolar disorder. *Journal of the American Academy of Child and Adolescent Psychiatry, 39*(6), 713–720.

Ladenson, P. W., Singer, P. A., Bagchi, N., Bigos, S., Levy, E., Smith, S., et al. (2000). American Thyroid Association guidelines for detection of thyroid dysfunction. *Archives of Internal Medicine, 160*(11), 1573–1575.

Langley, M., & Sorkin, E. (1989). Nimodipine: A review of its pharmacodynamic and pharmacokinetic properties and therapeutic potential in cerebrovascular disease. *Drugs, 37*, 669–699.

Lazar, L., Kalter-Leibovici, O., Pertzelan, A., Weintrob, N., Josefsberg, Z., & Phillip, M. (2000). Thyrotoxicosis in prepubertal children compared with pubertal and postpubertal patients. *Journal of Clinical Endocrinology and Metabolism, 85*, 3678–3682.

Leigh, H., & Kramer, S. (1984). The psychiatric manifestations of endocrine disorders. *Advances in Internal Medicine, 29*, 413–445.

Leiva, D. (1990). The neurochemistry of mania: A hypothesis of etiology and a rationale for treatment. *Progress in Neuro-Psychopharmacology and Biological Psychiatry, 14*, 423–429.

Lenox, R., & Manji, H. (1998). *Lithium*. Washington, DC: American Psychiatric Press.

Lenzi, A., Marazziti, S., Raffaelli, S., & Cassano, G. (1995). Effectiveness of the combination verapamil and chlorpromazine in the treatment of severe manic or mixed patients. *Progress in Neuro-Psychopharmacology and Biological Psychiatry, 19*, 519–528.

MacPhee, G., McInnes, G., Thompson, G., & Brodie, M. (1986). Verapamil potentiates carbamazepine neurotoxicity: A clinically important inhibitory interaction. *Lancet, 29*, 700–703.

Manji, H., Etchenberrigaray, R., Chen, G., & Olds, J. (1993). Lithium decreases membrane-associated protein kinase C in hippocampus: Selectivity for the a isozyme. *Journal of Neurochemistry, 61*, 2303–2310.

Manji, H., Potter, W., & Lenox, R. (1995). Signal transduction pathways: Molecular targets for lithium's actions. *Archives of General Psychiatry, 52*, 531–543.

Manna, V. (1991). Bipolar affective disorders and role of intraneuronal calcium: Therapeutic effects of the treatment with lithium salts and/or calcium antagonist in patients with rapid polar inversion [in Italian]. *Minerva Medicina, 82*(11), 757–763.

Meyer, F., Cascino, G., Whisnant, J., Sharbrough, F., Invik, R., Gorman, D., et al. (1995). Nimodipine as an add-on therapy for intractable epilepsy. *Mayo Clinic Proceedings, 70*, 623–627.

Nishizuka, Y. (1992). Intracellular signaling by hydrolysis of phospholipids and activation of protein kinase C. *Science, 258*, 607–614.

Oomen, H., Schipperijin, A., & Drexhage, H. (1996). The prevalence of affective disorder and in particular of rapid cycling bipolar disorder in patients with abnormal thyroid function tests. *Endocrinology, 45*, 215–223.

Pahor, M., Guralnik, J., Ferrucci, L., Corti, M., Salive, M., Cerhan, J., et al. (1996). Calcium-channel blockade and incidence of cancer in aged populations. *Lancet, 348*, 493–498.

Pazzaglia, P., George, M., Post, R., Rubinow, D., & Davis, C. (1995). Nimodipine increases CSF somatostatin in affectively ill patients. *Neuropsychopharmacology, 13*, 75–83.

Pazzaglia, P. J., Post, R. M., Ketter, T., Callahan, A., Marangell, L., Frye, M., et al. (1998). Nimodipine monotherapy and carbamazepine augmentation in patients with refractory recurrent affective illness. *Journal of Clinical Psychiatry, 18*(5), 404–413.

Pazzaglia, P., Post, R., Ketter, T., George, M., & Marangell, L. (1993). Preliminary controlled trial of nimodipine in ultra-rapid cycling affective dysregulation. *Psychiatry Research, 49*, 257–272.

Post, R. M., Frye, M. A., Denicoff, K., Leverich, G., Dunn, R., Osuch, E., et al. (2000). Emerging trends in the treatment of rapid cycling bipolar disorder: A selected review. *Bipolar Disorders, 2*, 305–315.

Price, W., & Giannini, A. (1986). Neurotoxicity caused by lithium-verapamil synergism. *Journal of Clinical Pharmacology, 26*, 717–719.

Prien, R., & Gelenberg, A. (1989). Alternatives to lithium for preventive treatment of bipolar disorder. *American Journal of Psychiatry, 146*, 840–848.

Prohaska, M., Stern, R. A., Mason, G. A., Nevels, C. T., & Prange, A. J., Jr. (1995). Thyroid hormone and lithium-related neuropsychological deficits: A preliminary test of the lithium-thyroid interactive hypothesis. *Journal of the International Neuropsychological Society, 1*, 134.

Ramasubbu, R. (2003). Thyroid hormone treatment for lithium-induced thyroid dysfunction in mood disorder. *Reviews in Psychiatry and Neuroscience, 28*(2), 134.

Sachs, G. (1989). Adjuncts and alternatives to lithium therapy for bipolar affective disorder. *Journal of Clinical Psychiatry, 50*(12, Suppl.), 31–39.

Safer, D., & Allen, R. (1971). The central effects of scopolamine in man. *Biological Psychiatry, 3*, 347–355.

Schaffer, A., Levitt, A., & Joffe, R. (2000). Mexitiline in treatment-resistant bipolar disorder. *Journal of Affective Disorders, 57*, 249–253.

Schreier, H. (1982). Mania responsive to lecithin in a 13-year-old girl. *American Journal of Psychiatry, 139*, 108–110.

Silverstone, P., & Birkett, L. (2000). Diltiazem as augmentation therapy in patients with treatment-resistant bipolar disorder: A retrospective study. *Journal of Psychiatry and Neuroscience, 25*(3), 276–280.

Silverstone, P., & Grahame-Smith, D. (1992). A review of the relationship between calcium channels and psychiatric disorders. *Journal of Psychopharmacology*, 6, 462–482.

Sokolov, S. T. H., Kutcher, S. P., & Joffe, R. T. (1994). Basal thyroid indices in adolescent depression and bipolar disorder. *Journal of the American Academy of Child and Adolescent Psychiatry*, 33(4), 469–475.

Sonino, N., Fava, G., Belluardo, P., Girelli, M., & Boscaro, M. (1993). Course of depression in Cushing's syndrome: Response to treatment and comparison with Graves' disease. *Hormone Research*, 39, 202–206.

Stanley, R. (1997). The calcium channel and the organization of the presynaptic transmitter release face. *Trends in Neuroscience*, 20, 404–409.

Stern, R., Legendre, S., Thorner, A., Solomon, D., Tremont, G., Arruda, M., et al. (2000). Exogenous thyroid hormone diminishes the amnestic side effects of electroconvulsive therapy. *Journal of the International Neuropsychological Society*, 6, 235.

Stern, R., Nevels, C., Shelhorse, M., Prohaska, M., Mason, G., & Prange, A. (1991). Antidepressant and memory effects of combined thyroid hormone treatment and electroconvulsive therapy: Preliminary findings. *Biological Psychiatry*, 30, 623–627.

Stoll, A., Cohen, B., Snyder, M., & Hanin, I. (1991). Erythrocyte choline concentrations in psychiatric disorders. *Biological Psychiatry*, 29, 309–321.

Stoll, A., Sachs, G., Cohen, B., Lafer, B., Christensen, J., & Renshaw, P. (1996). Choline in the treatment of rapid-cycling bipolar disorder: Clinical and neurochemical findings in lithium-treated patients. *Biological Psychiatry*, 40, 382–388.

Strober, M., Morrell, W., Burroughs, J., Lampert, C., Danforth, H., & Freeman, R. (1988). A family study of bipolar I disorder in adolescence: Early onset of symptoms linked to familial loading and lithium resistance. *Journal of Affective Disorders*, 15, 255–268.

Tremont, G., & Stern, R. A. (2000). Minimizing the cognitive effects of lithium therapy and electroconvulsive therapy using thyroid hormone. *International Journal of Neuropsychopharmacology*, 3, 175–186.

Triggle, D. (1992). *Biochemical and pharmacologic difference among calcium channel antagonists: Clinical implications*. Philadelphia: Hanley & Belfus.

Walton, S., Berk, M., & Brook, S. (1996). Superiority of lithium over verapamil in mania: A randomized, controlled, single-blind trial. *Journal of Clinical Psychiatry*, 57(11), 543–546.

Weeston, T. F., & Constantino, J. (1996). High-dose T4 for rapid-cycling bipolar disorder. *American Academy of Child and Adolescent Psychiatry*, 35(2), 131–132.

West, S. A., Sax, K. W., Stanton, S. P., Keck, P. E., McElroy, S. L., & Strakowski, S. M. (1996). Differences in thyroid function studies in acutely manic adolescents with and without attention deficit hyperactivity disorder (ADHD). *Psychopharmacology Bulletin*, 32(1), 63–66.

Willoughby, E. (1889). Pilocarpine in threatening mania. *Lancet*, 1, 1030.

Wisner, K., Peindl, K., Perel, J. M., Hanusa, B. H., Piontek, C. M., & Baab, S. (2002). Verapamil treatment of women with bipolar disorder. *Biological Psychiatry*, 51, 745–752.

Wright, B., & Jarrett, D. (1991). Lithium and calcium channel blockers: Possible neurotoxicity. *Biological Psychiatry*, 30, 635–636.

Yingling, D. R., Utter, G., Vengail, S., & Mason, B. (2002). Calcium channel blocker, nimodipine, for the treatment of bipolar disorder during pregnancy. *American Journal of Obstetrics and Gynecology*, 187(2), 1711–1712.

Zarate, C., Tohen, M., & Zarate, S. B. (1997). Thyroid function tests in first-episode bipolar disorder manic and mixed types. *Biological Psychiatry*, 42, 302–304.

CHAPTER 8

Nonpharmacological Biological Treatment for Pediatric Bipolar Disorder

Omega-3 Fatty Acids and Complementary and Alternative Medicine

RUSSELL E. SCHEFFER

Patients, and particularly parents of patients, are frequently interested in the use of complementary and alternative medicine (CAM) therapies. This is often because they view these "natural" therapies as less potentially harmful than standard Western medicine. There are difficulties with this perception. Just because a therapy is derived from nature does not mean that it is without adverse events. Cyanide is a naturally occurring chemical that is deadly. Vitamin supplementation can also be harmful (hypervitaminosis A). Products derived from natural products hold great promise for treating a variety of illnesses, but these potential treatments must be scrutinized by rigorous scientific methods.

The use of CAM in psychiatry appears to be growing. In a recently published study regarding the use of acupuncture for adults with bipolar disorder, the majority of the patients had used nonpharmacological treatments (Dennehy, Webb, & Suppes, 2002). This is true despite a paucity of data supporting the safety (or efficacy) of these treatments.

Another concern is that there are almost no empirical data regarding the use of these treatments. Standard medicinal therapies in pediatric psychiatry often have little evidence to support their use in children. The use of CAM suffers from an even greater lack of evidence and quality control. The contents of what one purchases from a health food store is not overseen by the Food and Drug Administration (FDA), and quantities of "active" ingredients may vary greatly.

The desire of parents and patients to obtain treatments without adverse events often leads to quackery. Many unscrupulous providers will charge exorbitant fees to provide treatments that are without documented benefits. Patients often endure great expense and suffer poor clinical outcomes as a result of these questionable practices. The flight to CAM by patients does result in questions regarding patient satisfaction with traditional Western medicine. Some CAM therapies have an explainable biological basis and may ultimately be proven to be clinically important. To date, there are no positive well-designed controlled trials of CAM for pediatric bipolar disorder.

Alternative medicine systems include homeopathic, naturopathic, traditional Chinese, and Ayurvedic medicine. Homeopathic treatments typically include giving small doses of potentially biologically active treatments. This is done in the hope that the subtle "bumps" will restore the body's natural state of homeostasis. Naturopathic treatments include biologically based (herbs and diet), manipulative (chiropractic manipulation, massage, and acupuncture) and energy (biofeedback and magnetic) therapies. In addition, there are a variety of mind–body interventions that include prayer, meditation, mental healing, and energy and creative therapies (art, music, and recreation).

A variety of nonpharmacological treatments are used for bipolar disorder. Some of these treatments possess face validity in that their use attempts to decrease stress and improve biological rhythms. These include regular exercise, avoidance of caffeine, light therapy, meditation, relaxation, and visual imagery. Other interventions that are unlikely to cause harm and that are commonly used include prayer, individual and group psychotherapies, and other therapies (art, music, crystal, aroma, and energy). Other commonly used nonpharmacological interventions can be harmful. These include: alcohol, recreational drugs, and misuse of prescription medications. However, one could argue that ineffective treatments actually cause harm just by being ineffective and by prolonging an affective episode.

Some evidence exists that CAM may be beneficial for conditions that are frequently concurrent with bipolar disorder. This remains a particularly promising area, as many of the traditional treatments for these conditions are liable to exacerbate mania, for example, selective serotonin reuptake inhibitors (SSRIs) for depression.

THE CASE FOR OMEGA-3 FATTY ACIDS

Essential long-chain polyunsaturated fatty acids (EPUFAs) are of great importance in development and brain function. These polyunsaturated fatty acids are considered essential because humans cannot modify fatty acids of less than 18 carbon backbones to longer fatty acids nor desaturate bonds closer to the noncarboxyl "tail" than omega 9. These fatty acids are named according to a variety of conventions. One convention is the dichotomous distribution into omega-3 and omega-6 fatty acids. This naming occurs because it is the site of the first carbon–carbon double-bound in the chain. The role of omega-3 fatty acids in biology is complex. The fatty-acid composition of membranes plays a large role in the determination of the tertiary and quaternary folding structure of proteins. This can have a dramatic impact on cell function. A genetically normal receptor can fail to function properly because of these conformational changes. A strong case can be made that a relative deficiency of membrane omega-3 fatty-acids abnormalities are associated with a variety of psychiatric illnesses. Whether these associations are causative, spurious, or epiphenomena is not determined.

Membrane omega-3 fatty acids in the central nervous system (CNS) and periphery have been shown to be deficient in patients with bipolar disorder and schizophrenia (Chiu et al., 2003). In addition, an increase in membrane lipid peroxidation products (a marker of fatty-acid damage) has been demonstrated *in vivo* by spectroscopy (Yao, Stanley, Reddy, Keshavan, & Pettegrew, 2002). Ethane, one of the oxidation products of EPUFAs, was reported to be elevated in the breath of children with attention-deficit/hyperactivity disorder (ADHD; Ross, McKenzie, Glen, & Bennett, 2003).

Although oxidative stress and most of the possible causes of fatty-acid depletion can occur throughout the body, the brain is particularly vulnerable (Ranjekar et al., 2003). This vulnerability is due to three main processes. First, the brain contains a high concentration of polyunsaturated fatty acids, proteins, and DNA. These serve as ready substrate for damage due to oxidative stress. There is little intrinsic ability to repair senescent neurons. Second, therefore, neurons are more vulnerable to free radical damage than many other cell types. Third, high oxygen consumption, leading to high concentration of oxygen free radicals, is a hallmark of the brain. Conservatively, the brain uses 20% of the total body consumption of oxygen.

Why would omega-3 fatty acids be low in patients with bipolar disorder? Decreased dietary intake is one possibility. The distribution of omega-3 to omega-6 fatty acids in traditional hunting and gathering diets was 1:1. Currently the ratio is frequently 1:100 or greater. Low dietary consumption of seafood, which is high in omega-3 fatty acids, is correlated with higher rates of bipolar disorder (Noaghiul & Hibbeln, 2003). This reflects a significant change in diet away from one rich in vegetables and fruit to one high in polyunsaturated fatty acids. Refrigeration and food preservation may account for much of this change. Children are particularly vulnerable to these dietary influences. Less than 10% of adult Americans obtain enough omega-3 fatty acids in their diet. No one questions that the percentage is worse in children.

Decreased absorption from the gastrointestinal system into the bloodstream is another potential cause of decreased omega-3 fatty acids. There are a number of passive and active absorption mechanisms. Fatty acids predominantly are brought into the bloodstream via transporters. It is possible that genetic problems or environment can have a large impact on absorption. Further, there are specific enzymes that incorporate fatty acids into membranes. If there is either deficiency of substrate or an enzyme abnormality, not enough of that particular fatty acid will be incorporated.

Damage to fatty acids can also lead to deficiencies; for example, oxidative stress could result from increased oxygen turnover of nonspecific stress or catecholamine turnover related to severe mental illnesses (Mahadik, Mukherjee, Scheffer, Correnti, & Mahadik, 1998; Khan et al., 2002). Cigarettes, which have a dopamine effect downstream, are also known to cause lipid damage. There are intrinsic and extrinsic antioxidant defense systems that effect the membrane status of omega-3 fatty acids (Mahadik & Scheffer, 1996). The intrinsic system consists of the enzymes superoxide dismutase (SOD), catalase (CAT), glutathione peroxidase (GPx), uric acid, and other components. The extrinsic system includes dietary sources such as vitamins E and C and beta-carotene. Foods that are rich in these antioxidants are often also rich in omega-3 fatty acids.

Increased fatty-acid turnover in membranes could also be responsible. Phospholipase A_2 exists at the membrane and in the cytosol. This enzyme is in part responsible for the turnover that usually assists in removing damaged fatty acids. This enzyme has been reported in higher than normal amounts in patients with schizophrenia. It has been implicated in a variety of psychiatric disorders (Bennett & Horrobin, 2000).

Genetics may play a role, for example, phospholipase A_2 and other incorporation-related enzymes could be genetically abnormal. Another genetic anomaly could be in the elongase and desaturase enzymes that alternatively add a carbon, then form a double bond, and then repeat the process to form longer biologically active fatty acids, such as arachadonic acid (AA) and docosahexanoic acid (DHA). Figure 8.1 delineates the primary means by which longer essential fatty acids are converted. Recently a genetic association was reported between ADHD and the enzyme fatty acid desaturase 1 (FASD1). This finding suggests that psychopathology may be in part explained by some individuals' inability to efficiently make longer essential fatty acids from shorter ones (Brookes, Chen, Xu, Taylor, & Asherson, 2006).

AA and DHA serve as second messengers in signal transduction. When

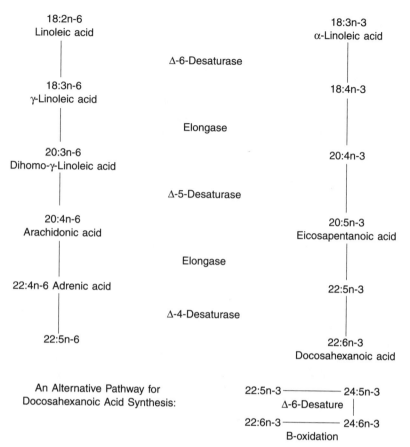

FIGURE 8.1. Metabolic pathways of essential fatty acids.

receptors are stimulated, they change their form and, in a variety of different ways, release second messengers. If these second messengers (AA and DHA) are not available for any of the preceding reasons, a signal may not be generated at the membrane level, and the nucleus will not receive a signal.

Brain development is dependent on omega-3 and omega-6 fatty acids. DHA is highly concentrated in the normal mammalian brain. There are only two conditions in which the mammalian brain readily releases DHA. These are during gestation and lactation. The mother's brain will "donate" DHA to the fetus if it is not obtained in sufficient dietary quantities. This may have implications for both the mother (significant depletion) and the fetus, if there is not enough DHA available to transfer for normal brain development. This donation appears to depend on interpersonal signaling factors. During normal lactation, bovine mothers secrete significant amounts of DHA to calves. However, when they are mechanically milked, their milk does not contain substantial amounts of DHA. Michael Crawford has written on the hazards of DHA deficiencies in earlier milk formulas (Cunnane, Francescutti, Brenna, & Crawford, 2000). Breast feeding in humans is associated with a 20-point IQ advantage when compared with formula feeding. This may in part be related to DHA transfer. Theoretically, if a child is born with low levels of EPUFAs, a failure of normal development may have already occurred. It is uncertain whether later supplementation would correct these abnormalities. In addition, a child with low levels of these fatty acids might be more susceptible to psychiatric (brain) illnesses.

The role of antioxidants in fatty-acid utilization (protection) has been underplayed in intervention studies. It has been demonstrated that adding polyunsaturated fatty acids to a free-radical-rich environment can exacerbate lipid peroxidation (Song & Miyazawa, 2001; Vericel, Polette, Bacot, Calzada, & Lagarde, 2003). Thus supplementation with EPUFAs could worsen a pathological condition. To date, the majority of clinical intervention trials with EPUFAs in psychiatric illnesses have not included antioxidants. Thus may explain some of the discrepant results. At a minimum, lipid peroxidation products should be measured to allow a better understanding of the ongoing damage to lipids (Mahadik & Scheffer, 1996).

Omega-3 fatty acids have been reported efficacious and effective in a variety of controlled studies in psychiatric illnesses. In schizophrenia, a series of trials have shown positive results. There is also a recent positive report in patients with autism (Amminger et al., 2007). In adult bipolar disorder, two open-label trials (Osher, Bersudsky, & Belmaker, 2005; Sagduyu et al., 2005) and two of three controlled studies have demonstrated an improvement in depressive symptoms and an increase in interepisode euthymic periods (Stoll et al., 1999; Frangou, Lewis, & McCrone, 2006). The Stanley Bipolar Network reported a negative trial with relatively high-dose ethyl-EPA (Keck et al., 2006). (See Table 8.1.)

Confounds in these studies may include the very high doses used in all but the Frangou et al. (2006) study (1 or 2 g). These include 9.6 g (Stoll et al., 1999), 6 g (Keck et al., 2006). The use of olive oil as a placebo may also confound studies. Olive oil is a monounsaturated fat that is known to improve cardiovascular health, likely by improving membrane dynamics. This may improve neuronal functioning as well.

Gracious, Chirieac, and Youngstrom (2006) recently completed the first large-scale controlled study of omega-3 fatty acids in youths with bipolar disorder. The study investigated flaxseed oil, which is rich in alpha-linolenic acid (ALA), to treating bipolar patients 6–18 years of age. This study has been orally reported as negative and is submitted for publication. In this study up to 12 grams per day of ALA was compared with olive oil.

TABLE 8.1. A Summary of Controlled Omega-3 Fatty-Acid Clinical Trials in Participants with Bipolar Disorder

Author (year)	Stoll et al. (1999)	Keck et al. (2006)	Frangou et al. (2006)	Gracious et al. (2006)
Agent	Fish oil (EPA and DHA)	Ethyl-EPA	Ethyl-EPA	Flax oil (alpha-linoleic acid)
Dose	9.6 grams	6 grams	1 or 2 grams	6–12 grams
Comparator	Olive oil	Liquid paraffin	Liquid paraffin	Olive oil
Number/ages	30 (18–65)	120 (18–70)	75 (18–70)	40 (6–18)
Duration of trial	4 months	4 months	12 weeks	16 weeks
Result	Positive	Negative	Positive—bipolar depression	Negative[a]

Note. None of these studies included adjunctive antioxidants to prevent increases in oxidative stress.
[a]The primary outcome measure was negative. However, participants on ALA remained in the study longer and had delays to adverse events compared with those on olive oil.

One potential issue with this study is that some patients may not be able to transform ALA to eicosapentaenoic acid (EPA) and DHA, the more biologically active omega-3s (see Figure 8.1). The elongase and desaturase enzymes needed to accomplish this transformation have been considered potential genetic abnormalities in patients with serious mental illnesses.

A second concern with this study is that the use of olive oil as a placebo may also confound results. Olive oil is a monounsaturated fat and likely has positive effects on cell membrane dynamics and possibly, in turn, brain function.

Third, there is some evidence that there is a therapeutic window for omega-3 fatty acids of between 1 and 2 grams per day. Higher doses, without the benefit of antioxidants, have been shown to be pro-oxidant (Song & Miyazawa, 2001; Vericel et al., 2003). This means that high doses may actually worsen the fatty-acid metabolism status of a patient. Previous studies had found 2 g/day of ethyl-EPA to be the optimal dose for schizophrenia (Peet & Horrobin, 2002) and 1 g/day for unipolar depression (Peet, Horrobin, & Ethyl-Eicosapentaenoate Multicentre Study Group, 2002).

A fourth potential issue is the low levels of symptoms needed to enter the trial. This may have made it more difficult to demonstrate a difference between the groups.

In a recently published open label trial to test the effectiveness and safety of omega-3 fatty acids [Omegabrite (R)] in the treatment of pediatric bipolar disorder (BPD) (Wozniak et al., 2007), twenty subjects ages 6 to 17 years with YMRS scores of >15 were treated for 8 weeks with omega-3 fatty acids 1290 mg–4300 combined EPA (eicosapentaenoic acid) and

DHA (docosahexaenoic acid). These subjects experienced a statistically significant but modest 8.9 ± 2.9 point reduction in the YMRS scores (baseline YMRS = 28.9 ± 10.1; endpoint YMRS = 19.1 ± 2.6, $p < .001$). Adverse events were few and mild. Red blood cell membrane levels of EPA and DHA increased in treated subjects. Thirty-five percent of these subjects had a response by the usual accepted criteria of >50% decrease on the YMRS. Therefore, omega-3 fatty acids treatment was associated with a very modest improvement in manic symptoms in children with BPD.

In ADHD, the results with omega-3 fatty acids have been less robust. Small primates are typically fed Monkey Chow in animal care facilities. Because this is made from fruit and vegetables, it is very high in omega-3 fatty acids and antioxidants. When the feed is depleted of omega-3 fatty acids, the animals become behaviorally irritable and are less able to learn on a variety of cognitive tasks. The monkeys show some symptoms that are similar to those of ADHD. When these animals are refed appropriate diets, these abnormalities reverse. Of five trials in children, results were inconsistent. The two using gamma-linolenic acid (GLA) of the omega-6 series were equivocal (Arnold et al., 1989; Arnold, Kleykahmp, Votolato, Gibson, & Horrocks, 1994). One trial with DHA failed. Two trials using a combination of omega-3 and GLA reported positive results with a weak signal. The aforementioned finding of an association between FASD1 and ADHD may ultimately help to explain the discrepant results. Omega-6 fatty acids are ubiquitous in the typical Western diet, and their use as supplements seems to be of unlikely benefit.

Prolonged bleeding times have been reported in those consuming high doses of omega-3 fatty acids. This finding is somewhat controversial as longer but not pathological bleeding times may be beneficial and normal given the preindustrial human diet. Nonetheless, bleeding times may lengthen in those treated with omega-3 fatty acids. Native people in Arctic areas consume huge quantities of omega-3 fatty acids from cold-water fish. Although their bleeding times are prolonged compared with the times of those eating a typical Western diet, there is no evidence that this is pathological.

CAM FOR DEPRESSION

In adults with bipolar disorder, the depressed phase of the illness is often the most treatment-resistant (Judd et al., 2003). Children with bipolar disorder often have serious depressions as well. Unfortunately, the addition of a conventional antidepressant can result in switches into frank mania (~20% in recently reported adult trials) and an increased frequency of mood cycling. Clinically, this conversion rate appears to be somewhat higher in youths treated with SSRIs.

The SSRI antidepressants are generally thought of as first-line treatments for major depressive disorder and anxiety disorders. When these conditions are concurrent with bipolar disorder, the risk of switches to mania with antidepressants is high.

There are a variety of CAM alternatives for depression that may prove useful. These include biological therapy with omega-3 fatty acids, Saint-John's-wort, S-adenosyl-L-methionine (SAM-e), folate, 5-hydroxytryptophan, and lavandula.

In adults, omega-3 fatty acids have been shown in two of three studies to improve depression associated with bipolar disorder. In the two positive studies, omega-3 fatty acids had general results similar to lamotrigine, including longer periods without mood cycling and delay of relapse of depression and mania. As reviewed recently by Sontrop and Campbell (2006), there have been positive studies in major depressive disorder, as well (Peet et al., 2002).

Saint-John's-wort has a mechanism of action similar to those of SSRIs and monoamine-oxidase inhibitors (MAOIs) and therefore should be considered to have risks similar to those of these antidepressants. Three percent hypericin dosed 300 mg by mouth three times per day has been found to be roughly as effective as low-dose tricyclic antidepressants for mild to moderate depression. The risk of precipitation of mania should be considered when patients contemplate the use of Saint-John's-wort. Findling et al. (2003) reported that 22 of 33 youths with major depression had significant improvement after 8 weeks of open-label treatment. It is important to remember that these were not patients with bipolar depression.

SAM-e is an essential component of cellular metabolism that is typically concentrated in liver and brain. It is thought to treat depression due to its transmethylation reactions that increase serotonin, dopamine, and norepinephrine. SAM-e increases the neuronal cell membrane uptake of phospholipids, which, in general, improve neuronal function. SAM-e is also required for synthesis of glutathione (an antioxidant enzyme), which is required to decrease damage from free radicals. SAM-e has been shown to be effective in adults with depression in doses of approximately 1,500 mg per day. There are no established dosing ranges for youths. Because of its effects on 5-HT, dopamine and norepinephrine the possibility exists that mania may be exacerbated by the use of SAM-e.

In adult women with mild to moderately severe major depressive disorder, a trial of acupuncture in a relatively small sample (38 women) demonstrated that specific acupuncture was better than nonspecific acupuncture and showed a trend for improvement in a wait-list control group (Gallagher, Allen, Hitt, Schnyer, & Manber, 2001). There are no published controlled trials of acupuncture for youths with bipolar disorder.

In addition, there are concerns regarding the standardization of acupuncture techniques, the lack of a placebo group, the difficulty in performing sham acupuncture for a placebo group, and other methodological issues that result in this being a treatment with some hope for being helpful but with little hard evidence.

A recent review found some evidence that acupuncture may be helpful in youths with nocturnal enuresis, but no definitive studies have been published (Bower, Diao, Tang, & Yeung, 2005). This condition can affect youths with bipolar disorder.

CAM FOR ADHD

As previously mentioned, animal behavior resulting from diets deficient in omega-3 fatty acids includes inattention and poor learning. Based on these considerations, essential fatty-acid supplementation has been attempted in patients with ADHD. Stevens et al. (2003) reported that both omega-3 and omega-6 were lower in participants with ADHD than in controls. Essential fatty-acid supplementation has promising systematic case-control data, but clinical trials are equivocal. Joshi et al. (2006) reported a positive clinical trial, whereas Voigt et al. (2006) had a negative result.

A previous review of alternative treatments summarized the status of alternative therapies for adults with ADHD (Arnold, 2001) and found many alternative treatment approaches. These ranged from mere hypotheses to positive controlled double-blind clinical trials. Zinc supplementation has been supported by systematic case-control data but not by systematic clinical trials (Arnold, Pinkham, & Votolato, 2000; Bekaroglu et al., 1996). Vitamin supplementation, non-Chinese herbals, homeopathic remedies, and antifungal therapy have no systematic data in ADHD. Megadose multivitamin combinations are probably ineffective for most patients and are potentially dangerous. Simple sugar restriction seems ineffective. Amino-acid supplementation is mildly effective in the short term, but not beyond 2–3 months. Thyroid treatment has been effective in the presence of documented thyroid abnormality. Many have failed to prove effective in controlled trials. It is uncertain whether these treatments will hold up to further scrutiny or be applicable to ADHD symptoms associated with bipolar disorder.

CONCLUSIONS

Alterations in omega-3 fatty-acid levels are likely play a large role in neuronal biology. It is likely that these abnormalities have significant impact on psychiatric illnesses. There is mounting clinical research to support their use in serious mental illnesses. It is important to remember methodological issues when conducting these trials. Antioxidant supplementation may be required to control oxidative stress. Further study is required to determine to what extent supplementation can have modifying effects on psychiatric illness.

CAM therapies may hold promise for the treatment of youths with bipolar disorder. This is particularly true when current treatments pose risks of exacerbating the underlying illness. Additional rigorous studies are needed to determine what role they may play.

REFERENCES

Amminger, G. P., Berger, G. E., Schäfer, M. R., Klier, C., Friedrich, M. H., & Feucht, M. (2007). Omega-3 fatty acids supplementation in children with autism: A double-blind, randomized, placebo-controlled pilot study. *Biological Psychiatry, 61*(4), 551–553.

Arnold, L. E. (2001). Alternative treatments for adults with attention-deficit hyperactivity disorder (ADHD). *Annals of the New York Academy of Sciences, 931,* 310–341.

Arnold, L. E., Kleykamp, D., Votolato, N., Gibson, R. A., & Horrocks, L. (1994). Potential link between dietary intake of fatty acids and behavior: Pilot exploration of serum lipids in ADHD. *Journal of Child and Adolescent Psychopharmacology, 4*(3), 171–180.

Arnold, L. E., Kleykamp, D., Votolato, N. A., Taylor, W. A., Kontras, S. B., Tobin, K. (1989). Gamma-linolenic acid for attention-deficit hyperactivity disorder: Placebo-controlled comparison to d-amphetamine. *Biological Psychiatry, 25,* 222–228.

Arnold, L. E., Pinkham, S. M., & Votolato, N. (2000). Does zinc moderate essential fatty acid and amphetamine treatment of attention-deficit/hyperactivity disorder? *Journal of Child and Adolescent Psychopharmacology, 10*(2), 111–117.

Bekaroglu, M., Aslan, Y., Gedik, Y., Deger, O., Mocan, H., Erduran, E., et al. (1996). Relationships between serum free fatty acids and zinc, and attention deficit hyperactivity disorder: A research note. *Journal of Child Psychology and Psychiatry and Allied Disciplines, 37*(2), 225–227.

Bennett, C. N., & Horrobin, D. F. (2000). Gene targets related to phospholipid and fatty acid metabolism in schizophrenia and other psychiatric disorders: An update. *Prostaglandins, Leukotrienes and Essential Fatty Acids, 63*(1–2), 47–59.

Bower, W. F., Diao, M., Tang, J. L., & Yeung, C. K. (2005). Acupuncture for nocturnal enuresis in children: A systematic review and exploration of rationale. *Neurourology and Urodynamics, 24*(3), 267–272.

Brookes, K. J., Chen, W., Xu, X., Taylor, E., & Asherson, P. (2005). Association of fatty acid desaturase genes with attention-deficit/hyperactivity disorder. *Biological Psychiatry, 60*(10), 1053–1061.

Chiu, C. C., Huang, S. Y., Su, K. P., Lu, M. L., Huang, M. C., Chen, C. C., et al. (2003). Polyunsaturated fatty acid deficit in patients with bipolar mania. *European Neuropsychopharmacology, 13*(2), 99–103.

Cunnane, S. C., Francescutti, V., Brenna, J. T., & Crawford, M. A. (2000). Breast-fed infants achieve a higher rate of brain and whole body docosahexaenoate accumulation than formula-fed infants not consuming dietary docosahexaenoate. *Lipids, 35*(1), 105–111.

Dennehy, E. B., Webb, A., & Suppes, T. (2002). Assessment of beliefs in the effectiveness of acupuncture for treatment of psychiatric symptoms. *Journal of Alternative and Complementary Medicine, 8*(4), 421–425.

Findling, R. L., McNamara, N. K., O'Riordan, M. A., Reed, M. D., Demeter, C. A., Branicky, L. A., et al. (2003). An open-label pilot study of St. John's wort in juvenile depression. *Journal of the American Academy of Child and Adolescent Psychiatry, 42*(8), 908–914.

Frangou, S., Lewis, M., & McCrone, P. (2006). Efficacy of ethyl-eicosapentaenoic acid in bipolar depression: Randomised double-blind placebo-controlled study. *British Journal of Psychiatry, 188*, 46–50.

Gallagher, S. M., Allen, J. J., Hitt, S. K., Schnyer, R. N., & Manber, R. (2001). Six-month depression relapse rates among women treated with acupuncture. *Complementary Therapies in Medicine, 9*(4), 216–218.

Gracious, B. L., Chirieac, M. C., & Youngstrom, E. A. (2006). *Randomized, placebo-controlled trial of flax oil in pediatric bipolar disorder.* Manuscript submitted for publication.

Joshi, K., Lad, S., Kale, M., Patwardhan, B., Mahadik, S. P., Patni, B., et al. (2006). Supplementation with flax oil and vitamin C improves the outcome of attention deficit hyperactivity disorder (ADHD). *Prostaglandins, Leukotrienes and Essential Fatty Acids, 74*(1), 17–21.

Judd, L. L., Schettler, P. J., Akiskal, H. S., Maser, J., Coryell, W,. Solomon, D., et al. (2003). Long-term symptomatic status of bipolar I vs. bipolar II disorders. *International Journal of Neuropsychopharmacology, 6*(2), 127–137.

Keck, P. E., Mintz, J., McElroy, S. L., Freeman, M. P., Suppes, T., Frye, M. A., et al. (2006). Double-blind, randomized, placebo-controlled trials of ethyl-eicosapentaenoate in the treatment of bipolar depression and rapid cycling bipolar disorder. *Biological Psychiatry, 60*(9), 1020–1022.

Khan, M. K., Evans, D. R., Gunna, V., Scheffer, R. E., Parikh, V. V., & Mahadik, S. P. (2002). Reduced erythrocyte membrane fatty acids and increased lipid peroxides in schizophrenia at the never-medicated first episode of psychosis and after years of treatment with antipsychotics. *Schizophrenia Research, 58*, 1–10.

Mahadik, S. P., Mukherjee, S., Scheffer, R. E., Correnti, E. E., & Mahadik, J. S. (1998). Elevated plasma lipid peroxides at the onset of nonaffective psychosis. *Biological Psychiatry, 43*, 674–679.

Mahadik, S., & Scheffer, R. E. (1996). Oxidative injury and potential use of antioxidants in schizophrenia. *Prostaglandins, Leukotrienes, and Essential Fatty Acids, 1*(2), 45–54.

Noaghiul, S., & Hibbeln, J. R. (2003). Cross-national comparisons of seafood consumption and rates of bipolar disorders. *American Journal of Psychiatry, 160*(12), 2222–2227.

Osher, Y., Bersudsky, Y., & Belmaker, R. H. (2005). Omega-3 eicosapentaenoic acid in bipolar depression: Report of a small open-label study. *Journal of Clinical Psychiatry, 66*(6), 726–729.

Peet, M., & Horrobin, D. F. (2002). A dose-ranging study of the effects of ethyl-eicosapentaenoate in patients with ongoing depression despite apparently adequate treatment with standard drugs. *Archives of General Psychiatry, 59*(10), 913–919.

Peet, M., Horrobin, D. F., & Ethyl-Eicosapentaenoate Multicentre Study Group. (2002). A dose-ranging exploratory study of the effects of ethyl-eicosapentaenoate in patients with persistent schizophrenic symptoms. *Journal of Psychiatric Research, 36*(1), 7–18.

Ranjekar, P. K., Hinge, A., Hegde, M. V., Ghate, M., Kale, A., Sitasawad, S., et al. (2003). Decreased antioxidant enzymes and membrane essential polyunsaturated fatty acids in schizophrenic and bipolar mood disorder patients. *Psychiatry Research, 121*(2), 109–122.

Ross, B. M., McKenzie, I., Glen, I., & Bennett, C. P. (2003). Increased levels of ethane, a non-invasive marker of n-3 fatty acid oxidation, in breath of children with attention deficit hyperactivity disorder. *Nutritional Neuroscience, 6*(5), 277–281.

Sagduyu, K., Dokucu, M. E., Eddy, B. A., Craigen, G., Baldassano, C. F., & Yildiz, A. (2005). Omega-3 fatty acids decreased irritability of patients with bipolar disorder in an add-on, open label study. *Nutrition Journal, 4*, 6.

Song, J. H., & Miyazawa, T. (2001), Enhanced level of n-3 fatty acid in membrane phospholipids induces lipid peroxidation in rats fed dietary docosahexaenoic acid oil. *Atherosclerosis, 155*(1), 9–18.

Sontrop, J., & Campbell, M. K. (2006). Omega-3 polyunsaturated fatty acids and depression: A review of the evidence and a methodological critique. *Preventive Medicine, 42*(1), 4–13.

Stevens, L., Zhang, W., Peck, L., Kuczek, T., Grevstad, N., Mahon, A., et al. (2003). Polyunsaturated fatty acid supplementation in children with inattention, hyperactivity and other dis-ruptive behaviors. *Lipids, 38,* 1007–1021.

Stoll, A. L., Severus, W. E., Freeman, M. P., Rueter, S., Zboyan, H. A., Diamond, E., et al. (1999). Omega 3 fatty acids in bipolar disorder: A preliminary double-blind, placebo-controlled trial. *Archives of General Psychiatry, 56*(5), 407–412.

Vericel, E., Polette, A., Bacot, S., Calzada, C., & Lagarde, M. (2003). Pro- and antioxidant activi-ties of docosahexaenoic acid on human blood platelets. *Journal of Thrombosis and Haemostasis, 1*(3), 566–572.

Voigt, R. G., Llorente, A. M., Jensen, C. L., Fraley, J. K., Berretta, M. C., & Heird, W. C. (2006). A randomized, double-blind, placebo-controlled trial of docosahexaenoic acid supple-mentation in children with attention-deficit/hyperactivity disorder. *Journal of Pediatrics, 139*(2), 189–196.

Wozniak, J., Biederman, J., Mick, E., Waxmonsky, J., Hantsoo, L., Best, C., et al. (2007). Omega-3 fatty acid monotherapy for pediatric bipolar disorder: A prospective open-label trial. *European Neuropsychopharmcology, 17*(6–7), 440–447.

Yao, J., Stanley, J. A., Reddy, R. D., Keshavan, M. S., & Pettegrew, J. W. (2002). Correlations be-tween peripheral polyunsaturated fatty acid content and in vivo membrane phospholipid metabolites. *Biological Psychiatry, 52*(8), 823–830.

CHAPTER 9

Family-Focused Treatment for Bipolar Disorder in Adolescence

DAVID J. MIKLOWITZ, KIMBERLEY L. MULLEN,
and KIKI D. CHANG

Bipolar disorder is a chronic, recurrent disorder carrying high morbidity and mortality, leading to health costs of more than $45 billion per year (Kleinman et al., 2003). It is the sixth leading cause of disability among all illnesses (Murray & Lopez, 1996). Up to 4% of the U.S. population is affected by bipolar I or II disorder (Kessler, Berglund, Demler, Jin, & Walters, 2005). Twenty-five to 50% of individuals with bipolar disorder attempt suicide at least once, and 8.6% to 18.9% die by suicide (Chen & Dilsaver, 1996). Suicidal risk, along with increased substance use and psychiatric comorbidity, is highest in childhood-onset bipolar disorder (Bellivier, Golmard, Henry, Leboyer, & Schurhoff, 2001; Brent et al.,1988; Carter, Mundo, Parikh, & Kennedy, 2003). Families are significantly affected by bipolar disorder in an offspring, with high levels of emotional, economic, and practical burden and distress (Perlick, Hohenstein, Clarkin, Kaczynski, & Rosenheck, 2005; Chang, Blaser, Ketter, & Steiner, 2001).

Between 15 and 28% of adults with bipolar disorder experience illness onset before the age of 13, and between 50 and 66% before the age of 19 (Perlis et al., 2004; Leverich et al., 2002, 2003). The exact prevalence in children is unknown, but estimates range from 420,000 to 2,072,000 among U.S. children alone (Post & Kowatch, 2006). Persons with onset of bipolar disorder in childhood or adolescence have a more severe, adverse, and continuously cycling course of illness than adults, often with a preponderance of mixed episodes, psychosis, and suicidal ideation or behaviors (Geller et al., 2002). They have high rates of comorbidity with attention-deficit/hyperactivity disorder (ADHD), conduct disorder, alcoholism, drug abuse, and anxiety disorders and—in part because of these complicated presentations—are more treatment-refractory than adults (Biederman, Mick, Faraone, et al., 2003; Biederman, Mick, Wozniak, et al., 2003; Perlis et al., 2004; Leverich et al., 2002; Leverich et al., 2003; Findling et al., 2005). Without early intervention, patients with early-onset bipolar disorder can be derailed, sometimes irrevocably, in social, intellectual, and emotional development.

Much disagreement exists about the boundaries between pediatric-onset bipolar disorder and other childhood psychiatric disorders; the continuity between the pediatric, adolescent, and adult forms of the illness; the population prevalence of the childhood-onset forms; and the pharmacological strategies that are appropriate in younger age groups (McClellan, 2005; Leibenluft, Charney, Towbin, Bhangoo, & Pine, 2003; National Institute of Mental Health, 2001). Nonetheless, resolving these disagreements should not stall efforts to develop and test effective early intervention programs. Given the severe morbidity and mortality associated with bipolar disorder and bipolar spectrum presentations, it is imperative to develop interventions designed to reduce the likelihood of recurrence among individuals with bipolar disorder or to prevent the progression from prodromal or spectrum forms (bipolar disorder not otherwise specified or cyclothymia) to bipolar I or II disorder (Post & Kowatch, 2006; Faedda et al., 1995). Intervening early in the illness may also help prevent inappropriate interventions that may worsen symptoms.

KINDLING AND PSYCHOSOCIAL STRESS

The theory of kindling, although controversial, is important to the assumptions of early psychosocial intervention. First applied to seizure disorders, the theory holds that the combination of stress and genetic vulnerability leads to greater destabilization until there is onset of a full mood-disorder episode (Post, 1992). Then with each episode the brain becomes sensitized until spontaneous episodes occur without being triggered by psychosocial stress. Thus patients with improperly treated bipolar disorder will develop episodes closer to one another and with more severity, leading to rapid cycling and treatment resistance (Post & Weiss, 1996). Conversely, early intervention aimed at controlling symptoms may arrest this process.

It is becoming clearer that areas in the prefrontal cortex, as well as other limbic areas, suffer neurodegeneration with prolonged bipolar illness (Strakowski et al., 2002; Rajkowska, Halaris, & Selemon, 2001; Gallelli et al., 2005; Manji & Duman, 2001). Stress from repeated mood episodes has been postulated to be causal to this process (Hashimoto, Shimizu, & Iyo, 2004; Rajkowska, 2000), leading to less prefrontal mood regulation and greater cycling (Chang et al., 2004). The developing juvenile brain may be especially susceptible to neuronal cell loss with repeated manic episodes (Chang et al., 2004; Kochman et al., 2005). Thus an intervention that decreases stress and improves cognitive control of mood could have a combined effect on preserving prefrontal function and neuronal integrity.

There is controversy regarding the kindling model in explaining the progressive course of bipolar disorder. Not all studies find shorter cycle lengths over time (Turvey et al., 1999) or that life events are more potent in provoking initial episodes than later episodes (Hammen & Gitlin, 1997; Hlastala et al., 2000). Nevertheless, retrospective reporting from patient histories (Roy-Byrne, Post, Uhde, Porcu, & Davis, 1985) and research at the level of the cell (Post, 1992) support this hypothesis. A review of longitudinal bipolar disorder studies concluded that multiple affective recurrences are linked with subsequent treatment resistance, disability, and functional neuroanatomic changes and that effective treatment early in the illness may have protective effects on subsequent illness course (Goldberg, Garno, & Harrow, 2005).

THE ROLE OF EARLY PSYCHOSOCIAL INTERVENTION IN BIPOLAR DISORDER

Interventions early in the course of bipolar disorder may alter the subsequent course of the disorder. Some of these interventions are likely to be pharmacological and aimed at decreasing biological vulnerabilities to stressors (Post, 2002). However, medications will probably have little effect on the intensity of external stressors and will not buffer the at-risk person against stress once he or she has discontinued taking them. In contrast, psychosocial interventions have two interrelated goals: decreasing the intensity of environmental stressors and increasing the at-risk person's resiliency and coping skills. More specifically, family-focused therapy (FFT) has two objectives: (1) to decrease family interactions characterized by high expressed emotion (EE; criticism and hostility) and (2) to enhance ability of the person with bipolar disorder to cope with emotionally charged or stressful family interactions.

Family interventions begin with the assumption that negativity in the family environment, even though often a product of the stress and burden of caregiving for an ill relative, is a risk factor for subsequent episodes of bipolar illness. Adults with bipolar disorder who have parents or spouses who express high levels of criticism, hostility, or emotional overinvolvement have earlier recurrences and poorer symptom outcomes than patients with bipolar disorder who have environments with lower conflict and lower EE (Honig, Hofman, Rozendaal, & Dingemanns, 1997; Miklowitz, Goldstein, Nuechterlein, Snyder, & Mintz, 1988; Miklowitz et al., 2000; O'Connell, Mayo, Flatow, Cuthbertson, & O'Brien, 1991; Yan, Hammen, Cohen, Daley, & Henry, 2004). In parallel, family environments characterized by high EE attitudes (Miklowitz, Biuckians, & Richards, 2006) or low maternal warmth (Geller, Tillman, Craney, & Bolhofner, 2004) are associated with poorer outcomes of pediatric bipolar disorder over 2- to 4-year follow-ups. In one sample of children of mothers with bipolar disorder (Meyer et al., 2006), maternal negativity contributed to risk for offspring bipolar disorder through its negative association with frontal lobe functioning.

EE is not the only risk process targeted by early family interventions. Medication noncompliance, the lack of ability to recognize and intervene early with prodromal symptoms, and the inability to cope with stressors that precipitate illness episodes are related to relapse in many individuals with bipolar disorder (Johnson, 2005; Lam, Wright, & Sham, 2005; Miklowitz, George, Richards, Simoneau, & Suddath, 2003; Vieta & Colom, 2004). Psychosocial stressors are believed to interact with genetic predispositions to induce the full expression of bipolar disorder (Post, Leverich, Xing, & Weiss, 2001; Miklowitz & Johnson, 2006). The mechanisms by which environmental threats affect the course of bipolar disorder may involve psychological vulnerability factors (e.g., negative cognitive styles; for review, see Miklowitz & Johnson, 2006) and activation of brain circuitry involved in emotional self-regulation (Chang et al., 2004).

Specific psychotherapeutic interventions for individuals with bipolar disorder should reduce the severity of psychosocial vulnerability factors and enhance the child's coping capacities to prevent or delay bipolar disorder recurrences. Data strongly support the efficacy of psychosocial interventions for the prevention of relapse of adult bipolar disorder (Miklowitz & Otto, 2006; Miklowitz, 2006). Current treatment guidelines recommend that patients with bipolar disorder receive medication and adjunctive psychotherapy (Keller, 2004; Kowatch et al., 2005). The various psychotherapeutic modalities available all share a focus on psychoeducation, enhancing medication adherence, early symptom recognition and management, and problem solving (Otto, Reilly-Harrington, & Sachs, 2003; Scott & Gutierrez, 2004).

INVOLVING THE FAMILY IN TREATMENT

Focusing psychosocial treatment on the family unit is essential for youths with bipolar disorder because they usually live with their parents and are more dependent on their families than are adults. High levels of family criticism are correlated with recurrences of both unipolar and bipolar mood disorders (see the meta-analysis of Butzlaff and Hooley, 1998), and when several individuals are struggling with mood dysregulation, the likelihood of a chaotic and potentially stressful family environment increases greatly. Also, many children with bipolar disorder are already on complicated medication regimens, which can be hard to maintain in a chaotic family environment. In order to delay recurrences of pediatric bipolar disorder, or at least reduce its severity and associated impairments, it is important to educate family members about the signs and symptoms of the illness, to develop emergency intervention plans, to manage environmental stressors, and to promote a family environment conducive to mood stability.

Randomized clinical trials with adults with bipolar disorder have shown that FFT, when given adjunctively with pharmacotherapy, delays recurrences of mania or depression, enhances stabilization of manic and depressive symptoms, improves medication compliance, and decreases stressful family interactions when compared with adjunctive brief psychoeducation or individual therapy (Miklowitz, George, et al., 2003; Miklowitz, Richards, et al., 2003; Rea et al., 2003; Miklowitz, Otto, et al., 2006; Simoneau, Miklowitz, Richards, Saleem, & George, 1999). FFT for bipolar adolescents (FFT-A; Miklowitz et al., 2004), multi-family psychoeducation groups (Fristad, Gavazzi, & Mackinaw-Koons, 2003), and the combination of cognitive behavior therapy and FFT (Pavuluri et al., 2004) have shown initial success in decreasing symptom severity in children with bipolar disorder. FFT-A is a modification of the adult version of FFT, addressing the developmental issues and unique clinical presentations of adolescents with bipolar disorder (Miklowitz et al., 2004). It consists of three phases: psychoeducation about mood dysregulation and ways to enhance mood stability, communication training, and problem-solving skills training.

EMPIRICAL STUDIES OF FFT

The first trial of FFT was conducted at the University of Colorado between 1990 and 1997 (Miklowitz et al., 2000; Miklowitz, George, et al., 2003). We randomly assigned 101 adult patients with bipolar I (mean = 36 years) to a 9-month, 21-session FFT plus standard pharmacotherapy or a usual care comparison condition called crisis management (CM) plus standard pharmacotherapy. Patients in CM received two family educational sessions plus crisis intervention sessions over 2 years. Patients assigned to FFT had a 2-year rate of survival without disease relapse of 52%, three times higher than patients assigned to CM (17%; $p = .003$). The mean survival duration for patients in FFT was 73.5 weeks, and for patients in CM, 53.2 weeks. FFT was superior to CM in reducing depressive symptoms ($p = .005$; Cohen's $d = 0.56$) and manic symptoms ($p < .05$; Cohen's $d = 0.40$) over 2 years. Analyses of mediating variables indicated that FFT operated through two mechanisms: improving the communication patterns of families from pre- to posttreatment (Simoneau et al., 1999) and enhancing the patients' adherence with medications (Miklowitz, George, et al., 2003).

A second trial conducted at the University of California, Los Angeles, involved 53 adult patients with bipolar I and mania, randomly assigned either to FFT plus medications or to individual psychoeducational therapy plus medications (Rea et al., 2003). The individual therapy was administered with the same frequency as FFT: 21 sessions over 9 months. Patients in FFT had fewer relapses during a 2- to 3-year follow-up (28%) than patients in individual therapy (60%; $p < .05$). Patients in FFT also had substantially fewer rehospitalizations at follow-up (12% in FFT vs. 60% in individual therapy; $p < .01$). FFT appeared to prevent rehospitalizations in part through teaching families to recognize relapses early and obtain emergency treatment (Rea et al., 2003).

Early open-trial results ($N = 20$) indicate that adolescent patients with bipolar disorder undergoing FFT-A and pharmacotherapy showed significant improvements over 24 months (Miklowitz et al., 2006). The improvements were observed in Kiddie Schedule for Affective Disorders and Schizophrenia (K-SADS) Depression Rating Scale Scores ($p < .002$; Cohen's $d = 0.87$), K-SADS mania scores ($p < .0001$; $d = 1.19$), and total mood scores ($p < .0001$; $d = 1.05$) over time. We also observed substantial improvements in parent-rated Child Behavior Checklist (CBCL) total problem behavior scores ($p < .0001$; $d = 0.99$), externalizing T-scores ($p < .0001$, $d = 1.02$) and internalizing T-scores ($p < .0005$, $d = 0.70$) over 2 years. So it would appear that FFT has a promising record of enhancing symptom stabilization among youths and adults with diagnosed bipolar disorder.

The remainder of this chapter is devoted to describing the FFT model as applied to adolescents with bipolar disorder (ages 13–17). We have not yet applied FFT to school-age children with bipolar disorder, although a version for children at risk for bipolar disorder (ages 9–17) is currently being designed and evaluated (Miklowitz & Chang, in press). We describe the three phases of the treatment and then present a case study.

OBJECTIVES OF FFT FOR ADOLESCENTS WITH BIPOLAR DISORDER (FFT-A)

FFT-A is given in 21 sessions over 9 months (weekly for 3 months, biweekly for 3 months, and monthly for 3 months), followed by maintenance sessions every 3 months for the next 15 months (up to 24 months) for up to 26 meetings. The objectives are to assist the adolescent and his or her parents and siblings to:

1. Understand the nature, pattern, and biopsychosocial context of the adolescent's recent mood cycling.
2. Recognize the adolescent's vulnerability to the disease and develop plans to minimize future symptoms.
3. Accept the role of psychotropic medications in managing mood states.
4. Distinguish the disorder from stable personality attributes or age-normative adolescent behaviors.
5. Identify stress triggers or daily hassles that provoke swings of mood.
6. Implement strategies for maintaining stability during euthymic periods (e.g., sleep/wake cycle stabilization).
7. Promote a family environment whose communication and problem-solving practices enhance the adolescent's and parents' stability and functioning.

The *psychoeducation module* (sessions 1–9) gives adolescents, their parents, and siblings concrete, didactic information about the symptoms, differential diagnosis, comorbidity, course, treatment, and self-management of bipolar disorder. Handouts and self-guided homework (e.g., keeping a daily mood and sleep chart) are provided about these topics. First, the clinician reviews the symptoms of bipolar disorder and distinguishes them from symptoms of anxiety, psychosis, or disruptive behavior disorders. Families watch a portion of the video *Teens with Bipolar Disorder* (Josselyn Foundation, 2000) and take home a copy to discuss. The clinician explains the interactive roles of genetic and biological vulnerability, stress, and coping in the disorder's onset and the role of risk factors (i.e., disruptions in sleep/wake rhythms, sudden discontinuance of medications, substance misuse, escalating family conflicts) and protective factors (i.e., consistency with medications and pharmacotherapy visits; stable sleep/wake patterns; structured, low-conflict family routines). Clinicians point out that "genetics is not destiny" and that the trajectory the child follows will depend on the balance over time of risk and protective factors.

Participants identify stressors that are currently affecting the child—family conflicts; sibling rivalries; peer or romantic relationships; or school, neighborhood, or extended family stressors—and the effects of these stressors on mood states. The impact of the disorder on family functioning is discussed. Care is taken to avoid any implication of blame to the parents, and therapists clarify that many of the adolescent's aversive behaviors are due to a biologically based illness rather than to willful intention.

A key component of psychoeducation is the "relapse drill," that is, planning during periods of stability for emergency intervention (medical or behavioral) when the adolescent's moods start to deteriorate or when he or she becomes suicidal. With the aid of a flip chart, families recall previous periods of mood instability and identify sequences consisting of triggers, early warning signs of relapse, and palliative measures. Where relevant, the discussion includes symptoms of emergent psychosis as prodromal signs (e.g., ideas of reference), and methods to manage decompensation. A prevention plan is developed (e.g., no-suicide/no-harm contracts, notifying the physician to arrange medication changes, reducing stress triggers at home, stabilizing sleep/wake rhythms). The plan is typed up and presented for the participants' signature in the next session.

Psychoeducation ends with a discussion of a handout titled "How the Family Can Help." Emphasis is placed on keeping regular family routines (e.g., mealtimes, bedtimes) and stress reduction strategies (e.g., maintaining a tolerant and low-key family atmosphere, using emotional self-regulation techniques). Methods to improve medication adherence and prevent behaviors that put the child at even higher risk for adverse outcomes (substance abuse, drunk driving, unsafe sex) take center stage with middle to late adolescents.

During psychoeducation and other phases of FFT, clinicians provide emotional support for parents and clinical referrals as appropriate (including pharmacotherapy). They teach parents to identify and cope with triggers for their own mood cycling (including high-intensity interactions with the bipolar offspring) and emphasize communication strategies (see the next discussion) to help preserve marital relationships and relations between parents and the affected and nonaffected offspring.

The *communication enhancement training module* (sessions 10–15) is designed to reduce unproductive interactions among family members and improve the quality of verbal and nonverbal exchanges. It is guided by the assumption that aversive communication reflects distress in the family's attempts to cope with bipolar disorder. It uses a role-playing format to teach adolescents and their family members four skills: expressing positive feelings, active listening, making positive requests for changes in each others' behaviors, and constructive negative feedback.

The clinician first emphasizes the link between effective family communication and mood stability (Simoneau et al., 1999; Snyder, Castellani, & Whisman, 2006). As each skill is introduced, the family is taken through six steps: (1) learning the components of the skill with the aid of a handout (e.g., for active listening: paraphrasing, keeping eye contact), (2) observing the clinician modeling the skill, (3) practicing the skill with each other, (4) obtaining feedback from the paired partner, (5) practicing the skill again with the same or a different family member, and (6) completing a between-session homework task involving practicing the skill. Communication training is done less formally with adolescents than with adults, capitalizing as much as possible on spontaneous interactions.

The *problem-solving module* (sessions 16–21) encourages families to discuss difficult problem topics, to break down large problems (i.e., "we don't get along") into smaller ones ("we need to use lower tones of voice"), to generate and evaluate various solutions, to agree on a best set of solutions, and to choose one or more solutions to implement (e.g., alerting each other when tones of voice become aggressive). Families practice problem solving between sessions using a self-guided homework sheet and report on their attempts in the next session.

Problem solving focuses on enhancing functional capacities and quality of life, as well as symptom control. Examples of issues covered in problem-solving include strategies for increasing consistency with medications, completing school homework, decreasing family arguments, getting along with teachers, and reducing overstimulation before bedtime. It can also focus on behavior management strategies that parents can employ without interfering with the adolescent's normal developmental quest for independence. Problem solving also includes strategies for the parents or siblings to use to manage their own tempers or emotions (e.g., using self-talk or relaxation techniques).

Toward the end of FFT, sessions are tapered to trimonthly (months 10–24). *Maintenance sessions* revisit the seven objectives of FFT. Has the family gained an understanding of the cyclic nature of the disorder? Is consistency of medication treatment in place? Has the family developed (and, where necessary, implemented) a relapse prevention plan? These sessions usually involve problem solving and rehearsal of communication skills.

CASE STUDY: FFT WITH AN ADOLESCENT WITH BIPOLAR DISORDER

Carl was a 15-year-old Caucasian male who lived with his parents and 18-year-old sister. The family came to our university-based outpatient clinic seeking psychosocial treatment and pharmacotherapy. Carl had received a diagnosis of bipolar disorder 5 years earlier and was taking a mood stabilizer (lithium) and antipsychotic (risperidone), although he did not like his current psychiatrist. After an extensive diagnostic evaluation (the Kiddie Schedule for Affective Disorders and Schizophrenia for School-Age Children, Present and Lifetime Version, or K-SADS-PL; Chambers et al., 1985; Kaufman et al., 1997) and the confirmation of Carl's diagnosis of bipolar I disorder, manic episode, he began treatment with a university-affiliated psychiatrist.

Despite Carl's reported aversion to mental health professionals, he was open and honest during the pretreatment assessment phase. In addition to his most recent manic episode, he reported experiencing ongoing, debilitating depression and anxiety, and he no longer attended school. Carl reported thoughts of suicide and past suicide attempts, but his mother felt that he made only manipulative gestures (e.g., tying a string around his neck). His mother was more concerned about Carl's affinity for climbing out his window and sitting on the roof when upset, but Carl reported that this was his way of calming down and not a suicidal gesture.

Carl also had episodes of extreme rage, often in response to seemingly mild frustrations, in which he would destroy property and threaten to harm his family and himself. Carl's most recent episode of mania, which began approximately 2 months prior to the K-SADS-PL interview, included several severe anger outbursts that resulted in his first psychiatric hospitalization. Furthermore, a week prior to his hospitalization, Carl had begun, but not finished, two ambitious projects: the construction of a life-sized space capsule and a motorized go-kart. At that time, Carl's mood was giddy and silly, but rather than recognizing this as a symptom of mania, his mother felt these moods were a welcome departure from Carl's depression. It was not until Carl attempted to telephone the president to demand the removal of troops from Iraq that Carl's parents began to question whether he had become manic. His mother's questioning directly preceded Carl's episodes of rage.

Two clinicians served as cotherapists for Carl's family. Although not ideal, due to scheduling conflicts, only Carl and his mother attended sessions. The therapists pointed out the importance of the involvement of the whole family. Carl's mother agreed that she would share handouts and the content of the therapy sessions with Carl's father and sister. Carl and his mother were very close and generally able to communicate openly, but they disagreed on many things. For example, during the initial psychoeducation sessions, when the symptoms of bipolar disorder were being reviewed, they agreed on the nature and duration of his depressive symptoms. During the third session, however, when reviewing his manic symptoms, significant conflict arose. Carl viewed his periods of intense, uncontrollable anger as normal reactions to unfair treatment from his family. When his mother explained that his reactions were disproportionate to the situation, Carl became angry and agitated. The clinicians labeled maternal criticism, coupled with Carl's view that he was being treated unfairly, as a sequence that led to Carl's rages. Carl appeared to feel validated by this observation and became calmer.

The therapists continued to review and describe the symptoms of mania. On hearing the definition and age-appropriate examples of grandiosity, Carl's mother correctly identified Carl's call to the president as grandiosity. The therapists asked Carl's mother about any other symptoms that were present at that time, and she described her joy that he was finally cheerful and making jokes "like a normal kid." She had wondered whether Carl was taking illicit drugs when his mood shifted so drastically, but, after searching his room and backpack while he was out, she decided her concerns were unfounded. Further, his mother reported feeling relieved that Carl had taken an interest in starting new projects but admitted that the 6-

foot-high space capsule took up the majority of the living room and, given Carl's current lack of interest, appeared as if it would never be finished. Carl described feeling like he was "on a mission" when he began constructing the space capsule and go-kart but that he didn't finish them because "the channels kept getting changed."

After obtaining more information about Carl's symptoms, the clinicians determined that Carl experienced racing thoughts and decreased need for sleep as well. The identification of Carl's mania symptoms aided in the development of a relapse prevention plan that focused on early identification of symptoms, symptom triggers, and emergency treatment/preventative measures.

The therapists introduced the communication enhancement module at session 8. Carl and his mother exchanged positive feedback sensitively and kindly. Carl told his mother that he appreciated all of her help with his mood disorder, including taking him to all of his therapy and medication appointments. Carl's mother spoke of her admiration for Carl's continued efforts to learn to control his anger and cope with bipolar disorder. Thus communication training began on a positive note.

When practicing the second skill, active listening, it became apparent that both Carl and his mother had a hard time waiting for their turn to speak and would often talk over one another "to help the conversation flow." However, each ultimately felt that the other was not listening. Not surprisingly, both were especially prone to this communication style when Carl was manic or hypomanic. The therapists highlighted this pattern of interaction and explored ways in which the therapists could stop the pattern within sessions. Carl and his mother both agreed that the therapists could simply stop the conversation and remind them to paraphrase each other (a component of active listening) before making their next argument. Throughout the remaining treatment, Carl and his mother both became more aware of their "punch–counterpunch" style and would often stop themselves before the therapists intervened. The clinicians then emphasized exporting this skill to the home setting, with the help of communication-oriented homework tasks (see examples in Miklowitz & Goldstein, 1997).

When making positive requests for change in session 12, Carl asked his mother to be more understanding and willing to help when he wanted to see his friends. Once again, the therapists asked the pair to focus on using active listening skills while discussing this emotionally charged topic. Carl felt very isolated because he no longer attended school and would become agitated and anxious in anticipation of his friends' return from school. His closest friends were engaged in extracurricular activities, further limiting their availability to him. He was beginning to panic that he would lose his friends if he did not immediately respond to their invitations. Carl's mother felt that his requests were often abrupt and demanded her immediate attention, which inconvenienced her. The therapists took this opportunity to introduce problem solving. It is generally better to initially practice problem solving with a low-key issue, but Carl and his mother's close relationship and ability to speak openly and respectfully seemed a good indicator of their ability to tackle the issue.

First, the problem was specifically defined as "Carl makes last-minute plans with friends and gets frustrated when his mother cannot accommodate him." Next, Carl and his mother "brainstormed" as many possible solutions to the problem as they could without judging the utility of any option. The therapists coached the family first by asking each of them what their ideal solution would be and then asking for "middle ground" solutions. This activity continued into the following session.

After evaluating the possible solutions, the pair agreed to try a solution that combined several ideas: Carl would discuss with his mother plans to invite friends over at least 1 day in advance. If his friends extended an invitation (e.g., going to Carl's favorite gaming store), he would immediately discuss it with his mother and try to find a ride with her, his older sister, or one of his friends. He was also to be aware of his propensity to react with his impulsive anger if he did not get his way. Carl's mom stipulated that she would not pick him up later than 9 P.M., a restriction that supported Carl's need for a regular sleep schedule. The family agreed that the determinant of success would be each feeling as if their needs were being met and their individual limits observed without either becoming angry with the other.

At this point, the therapists might have evaluated Carl's ability to regulate his emotions in response to not being able to see his friends. However, Carl had not had an outburst of rage in some time. They chose to set this issue aside for later problem solving and returned to the communication module by introducing the last skill, expressing negative feedback. Carl's mom began by telling Carl how it made her feel when he constantly questioned her regarding his chores. She felt that Carl was trying to determine how long he could procrastinate and how little effort he could apply and still stay out of trouble. After paraphrasing her, Carl stated that he wasn't trying to "get away with anything" but felt as if he needed each step of the chore laid out for him in a very concrete way. Noticing the similarity between this disagreement and Carl's anxiety regarding seeing his friends, the therapist explored Carl's attitudes about household chores. This discussion resulted in the discovery that Carl's questioning stemmed from anxiety due to a desire to do things right rather than to get out of chores. Carl's mother pointed out how this pattern related to Carl's difficulties at school as well.

The family engaged in problem solving to determine how best to structure Carl's chores so that he fully understood what was expected of him. Carl felt that his mother's frequent reminders to complete his chores were intolerable and triggered his anger. Therefore, they agreed that his mother would make a list of chores with times of expected completion each day.

After review at a later session, the pair agreed that this solution had been a success.

Carl's mother reported that she had discussed with Carl's father and sister this new conceptualization of Carl's anxiety. She felt that this renewed understanding contributed to a reduction in tension within the household.

The family still had problems to solve during the last phase of treatment, including evaluation of Carl's academic plans and his irregular sleep patterns, which were clearly affecting his mood. These problems were systematically addressed using the problem-solving skills worksheets. As the treatment drew to a close, the clinicians encouraged more and more autonomy in the use of problem solving by the family, such that Carl and his mother were able to conduct entire problem-solving exercises with little intervention from the clinicians.

At the end of the 9-month family treatment, Carl's moods were more stable due to his continuing adherence to his lithium, risperidone, and antidepressant (added by his psychiatrist mid-treatment) regimen, his efforts to apply new self-management techniques and skills, and his and his mother's willingness to incorporate communication and problem-solving skills and to encourage the rest of the family to do the same. Because he was about to begin a new vocational program that would be challenging for him, one of the clinicians offered to continue with Carl in individual treatment to help coach him through the stress of this program. A secondary goal was to work more comprehensively with Carl's emotional self-regulation skills so that he became less reliant on his mother when coping with mood fluctuations.

At 6-month follow-up, Carl had not had any further episodes of mania since the original episode that brought him into treatment 15 months earlier. He continued to struggle with anxiety and depressive symptoms, particularly in response to the pressures of returning to school. He continued to engage in biweekly individual therapy and was learning coping strategies, including mindfulness techniques, for use at school.

CONCLUSIONS AND FUTURE DIRECTIONS

Progress is rapidly being made in the application of adjunctive psychosocial interventions for children and adolescents with bipolar disorder. One approach, FFT, combines psychoeducation, communication enhancement, and problem-solving strategies to manage the postepisode phases of bipolar mania or depression. This chapter has clarified the core therapeutic techniques of FFT and the existing empirical studies with adults and adolescents and concluded with a case study illustrating the approach. FFT is now being tested in a large-scale ($N = 150$) multicenter study (Miklowitz,

2006b), which will examine overall effectiveness, hypothesized treatment mediators (e.g., changes in family EE), and treatment moderators (e.g., severity of illness at baseline).

Many questions remain unanswered. Notable among these is the role of psychosocial stressors—both intrafamilial and extrafamilial—in eliciting episodes of pediatric mania or depression. The kindling model offers a framework for understanding the interface between stress, neurochemical changes, and neuroanatomical changes across different phases of development. However, there are other models that may apply to the role of stress in bipolar disorder. For example, Hammen (1991) has described a stress-generation model in which teens with mood disorder create negative life stressors, which then have an impact on subsequent mood cycling and stress and contribute to the long-term chronicity of the disorder. One could easily imagine how such a stress-generation cycle could operate within a distressed family environment. The role of stress generation in bipolar illness and its association with progressive changes in the developing juvenile brain are fruitful areas for future research.

Another important focus is the potential application of early psychosocial intervention for children at risk for bipolar disorder. Miklowitz and Chang (in press) have initiated a study that begins by identifying children at high risk for bipolar disorder: those with a first-degree relative with bipolar I or II disorder and who have early subsyndromal symptoms of mania, hypomania, or depression. These children will be randomized to a version of FFT for high-risk children (FFT-HR) or a treatment-as-usual comparison group. Key outcome variables will include the severity of manic or depressive symptoms at follow-up, time to first onset of a manic or mixed episode, and academic and social functioning. In our view, early intervention studies are going to be critical in the next generation of research on juvenile-onset bipolar disorder.

REFERENCES

Bellivier, F., Golmard, J. L., Henry, C., Leboyer, M., & Schurhoff, F. (2001). Admixture analysis of age at onset in bipolar I affective disorder. *Archives of General Psychiatry, 58,* 510–512.

Biederman, J., Mick, E., Faraone, S. V., Spencer, T., Wilens, T. E., & Wozniak, J. (2003). Current concepts in the validity, diagnosis and treatment of paediatric bipolar disorder. *International Journal of Neuropsychopharmacology, 6,* 293–300.

Biederman, J., Mick, E., Wozniak, J., Monuteau, M. C., Galdo, M., & Faraone, S. V. (2003). Can a subtype of conduct disorder linked to bipolar disorder be identified? Integration of findings from the Massachusetts General Hospital Pediatric Psychopharmacology Research Program. *Biological Psychiatry, 53,* 952–960.

Brent, D. A., Perper, J. A., Goldstein, C. E., Kolko, D. J., Allan, M. J., Allman, G. J., et al. (1988). Risk factors for adolescent suicide: A comparison of adolescent suicide victims with suicidal inpatients. *Archives of General Psychiatry, 45,* 581–588.

Butzlaff, R. L., & Hooley, J. M. (1998). Expressed emotion and psychiatric relapse: A meta-analysis. *Archives of General Psychiatry, 55,* 547–552.

Carter, T. D., Mundo, E., Parikh, S. V., & Kennedy, J. L. (2003). Early age at onset as a risk factor for poor outcome of bipolar disorder. *Journal of Psychiatric Research, 37,* 297–303.

Chambers, W. J., Puig-Antich, J., Hirsch, M., Paez, P., Ambrosini, P. J., Tabrizi, M. A., et al. (1985). The assessment of affective disorders in children and adolescents by semi-structured interview: Test-retest reliability. *Archives of General Psychiatry, 42,* 696–702.

Chang, K., Adleman, N. E., Dienes, K., Simeonova, D. I., Menon, V., & Reiss, A. (2004). Anomalous prefrontal-subcortical activation in familial pediatric bipolar disorder: A functional magnetic resonance imaging investigation. *Archives of General Psychiatry, 61,* 781–792.

Chang, K. D., Blaser, C., Ketter, T. A., & Steiner, H. (2001). Family environment of children and adolescents with bipolar parents. *Bipolar Disorders, 3,* 73–78.

Chen, Y. W., & Dilsaver, S. C. (1996). Lifetime rates of suicide attempts among subjects with bipolar and unipolar disorders relative to subjects with other Axis I disorders. *Biological Psychiatry, 39,* 896–899.

Faedda, G. L., Baldessarini, R. J., Suppes, T., Tondo, L., Becker, I., & Lipschitz, D. S. (1995). Pediatric-onset bipolar disorder: A neglected clinical and public health problem. *Harvard Review of Psychiatry, 3,* 171–195.

Findling, R. L., Youngstrom, E. A., McNamara, N. K., Stansbrey, R. J., Demeter, C., Bedoya, D., et al. (2005). Early symptoms of mania and the role of parental risk. *Bipolar Disorders, 7,* 623–634.

Fristad, M. A., Gavazzi, S. M., & Mackinaw-Koons, B. (2003). Family psychoeducation: An adjunctive intervention for children with bipolar disorder. *Biological Psychiatry, 53,* 1000–1009.

Gallelli, K. A., Wagner, C. M., Karchemskiy, A., Howe, M., Spielman, D., Reiss, A., et al. (2005). N-acetylaspartate levels in bipolar offspring with and at high-risk for bipolar disorder. *Bipolar Disorders, 7,* 589–597.

Geller, B., Craney, J. L., Bolhofner, K., Nickelsburg, M. J., Williams, M., & Zimerman, B (2002): Two-year prospective follow-up of children with a prepubertal and early adolescent bipolar disorder phenotype. *American Journal of Psychiatry, 159,* 927–933.

Geller, B., Tillman, R., Craney, J. L., & Bolhofner, K. (2004). Four-year prospective outcome and natural history of mania in children with a prepubertal and early adolescent bipolar disorder phenotype. *Archives of General Psychiatry, 61,* 459–467.

Goldberg, J. F., Garno, J. L., & Harrow, M. (2005). Long-term remission and recovery in bipolar illness: A review. *Current Psychiatric Reports, 7,* 456–461.

Hammen, C. (1991). Generation of stress in the course of unipolar depression. *Journal of Abnormal Psychology, 100,* 555–561.

Hammen, C., & Gitlin, M. J. (1997). Stress reactivity in bipolar patients and its relation to prior history of the disorder. *American Journal of Psychiatry, 154,* 856–857.

Hashimoto, K., Shimizu, E., & Iyo, M. (2004). Critical role of brain-derived neurotrophic factor in mood disorders. *Brain Research Review, 45,* 104–114.

Hlastala, S. A., Frank, E., Kowalski, J., Sherrill, J. T., To, X. M., Anderson, B., et al. (2000). Stressful life events, bipolar disorder, and the "kindling model." *Journal of Abnormal Psychology, 109,* 777–786.

Honig, A., Hofman, A., Rozendaal, N., & Dingemanns, P. (1997). Psychoeducation in bipolar disorder: Effect on expressed emotion. *Psychiatry Research, 72,* 17–22.

Johnson, S. L. (2005). Life events in bipolar disorder: Towards more specific models. *Clinical Psychology Review, 25,* 1008–1027.

Josselyn Foundation. (2000). *In their own words: Teens with bipolar disorder* [Videotape]. Chicago: Author.

Kaufman, J., Birmaher, B., Brent, D., Rao, U., Flynn, C., Moreci, P., et al. (1997). Schedule for Affective Disorders and Schizophrenia for School-Age Children—Present and Lifetime Version (K-SADS-PL): Initial reliability and validity data. *Journal of the American Academy of Child and Adolescent Psychiatry, 36*, 980–988.

Keller, M. B. (2004). Improving the course of illness and promoting continuation of treatment of bipolar disorder. *Journal of Clinical Psychiatry, 65*, 10–14.

Kessler, R. C., Berglund, P., Demler, O., Jin, R., & Walters, E. E. (2005). Lifetime prevalence and age-of-onset distributions of DSM-IV disorders in the National Comorbidity Survey Replication. *Archives of General Psychiatry, 62*, 593–602.

Kleinman, L., Lowin, A., Flood, E., Gandhi, G., Edgell, E., & Revicki, D. (2003). Costs of bipolar disorder. *Pharmacoeconomics, 21*, 601–622.

Kochman, F. J., Hantouche, E. G., Ferrari, P., Lancrenon, S., Bayart, D., & Akiskal, H. S. (2005). Cyclothymic temperament as a prospective predictor of bipolarity and suicidality in children and adolescents with major depressive disorder. *Journal of Affective Disorders, 85*, 181–189.

Kowatch, R. A., Fristad, M., Birmaher, B., Wagner, K. D., Findling, R. L., Hellander, M., et al. (2005). Treatment guidelines for children and adolescents with bipolar disorder. *Journal of the American Academy of Child and Adolescent Psychiatry, 44*, 213–235.

Lam, D., Wright, K., & Sham, P. (2005). Sense of hyper-positive self and response to cognitive therapy in bipolar disorder. *Psychological Medicine, 35*, 69–77.

Leibenluft, E., Charney, D. S., Towbin, K. E., Bhangoo, R. K., & Pine, D. S. (2003). Defining clinical phenotypes of juvenile mania. *American Journal of Psychiatry, 160*, 430–437.

Leverich, G. S., Altshuler, L. L., Frye, M. A., Suppes, T., Keck, P. E., Jr., McElroy, S. L., et al. (2003). Factors associated with suicide attempts in 648 patients with bipolar disorder in the Stanley Foundation Bipolar Network. *Journal of Clinical Psychiatry, 64*, 506–515.

Leverich, G. S., McElroy, S. L., Suppes, T., Keck, P. E., Jr., Denicoff, K. D., Nolen, W. A., et al. (2002). Early physical and sexual abuse associated with an adverse course of bipolar illness. *Biological Psychiatry, 51*, 288–297.

Manji, H. K., & Duman, R. S. (2001). Impairments of neuroplasticity and cellular resilience in severe mood disorders: Implications for the development of novel therapeutics. *Psychopharmacology Bulletin, 35*, 5–49.

McClellan, J. (2005). Commentary: Treatment guidelines for child and adolescent bipolar disorder. *Journal of the American Academy of Child and Adolescent Psychiatry, 44*, 236–239.

Meyer, S. E., Carlson, G. A., Wiggs, E. A., Ronsqville, D. S., Martinez, P. E., Klimes-Douglan, B., et al. (2006). A prospective high-risk study of the association among maternal negativity, apparent frontal lobe dysfunction, and the development of bipolar disorder. *Development and Psychopathology, 18*, 573–589.

Miklowitz, D. J. (2006a). A review of evidence-based psychosocial interventions for bipolar disorder. *Journal of Clinical Psychiatry, 67*(Suppl. 11), 28–33.

Miklowitz, D. J. (2006b). *Family-focused treatment for bipolar adolescents* (National Institute of Mental Health Grant No. R01-MH073871). Unpublished manuscript.

Miklowitz, D. J., Biuckians, A., & Richards, J. A. (2006). Early-onset bipolar disorder: A family treatment perspective. *Development and Psychopathology, 18*, 1247–1265.

Miklowitz, D. J., & Chang, K. D. (in press). Prevention of bipolar disorder in at-risk children: Theoretical assumptions and empirical foundations. *Development and Psychopathology*.

Miklowitz, D. J., George, E. L., Axelson, D. A., Kim, E. Y., Birmaher, B., Schneck, C., et al. (2004). Family-focused treatment for adolescents with bipolar disorder. *Journal of Affective Disorders, 82*, 113–128.

Miklowitz, D. J., George, E. L., Richards, J. A., Simoneau, T. L., & Suddath, R. L. (2003). A randomized study of family-focused psychoeducation and pharmacotherapy in the outpatient management of bipolar disorder. *Archives of General Psychiatry, 60*, 904–912.

Miklowitz, D. J., & Goldstein, M. J. (1997). *Bipolar disorder: A family-focused treatment approach*. New York: Guilford Press.

Miklowitz, D. J., Goldstein, M. J., Nuechterlein, K. H., Snyder, K. S., & Mintz, J. (1988). Family factors and the course of bipolar affective disorder. *Archives of General Psychiatry, 45,* 225–231.

Miklowitz, D. J., & Johnson, S. L. (2006). The psychopathology and treatment of bipolar disorder. *Annual Review of Clinical Psychology, 2,* 199–235.

Miklowitz, D. J., & Otto, M. W. (2006). New psychosocial interventions for bipolar disorder: A review of literature and introduction of the Systematic Treatment Enhancement Program. *Journal of Cognitive Psychotherapy, 20,* 215–230.

Miklowitz, D. J., Otto, M. W., Frank, E., Reilly-Harrington, N. A., Wisniewski, S. R., Kogan, J. N., et al. (2006). Psychosocial treatments for bipolar depression: A 1-year randomized trial from the Systematic Treatment Enhancement Program. *Archives of General Psychiatry, 64,* 419–427.

Miklowitz, D. J., Richards, J. A., George, E. L., Frank, E., Suddath, R. L., Powell, K. B., et al. (2003). Integrated family and individual therapy for bipolar disorder: Results of a treatment development study. *Journal of Clinical Psychiatry, 64,* 182–191.

Miklowitz, D. J., Simoneau, T. L., George, E. L., Richards, J. A., Kalbag, A., Sachs-Ericsson, N., et al. (2000). Family-focused treatment of bipolar disorder: 1-year effects of a psychoeducational program in conjunction with pharmacotherapy. *Biological Psychiatry, 48,* 582–592.

Murray, C. J. L., & Lopez, A. D. (1996). *The global burden of disease: A comprehensive assessment of mortality and disability from diseases, injuries, and risk factors in 1990 and projected to 2020.* Boston: Harvard University Press.

National Institute of Mental Health. (2001). Research roundtable on prepubertal bipolar disorder. *Journal of the American Academy of Child and Adolescent Psychiatry, 40,* 871–878.

O'Connell, R. A., Mayo, J. A., Flatow, L., Cuthbertson, B., & O'Brien, B. E. (1991). Outcome of bipolar disorder on long-term treatment with lithium. *British Journal of Psychiatry, 159,* 123–129.

Otto, M. W., Reilly-Harrington, N., & Sachs, G. (2003). Psychoeducational and cognitive-behavioral strategies in the management of bipolar disorder. *Journal of Affective Disorders, 73,* 171–181.

Pavuluri, M. N., Graczyk, P. A., Henry, D. B., Carbray, J. A., Heidenreich, J., & Miklowitz, D. J. (2004). Child and family-focused cognitive behavioral therapy for pediatric bipolar disorder: development and preliminary results. *Journal of the American Academy of Child and Adolescent Psychiatry, 43,* 528–537.

Perlick, D. A., Hohenstein, J. M., Clarkin, J. F., Kaczynski, R., & Rosenheck, R. A. (2005). Use of mental health and primary care services by caregivers of patients with bipolar disorder: A preliminary study. *Bipolar Disorders, 7,* 126–135.

Perlis, R. H., Miyahara, S., Marangell, L. B., Wisniewski, S. R., Ostacher, M., DelBello, M. P., et al. (2004). Long-term implications of early onset in bipolar disorder: Data from the first 1000 participants in the systematic treatment enhancement program for bipolar disorder (STEP-BD). *Biological Psychiatry, 55,* 875–881.

Post, R. M. (1992). Transduction of psychosocial stress into the neurobiology of recurrent affective disorder. *American Journal of Psychiatry, 149,* 999–1010.

Post, R. M. (2002). Do the epilepsies, pain syndromes, and affective disorders share common kindling-like mechanisms? *Epilepsy Research, 50,* 203–219.

Post, R., & Kowatch, R. A. (2006). The health care crisis of childhood-onset bipolar illness: Some recommendations for its amelioration. *Journal of Clinical Psychiatry, 67,* 115–125.

Post, R. M., Leverich, G. S., Xing, G., & Weiss, R. B. (2001). Developmental vulnerabilities to the onset and course of bipolar disorder. *Developmental Psychopathology, 13,* 581–598.

Post, R. M., & Weiss, S. R. (1996). A speculative model of affective illness cyclicity based on patterns of drug tolerance observed in amygdala-kindled seizures. *Molecular Neurobiology, 13,* 33–60.

Rajkowska, G. (2000). Postmortem studies in mood disorders indicate altered numbers of neurons and glial cells. *Biological Psychiatry, 48,* 766–777.

Rajkowska, G., Halaris, A., & Selemon, L. D. (2001). Reductions in neuronal and glial density characterize the dorsolateral prefrontal cortex in bipolar disorder. *Biological Psychiatry, 49*, 741–752.

Rea, M. M., Tompson, M., Miklowitz, D. J., Goldstein, M. J., Hwang, S., & Mintz, J. (2003). Family focused treatment vs. individual treatment for bipolar disorder: Results of a randomized clinical trial. *Journal of Consulting and Clinical Psychology, 71*, 482–492.

Roy-Byrne, P., Post, R. M., Uhde, T. W., Porcu, T., & Davis, D. (1985): The longitudinal course of recurrent affective illness: Life chart data from research patients at the NIMH. *Acta Psychiatrica Scandinavica* (Suppl.), *317*, 1–34.

Scott, J., & Gutierrez, M. J. (2004). The current status of psychological treatments in bipolar disorders: A systematic review of relapse prevention. *Bipolar Disorders, 6*, 498–503.

Simoneau, T. L., Miklowitz, D. J., Richards, J. A., Saleem, R., & George, E. L. (1999). Bipolar disorder and family communication: Effects of a psychoeducational treatment program. *Journal of Abnormal Psychology, 108*, 588–597.

Snyder, D. K., Castellani, A. M., & Whisman, M. A. (2006). Current status and future directions in couple therapy. *Annual Review of Psychology, 57*, 314–344.

Strakowski, S. M., DelBello, M. P., Zimmerman, M. E., Getz, G. E., Mills, N. P., Ret, J., et al. (2002). Ventricular and periventricular structural volumes in first- versus multiple-episode bipolar disorder. *American Journal of Psychiatry, 159*, 1841–1847.

Turvey, C. L., Coryell, W. H., Solomon, D. A., Leon, A. C., Endicott, J., Keller, M. B., et al.(1999). Long-term prognosis of bipolar I disorder. *Acta Psychiatrica Scandinavica, 99*, 110–119.

Vieta, E., & Colom, F. (2004). Psychological interventions in bipolar disorder: From wishful thinking to an evidence-based approach. *Acta Psychiatrica Scandinavica* (Suppl.), *422*, 34–38.

Yan, L. J., Hammen, C., Cohen, A. N., Daley, S. E., & Henry, R. M. (2004). Expressed emotion versus relationship quality variables in the prediction of recurrence in bipolar patients. *Journal of Affective Disorders, 83*, 199–206.

CHAPTER 10

Psychoeducational
Psychotherapy

KRISTEN H. DAVIDSON *and* MARY A. FRISTAD

Psychoeducational psychotherapy for families of children with mood disorders addresses three main areas—education about the child's condition and its treatment, skill building to more effectively manage symptoms, and social support from other group members and clinical providers. Programs typically begin by forming a collaborative relationship between the therapeutic team and family members (Holder & Anderson, 1990) and may occur as a treatment for individual families or in the form of multifamily groups or workshops. Psychoeducation is an important model for intervention because it views psychiatric disorders from a "no fault" perspective (i.e., neither the patient nor the family is to blame). This approach helps to prevent family members from blaming and criticizing the patient and each other and allows them to work together to control and manage the patient's illness. One way that psychoeducation accomplishes this is by helping families recognize the separation between the individual and his or her symptoms (Fristad, Gavazzi, & Soldano, 1999). Family members are encouraged to "back off" to help the patient recuperate from his or her current episode and are also provided with support, validation, and recognition of the demands of living with a mentally ill family member. Family members are taught that patients are particularly vulnerable to stress and tension; thus therapists work with families to reduce the level of stress and tension in their homes. Therapists also emphasize the importance of setting limits in a matter-of-fact rather than a critical or hostile way (McFarlane, 1991). A unique aspect of psychoeducational interventions is that they are often used as adjuncts to other therapies (e.g., medication or individual psychotherapy).

In this chapter, we briefly review the origins of psychoeducational psychotherapy as a treatment for adults with schizophrenia and its recent adaptation for use in families of children with mood disorders. We also address evidence regarding the effectiveness of this form of treatment within these populations. We conclude with a discussion of the need for future research and the applications of psychoeducational psychotherapy for treating other childhood mental illness.

ORIGINS OF
PSYCHOEDUCATIONAL PSYCHOTHERAPY

Psychoeducational psychotherapy was first applied to patients with schizophrenia who came from families with high levels of expressed emotion (EE; Hogarty, Anderson, Reiss, & Kornbluth, 1991; see Table 10.1). The concept of EE emerged from a series of studies that found that critical comments, hostility, and emotional overinvolvement (i.e., high EE) predicted higher relapse rates in adults with schizophrenia (Brown, Birley, & Wing, 1972; Brown, Carstairs, & Topping, 1958; Brown, Monck, Carstairs, & Wing, 1962). As high EE is associated with relapse, it follows that lowering EE in families might improve the course of illness for patients and their families. With this in mind, Hogarty and colleagues investigated the impact of family psychoeducation on relapse rates for patients with schizophrenia. They found that after 2 years of treatment, patients with schizophrenia in the psychoeducation-plus-medication group had significantly lower relapse rates compared with the medication-only group (34 vs. 66%, respectively; Hogarty et al., 1991).

Recent studies have demonstrated that EE plays a similar role in families of adults with mood disorders (Hooley, 1998; Hooley, Orley, & Teasdale, 1986; Koenig, Sachs-Ericsson, & Miklowitz, 1997; Miklowitz, Goldstein, Nuechterlein, Snyder, & Mintz, 1988; Simoneau, Miklowitz, & Saleem, 1998), and several research groups have found psychoeducational interventions also to be effective in reducing relapse rates in adults with bipolar disorder. Colom et al. (2003) found lower relapse rates in participants receiving group psychoeducation compared with nonstructured group therapy, both during the acute treatment phase (38% relapse vs. 60%, respectively) and at 2-year follow-up (67% vs. 92%). Using an individual family format, Miklowitz and colleagues have found that psychoeducational treatments reduce relapse rates in adults with bipolar disorder (Miklowitz &

TABLE 10.1. Psychoeducational Studies in Adults

Authors	n	Age	Design	Diagnostic tools	Therapy manual type	Diagnoses	Outcome measures	Outcome statistics
Miklowitz & Goldstein (1990)	9 patients receiving treatment compared with 23 historical controls receiving TAU	Adults recently discharged from an inpatient unit	Open trial	Diagnosis of mania from inpatient stay	BFM and appropriate pharmacotherapy	Mania	Relapse	Lower relapse for patients in BFM group compared with patients from naturalistic outcome study (11% vs. 61%)
Hogarty et al. (1991)	108	Adult inpatients	All on medication. Random assignment to 1 of 4 psychotherapy conditions	RDC criteria	FT, SST, FT + SST, supportive therapy	Schizophrenia	Relapse	FT forestalls relapse by 2 years; SST does not
Honig et al. (1997)	52	Mean age of patients in treatment group = 43.8 years (SD = 13.0), for relatives, 47.1 years (SD = 13.7)	Wait-list control	Patients met DSM-IV criteria based on information from referring psychiatrist, medical record, and information gathered from family members	Group psychoeducation	BPD	FMSS	Significant decrease in level of EE for participants in the treatment group compared with the control group ($p < .03$)

Study	N	Age	Design	Assessment	Intervention	Diagnosis	Measures	Results
Colom et al. (2003)	120	18–65 years	Parallel two-group randomized single-blind trial	Lifetime diagnosis of BP-I or II by a trained psychiatrist	21-session group psychoeducation	BP-I BP-II	# of recurrences Time to recurrence Hospitalizations	Members of treatment group had fewer recurrences of manic/hypomanic episodes (log rank$_1$ = 7.79, $p < .006$) and depressive episodes (log rank$_1$ = 15.47, $p < .001$)
Miklowitz et al. (2003)	100	18–60 years	Open trial	SCID-P	IFIT	BP-I BP-II	Relapse Mood symptoms	Patients in IFIT had longer survival intervals until relapse compared with controls (42.5 vs. 34.5 weeks; χ^2 = 5.63, $p < .02$). IFIT patients had a greater decrease in depressive symptoms at 1 year (F = 5.44, $p < .0001$)

Note. TAU, treatment as usual; BPD, bipolar disorder; BP-I, bipolar I disorder; BP-II, bipolar II disorder; FMSS, 5-minute speech sample; EE, expressed emotion; SCID-P, Structured Clinical Interview for DSM-IV—Patient Version; IFIT, integrated family and individual therapy; RDC, research diagnostic criteria; BFM, behavioral family management; FT, family psychoeducation/management; SST, social skills training.

Goldstein, 1990: 11% relapse vs. 61% relapse in a 9-month period; Miklowitz et al., 2003: delays relapse by 21 weeks). Psychoeducation is also associated with high patient retention rates (Miklowitz, Goldstein, & Nuechterlein, 1995) and reduction of EE in relatives of bipolar patients (Honig, Hofman, Rozendaal, & Dingemanns, 1997). Specifically, Honig and colleagues found that 31% of relatives in the psychoeducation group moved from high-EE to low-EE status compared with 0% change in status for relatives in the wait-list control group.

PSYCHOEDUCATIONAL PSYCHOTHERAPY IN CHILDREN AND ADOLESCENTS

High EE levels in the family have been linked to symptom presentation, recovery, and relapse rates in children with mood disorders (Asarnow, Tompson, Hamilton, Goldstein, & Guthrie, 1994; Asarnow, Tompson, Woo, & Cantwell, 2000; Geller et al., 2003). Asarnow and colleagues found that high EE was related to a more insidious onset of major depressive disorder (MDD) and a slower course of recovery in children with depression. Similarly, in a sample of children and adolescents with BPD, Geller et al. (2003) found that relapse rates were 4.1 times more likely at 2-year follow up in families with low maternal–child warmth compared with those with high maternal–child warmth. These results were maintained at the 4-year follow-up, in which it was estimated that 85.9% of participants with low maternal warmth relapsed compared with 50.3% of patients with high maternal warmth (Geller, Tillman, Craney, & Bolhofner, 2004). Despite this evidence of the role of EE in families of children with mood disorders and the indication from the adult literature that psychoeducation reduces EE in families, examination of psychoeducation with families of mood-impaired children and adolescents has not reached the same level of empirical sophistication as studies in the adult population.

To date, four groups have investigated psychoeducational interventions for families of children with mood disorders (see Table 10.2). Of these, only one has conducted randomized clinical trials. Brent, Poling, McKain, and Baugher (1993) found that as a result of attending a 2-hour workshop, parents of adolescents with mood disorders significantly increased their knowledge and modified some dysfunctional beliefs about depression. Miklowitz and colleagues (2004) piloted an adolescent version of their functional family therapy (FFT), which includes psychoeducation and skill building, in an open trial with 20 adolescents diagnosed with bipolar disorder and their families. They found decreased ratings of depression and mania on the K-SADS, as well as lower scores on the Child Behavior Checklist (CBCL) Behavior Problems Scale following intervention.

Drawing from FFT, Pavuluri and colleagues (2004) created child- and

TABLE 10.2. Psychoeducational Studies in Children

Authors	n	Age	Design	Diagnostic tools	Therapy manual type	Diagnoses	Outcome measures	Outcome statistics
Brent et al. (1993)	62 parents of 34 teens	Mean age = 15.4 years	Open trial, no control group	Chart review	2-hour workshop	MDD, DD, BP-I, BP-II, cyclothymia, atypical affective disorder	Parental beliefs and knowledge about depression	Parents demonstrated increased knowledge about depression and modification of dysfunctional beliefs
Miklowitz et al. (2004)	20	13–17 years	Open trial, no control group	K-SADS	1 year of FFT-A	BP-I, BP-II, BP-NOS	K-SADS CBCL	38% improvement in K-SADS scores at 12 months (Cohen's $d = .65$). 46% improvement on mania subscale (Cohen's $d = .79$) Reduction in CBCL scores at 12 months (Cohen's $d = 1.7$)
Pavuluri et al. (2004)	34	5–17 years	Open trial, no control group	K-SADS	12-session RAINBOW program	BPD	Feasibility (treatment integrity, adherence to psychotherapy, consumer satisfaction) CGI-BP CGAS	Reduction of symptoms of mania ($t_{33} = 12.83$, $p < .0001$) and depression $t_{33} = 5.38$, $p < .0001$)

(continued)

TABLE 10.2. (continued)

Authors	n	Age	Design	Diagnostic tools	Therapy manual type	Diagnoses	Outcome measures	Outcome statistics
Fristad, Goldberg-Arnold, & Gavazzi (2002) Fristad, Goldberg-Arnold, & Gavazzi (2003)	35	8–12 years	RCT	ChIPS MRS CDRS-R	6-session MFPG	MDD, DD, BP-I, BP-II	UMDQ Social support Qualitative analysis of parent report	Immediate treatment group showed more knowledge about follow-up, $F(1,28) = 7.85$, $p < .009$, and more positive family interactions, $F(1,26) = 4.09$, $p < .05$
Fristad (2006)	165	8–12 years	RCT	ChIPS MRS CDRS-R	8-session MFPG	BP-I	Mood Severity Index Rage Index	Treatment group had lower mood severity at 6 and 12 months ($\chi^2 = 6.19$, $p < .02$)
Fristad (2006)	20	8–12 years	RCT	ChIPS MRS CDRS-R	16-session IFP	BP-I, BP-II, BP-NOS	Mood Severity Index Qualitative analysis of parent report	Children in treatment group had improved mood at 6- and 12-month follow-up (ES = .45 and .60, respectively)

Note. RCT, randomized controlled trial; K-SADS, Kiddie Schedule for Affective Disorders and Schizophrenia for School-Age Children; ChIPS, Children's Interview for Psychiatric Syndromes; MRS, Mania Rating Scale; CDRS-R, Child Depression Rating Scale—Revised; FFT-A, functional family therapy for adolescents; MFPG, multifamily psychoeducation groups; IFP, individual family psychoeducation; BPD, bipolar disorder; BP-I, bipolar I disorder; BP-II, bipolar II disorder; BP-NOS, bipolar disorder not otherwise specified; MDD, major depressive disorder; DD, dysthymic disorder; CBCL, Child Behavior Checklist; CGI-BP, Clinical Global Impression Scales for Bipolar Disorder; CGAS, Children's Global Assessment Scale; UMDQ, Understanding Mood Disorders Questionnaire; ES, effect size.

family-focused cognitive-behavioral therapy (CFF–CBT), also known as the RAINBOW program, as an adjunct to medication for children with bipolar disorder. This 12-session treatment program consisted of three phases. Goals of the first phase were to build a therapeutic alliance and to provide psychoeducation about mood disorders and the use of medication. The second phase focused on acquisition of cognitive-behavioral skills such as affect regulation, positive self-talk, reframing negative thoughts, and problem solving. In the third phase, emphasis was placed on social skills and parental support. The RAINBOW program was administered individually to families, which allowed the treatment to be tailored to each family's needs. A unique aspect of the RAINBOW program is the inclusion of the patients' siblings in treatment, which provided them with the opportunity to learn coping strategies for managing their own difficulties and dealing with the stressors associated with their sibling's illness.

In an exploratory investigation of this program, 34 youths ages 5–17 with bipolar disorder received specialty clinic medication management plus psychoeducational intervention. Results indicated that participants had significantly lower bipolar symptom severity and increased global functioning. Results also supported the feasibility of implementing this program and suggested high levels of participant satisfaction. Limitations included the lack of a control group and the fact that experimenters were not blind to treatment status. Thus, although the RAINBOW program showed promising results, future research is needed to establish its efficacy through randomized controlled trials. In addition, the pilot study was implemented with a wide age range of youths with bipolar disorder. Because symptom presentation and treatment needs differ based on the child's age and developmental level, further consideration is needed regarding the age range for which this treatment has been developed.

MULTIFAMILY PSYCHOEDUCATION GROUPS

As reviewed herein, psychoeducation has been shown to have many positive outcomes for adults with schizophrenia and mood disorders. Although a handful of programs have also been developed for families of children with mood disorders, conclusions regarding their efficacy are limited by methodological constraints. To improve the availability of family-focused treatment for children with bipolar disorder, our research group has developed and empirically validated multifamily psychoeducation group therapy (MFPG) as an effective treatment modality. To date, two randomized controlled trials (RCTs) have been implemented—a pilot study ($n = 35$; Fristad, Goldberg-Arnold, & Gavazzi, 2002; Fristad, Gavazzi, & Mackinaw-Koons, 2003; Fristad, Goldberg-Arnold, & Gavazzi, 2003) and a large-scale ($n = 165$) randomized control study on MFPG (Fristad, 2006). In this section, we briefly review the goals and content of MFPG and discuss research findings.

The MFPG treatment program was designed to be an *adjunctive* intervention for families of children ages 8–12. Therefore, children who are enrolled are often receiving concurrent mental health counseling and medication management from providers in the community, in addition to support services at school. Given the family component, we require that at least one parent or caregiver (preferably two, if available, or more, in the case of stepparents from two households) participate in the program along with their child. Groups are led by trained mental health professionals (i.e., clinical psychologists, licensed independent social workers). Though parents and children participate in separate groups, each session begins and ends with a family component. During the middle portion of each group, when parents and children meet separately, the content of children's and parents' sessions is thematically connected. Typically, parent groups are run by one leader, whereas child groups have two leaders, with the second child leader assisting with behavioral management of the group.

The main goals of MFPG are to provide parents and children with social support, information about the etiology and treatment of mood disorders, and skill building (i.e., communication skills, problem-solving skills, symptom management skills). During child groups there are opportunities for *in vivo* social skills training. Parents and children complete weekly home activity projects to practice the skills learned during that week (for specific information on group content and activities, see Davidson & Fristad, 2008; Fristad & Goldberg-Arnold, 2003; Goldberg-Arnold & Fristad, 2003). Thus far, we have implemented these groups in a medical center setting, though they likely can be easily transferred to other settings as well.

MFPG Pilot Randomized Controlled Trial

The MFPG pilot study included 35 children (ages 8–11) with major mood disorders and 47 of their parents (14 fathers, 33 mothers). Primary mood disorder diagnoses included: major depressive disorder ($n = 13$; 37%); dysthymic disorder ($n = 6$; 17%); bipolar I disorder ($n = 5$; 14%); and bipolar II disorder ($n = 11$; 31%). As MFPG is designed to be an adjunctive treatment, all families were encouraged to continue treatment-as-usual (TAU) during the study. Eighteen families were enrolled immediately into a six-session MFPG (IMM +TAU) condition. Seventeen families were enrolled into a 6-month wait-list condition (WLC + TAU), after which they received MFPG. Four assessments were conducted: time 1 (T1) at baseline; T2, 2 months after study enrollment (post-MFPG for IMM); T3, 6 months after study enrollment (pre-MFPG for WLC); and T4 for the WLC only, post-MFPG.

Results indicated that participation in MFPG led to gains in several areas. Specifically, parents in the immediate-treatment (IMM) group demonstrated significantly greater knowledge about mood disorders than wait-list (WLC) families immediately after treatment and at the 6-month follow-up (Fristad, Gavazzi, & Mackinaw-Koons, 2003). In addition, parents reported multiple benefits of having participated in treatment, including increased knowledge about mood disorders, increased social support, attitude changes, and acquisition of coping skills. Parents in the IMM group also reported an improvement in their ability to obtain appropriate services compared with parents in the WLC group (82% vs. 20%, respectively). Children in the IMM group reported a significant gain in perceived social support from their parents compared with children in the WLC group (Fristad, Goldberg-Arnold, & Gavazzi, 2003).

This study had several significant methodological constraints. First, the sample size was small, limiting the power to find significant results. Second, the use of a 6-month wait-list control meant that T1 and T3 assessments occurred at different times of the year (e.g., if T1 occurred during the summer, a relatively low-stress time, T3 would occur in the middle of the school year, a higher stress time). Third, interviewers were not consistently masked to group status. These methodological constraints were addressed in the large-scale MFPG study, which is described in greater detail in the next section.

Following study completion, a number of changes were made to the content and delivery of the MFPG program after reviewing anonymous posttreatment feedback from parents and children, reviewing transcripts of group sessions for fidelity and integrity of treatment delivery, and conducting a focus group of study participants and community mental health leaders. Based on this review, the number of sessions was increased from six to eight to allow more time for skill building and to increase the amount of information provided regarding working with school personnel and mental health professionals. Session lengths were increased from 75 to 90 minutes to allow greater time for discussion. Finally, the utilization of family projects within the MFPG program was increased.

MFPG Large-Scale Randomized Controlled Trial

As mentioned, several changes were made to the MFPG protocol based on the pilot study. A NIMH grant (MH61512, 5/1/01–4/30/07; PI: Mary A. Fristad; Fristad, 2006) allowed us to further assess the efficacy of the extended MFPG in 165 children ages 8–11 with mood disorders and their primary and secondary parents. Seventy-eight families were randomized into immediate treatment and 87 families into a 1-year wait-list condition. Four assessments were conducted over 18 months: baseline (T1), 6 months (T2), 12 months (T3), and 18 months (T4).

In its current format, MFPG consists of eight 90-minute sessions for children with bipolar and depressive spectrum illnesses and their parents (Fristad, Gavazzi, & Mackinaw-Koons, 2003). Each session begins with a brief "check-in" meeting of parents and children, during which the previous week's projects are discussed, except at week 1, when introductions are made. Children and parents then go to their respective groups and discuss that particular session's topics. One therapist leads the parent group, and a therapist and cotherapist lead the child group. The final 15–20 minutes of the children's session is spent in *in vivo* social skills training, in which children engage in recreational activities and noncompetitive group games to foster appropriate social interactions, develop friendships, and further extend the "lesson" of the day. Each session ends with the children rejoining the parent group, in which they explain their session's topic and discuss that particular week's family projects.

The session outlines for parent and child groups are shown in Table 10.3. Initial sessions are more didactic in nature. In these sessions, families learn about manic and depressive symptoms and comorbid conditions, how to differentiate the child from his or her symptoms using the "naming the enemy" exercise (Fristad et al., 1999), and medications and side-effect management. Families then set unique treatment goals for themselves. Next, parents learn about mental health, school, and community-based treatment teams and services as well as how to advocate for their child and work effectively with service care providers. Parent treatment then shifts to skill building with focus on communication and problem solving. Children's sessions address affect regulation and basic cognitive-behavioral principles, problem solving, and communication skills.

TABLE 10.3. The Eight-Session Outline of MFPG Parent and Child Groups

Session	Parent group	Child group
1	Learn about symptoms and disorders	Learn about symptoms and disorders
2	Learn about medications	Learn about medications
3	Learn about systems, school, and treatment teams	Develop a "tool kit" to manage emotions
4	Learn about the negative family cycle and wrap up first half of program	Learn the connection between thoughts, feelings, and actions (responsibility/choices)
5	Improve coping skills—problem solving	Improve problem-solving skills
6	Improve coping skills—communication	Improve nonverbal communication skills
7	Improve coping skills—symptom management	Improve verbal communication skills
8	Wrap up second half of program, graduate	Review and graduate

For the large-scale study, 225 families were screened via telephone. Of those, 203 (90%) passed the screen, and 171 (84%) arrived at the baseline assessment. Of those who completed the baseline assessment, 165 (96%) met study criteria. Referral sources included health care providers (62%), media (19%), and other means (i.e., library posters, word of mouth; 19%). Of the total sample, 115 (70%) met criteria for a bipolar spectrum disorder (bipolar disorder-I, bipolar disorder-II, cyclothymia, bipolar disorder not otherwise specified). Of these, 55 were randomly assigned to the immediate treatment group and 60 to the wait-list group.

Within the subset of families whose children had bipolar disorder, 16.5% of families were from rural or geographically remote (i.e., families traveled more than 50 miles each way to participate) areas, with the average round trip for these families being 70 miles (range, 14–344). Children were, on average, 9.8 years of age (study criteria required them to be ages 8–11 at study entry). A majority were boys (72%), white (91%), and from two-parent (including stepparent) families (65%). Family history of mood disorders was high, with 53% endorsing bipolar disorder in first- or second-degree relatives; 73%, depression; and 84%, depression and/or bipolar disorder. Cormorbidity was high for anxiety disorders (70%), attention-deficit/hyperactivity disorder (ADHD) (80%) and any behavior disorder (i.e., ADHD, oppositional defiant disorder, and/or conduct disorder, 95%). The immediate-treatment and 1-year wait-list control groups did not differ significantly on any demographic variables.

Two main outcome measures are the Mood Severity Index (MSI) and the Rage Index. The MSI combines participant scores on the Children's Depression Rating Scale—Revised (CDRS-R) and the Mania Rating Scale (MRS), giving equal weight to each. The MSI is calculated using the following equation: (CDRS-R score $-$ 17 $\times$ 11/17) + MRS. The Rage Index is the summation of the MRS Irritability and Disruptive–Aggressive items. This measure was chosen because irritability and aggression are associated with significant functional impairment across spheres of home, school, and peers for children with mood disorders. Using linear mixed-effects modeling, children who received MFPG had decreased MSI scores at 6 and 12 months compared with the wait-list children ($\chi^2 = 6.19$, $p < .02$), with MSI score differences of 3.9/6 months (Fristad, 2006). Similar differences were noted between groups on the Rage Index ($\chi^2 = 13.21$, $p < .002$), with scores differing 2 points, on average, per each 6-month interval.

INDIVIDUAL FAMILY PSYCHOEDUCATION

The results of the pilot and large-scale MFPG studies support its efficacy for increasing parents' and children's social support and knowledge about mood disorders and for reducing children's mood symptoms. However, limitations to the group format as described here led us to develop a more individualized treatment protocol, individual family psychoeducation (IFP). First, for many community-based providers, especially those in geographically remote areas, the low-base rate of bipolar disorder is not conducive to conducting group treatment. Second, MFPG groups are closed groups (i.e., new members cannot be added once the group has started); therefore, families of children who are newly diagnosed during the middle of a group cycle may have to wait longer than would be ideal to participate in treatment. An individualized treatment allows the patient's treatment needs to be met in a timely manner. Finally, some families may be uncomfortable about sharing personal information in a group setting and prefer to discuss their clinical concerns in the privacy of a one-on-one relationship with their therapist. Given these concerns, IFP was designed to be an individualized version of MFPG for families of children with bipolar disorder. As it was initially designed, IFP contained sixteen 50-minute sessions, altering between parent-only sessions and child-only sessions (with parent check-in at the beginning; see Table 10.4). Within the framework of IFP, 15 sessions were designed to address a specific topic related to bipolar disorder, and one "in the bank" session was available for use at any time to address crises and/or review previous material. Methodology and results from the pilot RCT of IFP are described in the following section. In addition, we have recently extended IFP to include 24 sessions and are currently conducting a pilot study, which is described in greater detail in the next section.

16-Session IFP Pilot RCT

A pilot study of the efficacy of IFP in 20 children with bipolar disorder and their parents was funded by the Ohio Department of Mental Health (6/1/02–6/30/04; PI: Mary A. Fristad; Fristad, 2006). The methodology used in the IFP pilot was similar to that of the MFPG NIMH study, though assessments were less extensive and data were collected only from primary informants. Of the 20 families enrolled in the study, 10 were randomized to immediate IFP + TAU (IMM) and the other 10 into a 12-month wait-list control group (WLC + TAU). The families in the wait-list group participated in IFP after 1-year. As with MFPG, four assessments occurred over an 18-month period. IFP therapists included two clinical psychology postdoctoral study coordinators and one clinical psychology doctoral candidate who also served as a parent advocate for the Child and Adolescent Bipolar Foundation (CABF).

Thirty-four families with children ages 8–11 were screened for participation within a 6-month period. Of these, 28 (82%) passed the screen and came to the baseline assessment. Of these, 20 (71%) met study inclusion criteria. Recruitment resources included psychologists (40%), media (35%), psychiatrists (10%), school counselors (5%), library posters (5%), and the

TABLE 10.4. The 16 Sessions of IFP

Session	Who attends	Session content
1	Parent and child	Overview of IFP; depression, mania, and other symptoms
2	Parent only	Specifics about symptoms and diagnoses
3	Parent and child	Child's medications
4	Parent only	All about medications
5	Parent and child	Taking charge of the mad, bad, sad feelings
6	Parent only	Treatment and education teams
7	Parent and child	The relationship of thoughts, feelings, and behaviors
8	Parent only	Family conflicts
9	Parent and child	Problem solving for child
10	Parent only	Problem solving for parents
11	Parent and child	Healthy habits—sleep, diet, and exercise
12	Parent only	Improving communication
13	Parent and child	Nonverbal communication, feelings, and verbal communication
14	Parent only	Crisis management and family issues, review previous sessions, and discuss how to handle future problems
15	Parent and child	With child, review previous sessions and how to handle future problems; chip bank; and graduation
16	Parent and child	An "in the bank" extra session to be used at any time during treatment at the family's request to manage crises or focus more intensively on a specific problem area (e.g., school programming)

MFPG study (5%). Most children were male (85%), Caucasian (90%), and came from two-parent (including stepparent) families (65%). Incomes were equally distributed, with 20% below $39,000, 40% between $40,000 and $79,000, and 40% over $80,000. Many families (40%) traveled from rural or geographically remote areas to participate (average round trip: $M + SD =$ 70 miles ± 70 miles, range 14–344 miles).

Primary mood disorder diagnoses included: bipolar I disorder (40%: 10% manic; 30% mixed); bipolar II disorder (35%); and bipolar disorder not otherwise specified (BP-NOS: 25%). Children were, on average, impaired for a considerable length of time (manic episode, $M = 482.2$ days, $SD = 880.2$; major depressive disorder [MDD], $M = 73.5$ weeks, $SD = 121.8$; and dysthymic disorder [DD], $M = 85.3$ weeks, $SD = 145.7$). Family history was significant for bipolar disorder. Deleting from the analyses one adopted child for whom family history data were unattainable, 53% of children had first- and/or second-degree relatives with bipolar disorder; 79% had first- and/or second-degree relatives with depressive disorders; and 84% had first- and/or second-degree relatives with bipolar disorder and/or depressive disorders.

The sample size was small to begin with, and difficulties with participant retention further lowered the power to detect significant results. Seven families dropped out before study completion. Of four IMM families, two completed treatment, two did not; and of three WLC families, none completed treatment. Study dropouts were not statistically different from study completers on relevant baseline variables. Results revealed that children who participated in IFP showed improvement in their mood immediately following treatment and that the improvement continued for 12 months posttreatment. Though results were not statistically significant due to the small sample size and subsequent low power, power calculations (Cohen, 1988) using $\alpha = .05$ and power $= .80$ indicate that from baseline to 6 months an effect size of .45 was detected. From baseline to 12 months, an effect size of .60 was detected (see Fristad, 2006).

Other positive changes noted as a result of participation in IFP include reduced levels of EE and improved service utilization in IMM families compared with WLC families. Again, due to low sample size and limited power, these results were not statically significant. Although the initial results of IFP appear to be positive, further evaluation in a larger sample is warranted.

Qualitative analysis of parent and child reports indicated that reviews of IFP were positive and that participants were satisfied with the treatment. Parents reported that attending sessions helped them better understand their child's symptoms and treatment needs and feel less guilty about their child's difficulties. Children also reported better understanding of their symptoms and treatment needs, as well as feeling that sessions helped them learn ways to get along better at home and school. Both parents and children reported feeling comfortable sharing personal information and feeling supported by the therapist (Fristad, 2006).

24-Session IFP Pilot Randomized Controlled Trial

Our research group is currently conducting a pilot study on an extended 24-session IFP protocol that equalizes the amount of therapist contact time between MFPG and IFP. IFP-24 includes 20 set sessions and 4 "in the bank" sessions, as outlined in Table 10.5. The study is nearly complete. Although outcome data are still being collected, it appears that the session format is acceptable to families. In their final wrap-up session, parents and children are both asked to write "words of wisdom" for families who will receive treatment at a later date. In our IFP-24 pilot study, sample words of wisdom from parents include "Take a break when you need it, parents need time for themselves to regroup. . . . Don't be embarrassed, it's no one's fault. . . . Focus on the good things about your child," and children's words of wisdom include our motto, "It's not your fault but it's your challenge."

TABLE 10.5. Session Content for IFP-24

Session	Who attends	Session content
1	Parent and child	Overview of IFP, goals
2	Parent and child	Depression, mania, and other symptoms
3	Child only	Self vs. symptoms, medication side effects
4	Parent only	Medications
5	Child only	Tracking health habits
6	Parent only	Mental health services
7	Child only	Feelings and triggers, tool kit, taking charge of mad, sad, bad feelings
8	Parent only	Negative family cycles; thinking, feeling, doing
9	Child only	Thinking, feeling, doing
10	Parent only	Problem solving for parents
11	Child only	Problem-solving skills
12	Parent only	School services
13	Child only	Review healthy habits
14	Parent only	School professionals
15	Child only	Nonverbal communication
16	Parent and child	Communication
17	Child only	Verbal communication
18	Parent only	Symptom management
19	Sibling(s)	Sibling session
20	Parent and child	Wrap up, graduation

SUMMARY

The goal of psychoeducational psychotherapy is to increase knowledge about a disorder, improve family relationships, and decrease patient relapse rates. A number of psychoeducational treatments have been developed and empirically validated for adults with schizophrenia and bipolar disorder. Although treatments have also been developed to address childhood mood disorders, investigation of the efficacy of these treatments has not reached the same level of methodological sophistication as adult studies. To date, our research team has completed testing of two forms of psychoeducational psychotherapy: a group-based intervention, MFPG, in 165 children with mood disorders and a pilot individual family psychoeducation, IFP, in 20 children with bipolar disorder. These two clinical trials suggest that a combination of support, psychoeducation, and skill building is effective in: (1) reducing mood symptom severity; (2) improving family climate; (3) improving global functioning; (4) reducing irritability and aggression; and (5) improving treatment utilization. Both MFPG and IFP are well received by parents and children. Although MFPG offers the advantage of social support from adult and child peers, it will probably not be feasible to offer except in larger clinic settings; therefore, a large number of children and families will be deprived of this specialized care. IFP, on the other hand, is more readily provided regardless of community size, location, or treatment facility available for care. A more rigorous evaluation of IFP's efficacy and documentation of variables that mediate and moderate treatment outcome is warranted.

REFERENCES

Asarnow, J. R., Tompson, M., Hamilton, E. B., Goldstein, M. J., & Guthrie D. (1994). Family expressed emotion, childhood-onset depression, and childhood-onset schizophrenia spectrum disorders: Is expressed emotion a nonspecific correlate of child psychopathology or a specific risk factor for depression? *Journal of Abnormal Child Psychology, 22*(2), 129–146.

Asarnow, J. R., Tompson, M. C., Woo, S. M., & Cantwell, D. (2000). Is family expressed emotion a specific risk factor for depression in youth or a nonspecific correlate of youth psychopathology? *Journal of Abnormal Child Psychology, 29,* 573–583.

Brent, D. A., Poling, K., McKain, B., & Baugher, M. (1993). A psychoeducational program for families of affectively ill children and adolescents. *Journal of the American Academy of Child and Adolescent Psychiatry, 32*(4), 770–774.

Brown, G. W., Birley, J. L., & Wing, J. K. (1972). Influence of family life on the course of schizophrenic disorders: A replication. *British Journal of Psychiatry, 121*(562), 241–258.

Brown, G. W., Carstairs, G. M., & Topping, G. (1958). Post hospital adjustment of chronic mental patients. *Lancet, 2,* 685–689.

Brown, G. W., Monck, E. M., Carstairs, G. M., & Wing, J. K. (1962). Influence of family life on the course of schizophrenic illness. *British Journal of Preventive and Social Medicine, 16,* 55–68.

Cohen, J. (1988). *Statistical power analysis for the behavioral sciences.* Hillsdale, NJ: Erlbaum.

Colom, F., Vieta, E., Martínez-Arán, A., Reinares, M., Goikolea, J. M., Benabarre, A., et al. (2003). A randomized trial on the efficacy of group psychoeducation in the prophylaxis of recurrences in bipolar patients whose disease is in remission. *Archives of General Psychiatry, 60,* 402–407.

Davidson, K. H., & Fristad, M. A. (2008). Moodiness. In A. Eisen (Ed.), *Clinical handbook of childhood behavior problems.* New York: Guilford Press.

Fristad, M. A. (2006). Psychoeducational treatment for school-aged children with bipolar disorder. *Development and Psychopathology, 18,* 1289–1306.

Fristad, M. A., Gavazzi, S. M., & Mackinaw-Koons, B. (2003). Family psychoeducation: An adjunctive intervention for children with bipolar disorder. *Biological Psychiatry, 53*(11), 1000–1008.

Fristad, M. A., Gavazzi, S. M., & Soldano, K. W. (1999). Naming the enemy: Learning to differentiate mood disorder "symptoms" from the "self" that experiences them. *Journal of Family Psychotherapy, 10*(1), 81–88.

Fristad, M. A., & Goldberg-Arnold, J. S. (2003). Family interventions for early-onset bipolar disorder. In B. Geller & M. P. DelBello (Eds.), *Bipolar disorder in childhood and early adolescence* (pp. 295–313). New York: Guilford Press.

Fristad, M. A., Goldberg-Arnold, J. S., & Gavazzi, S. M. (2002). Multifamily psychoeducation groups (MFPG) for families of children with bipolar disorder. *Bipolar Disorder, 4*(4), 254–262.

Fristad, M. A., Goldberg-Arnold, J. S., & Gavazzi, S. M. (2003). Multifamily psychoeducation groups (MFPG) in the treatment of children with mood disorders. *Journal of Marital and Family Therapy, 29*(4), 491–504.

Geller, B., Craney, J. L., Bolhofner, K., DelBello, M. P., Axelson, D., & Luby, J. (2003). Phenomenology and longitudinal course of children with a prepubertal and early adolescent bipolar disorder phenotype. In B. Geller & M. P. DelBello (Eds.), *Bipolar disorder in childhood and early adolescence* (pp. 25–50). New York: Guilford Press.

Geller, B., Tillman, R., Craney, J. L., & Bolhofner, K. (2004). Four-year prospective outcome and natural history of mania in children with a prepubertal and early adolescent bipolar disorder phenotype. *Archives of General Psychiatry, 61,* 459–467.

Goldberg-Arnold, J. S., & Fristad, M A. (2003). Psychotherapy with children diagnosed with early-onset bipolar disorder. In B. Geller & M. DelBello (Eds.), *Bipolar disorder in childhood and early adolescence* (pp. 272–294). New York: Guilford Press.

Hogarty, G. E., Anderson, C. M., Reiss, D. J., & Kornbluth, S. J. (1991). Family psychoeducation, social skills training, and maintenance chemotherapy in the aftercare treatment of schizophrenia: II. Two-year effects of a controlled study on relapse and adjustment. *Archives of General Psychiatry, 48*(4), 340–347.

Holder, D., & Anderson, C. (1990). Psychoeducational family intervention for depressed patients and their families. In G. I. Keitner (Ed.), *Depression and families: Impact and treatment* (pp. 159–184). Washington, DC: American Psychiatric Press.

Honig, A., Hofman, A., Rozendaal, N., & Dingemanns, P. (1997). Psychoeducation in bipolar disorder: Effect on expressed emotion. *Psychiatry Research, 72,* 17–22.

Hooley, J. M. (1998). Expressed emotion and psychiatric illness: From empirical data to clinical practice. *Behavior Therapy, 29*(4), 631–646.

Hooley, J. M., Orley, J., & Teasdale, J. D. (1986). Levels of expressed emotion and relapse in depressed patients. *British Journal of Psychiatry, 148,* 642–647.

Koenig, J. E., Sachs-Ericsson, N., & Miklowitz, D. J. (1997). How do psychiatric patients experience interactions with their relatives? *Journal of Family Psychology, 11*(2), 251–256.

McFarlane, W. R. (1991). Family psychoeducational treatment. In A. S. Gurman & D. P. Kniskern (Eds.), *Handbook of family therapy* (2nd ed.). New York: Brunner/Mazel.

Miklowitz, D. J., George, E. L., Axelson, D. A., Kim, E. Y., Birmaher, B., Schneck, C., et al. (2004). Family-focused treatment for adolescents with bipolar disorder. *Journal of Affective Disorders, 82S,* S113–S128.

Miklowitz, D. J., & Goldstein, M. J. (1990). Behavioral family treatment for patients with bipolar affective disorder. *Behavior Modification, 14*(4), 457–489.

Miklowitz, D. J., Goldstein, M. J., & Nuechterlein, K. H. (1995). Verbal interactions in the families of schizophrenic and bipolar affective patients. *Journal of Abnormal Psychology, 104*(2), 268–276.

Miklowitz, D. J., Goldstein, M. J., Nuechterlein, K. H., Snyder, K. S., & Mintz, J. (1988). Family factors and the course of bipolar affective disorder. *Archives of General Psychiatry, 45*(3), 225–231.

Miklowitz, D. J., Richards, J. A., George, E. L., Frank, E., Suddath, R. L., Powell, K. B., et al. (2003). Integrated family and individual therapy for bipolar disorder: Results of a treatment development study. *Journal of Clinical Psychiatry, 64*(2), 182–191.

Pavuluri, M. N., Graczyk, P. A., Henry, D. B., Carbray, J. A., Heidenreich, J., & Miklowitz, D. J. (2004). Child- and family-focused cognitive behavioral therapy for pediatric bipolar disorder: Development and preliminary results. *Journal of the American Academy of Child and Adolescent Psychiatry, 43*(5), 528–537

Simoneau, T. L., Miklowitz, D. J., & Saleem, R. (1998). Expressed emotion and interactional patterns in the families of bipolar patients. *Journal of Abnormal Psychology, 107*(3), 497–507.

PART II

COMORBID DISORDERS AND SPECIAL POPULATIONS

CHAPTER 11

Pharmacotherapy for Attention-Deficit/Hyperactivity Disorder in Children with Mania

KAREN DINEEN WAGNER

Children with bipolar disorder frequently have comorbid attention-deficit/hyperactivity disorder (ADHD). The prevalence rates of comorbid ADHD and bipolar disorder in preschoolers has been reported to be 95% (Wilens et al., 2003) and as high as 98% in school-age children (Wozniak et al., 1995). Children with mania and ADHD have a more severe clinical course, including higher rates of psychosis, psychiatric hospitalization, and functional impairment, than children with ADHD alone. Furthermore, the clinical characteristics of ADHD in children with mania are severe, including a greater number of ADHD symptoms and higher rates of reading disability than children with ADHD alone (Wozniak et al., 1995).

Children with bipolar disorder and comorbid ADHD are often prescribed multiple medications. In a community sample of 111 children and adolescents with bipolar disorder, 56 (63%) had comorbid ADHD (Bhangoo et al., 2003). The mean number of medications used to treat these youths was 3.4, and the mean number of psychotropic medication trials in the past was 6.3. Of these youths, 98% had trials of a mood stabilizer/anticonvulsant, 76% had trials of an atypical antipsychotic, 68% had trials of a stimulant, and 76% had trials of a selective serotonin reuptake inhibitor (SSRI).

The medical records were reviewed for 83 children and adolescents with bipolar I disorder in a state mental health system (Jerrell & Shugart, 2004a). Of this sample, 83% received mood stabilizers, 40% received atypical antipsychotics, 61% received antidepressants, and 28% received stimulants.

Pharmacological treatment is often necessary to manage comorbid ADHD in children who have bipolar disorder. Because the age of onset of ADHD typically precedes the age of onset of bipolar disorder (Tillman et al., 2003), it is likely that children with bipolar disorder would have received stimulant treatment for ADHD. There is significant controversy about whether ADHD treatments, such as stimulants and antidepressants, will worsen mania in children with bipolar disorder. There are minimal controlled data to definitively resolve this controversy. However, case reports, chart reviews, open studies, and longitudinal follow-up provide some clinically useful information to address this issue. This chapter reviews available evidence on the question of whether pharmacological treatments for comorbid ADHD worsen the clinical course of mania in children with bipolar disorder.

MEDICATION TREATMENT FOR COMORBID ADHD WORSENS MANIA: EVIDENCE BASE

Case Reports

There have been a number of case reports of stimulant-associated mania. A 10-year-old boy with ADHD and a positive family history for bipolar disorder was treated with methylphenidate up to 45 mg/day by day 14 (Koehler-Troy, Strober, & Malenbaum, 1986). Between days 14 and 20, he developed a manic episode characterized by pressured speech, tangential thought, flight of ideas, severe hyperactivity, intrusiveness, belligerence, grandiose delusions, and sexually provocative comments. Methylphenidate was discontinued on day 24. Within 2 days, some improvement occurred in his condition. Treatment with lithium was initiated, with full remission of his manic symptoms.

An 8-year-old boy with bipolar disorder had a history of dysphoria associated with methylphenidate treatment and visual hallucinations associated with dexedrine (Weller, Weller, & Dogin, 1998).

A methylphenidate challenge induced manic symptoms (elevated mood, grandiosity, talkativeness, flight of ideas) in a 6-year-old boy suspected of having bipolar illness (Schmidt, Delaney, Jensen, Levinson, & Lewitt, 1986).

Stimulant rebound that mimicked symptoms of bipolar disorder (irritability, anger, moodiness, insomnia, agitation, distractibility) was reported in a 7-year-old girl diagnosed with attention-deficit/hyperactivity disorder (Sarampote, Efron, Robb, Pearl, & Stein, 2002).

A 17-year-old boy with narcolepsy who was treated with modafinil 400 mg per day developed symptoms of mania—for example, flight of ideas, sexual excitation, and increased irritability (Vorspan, Warot, Consoli, Cohen, & Mazet, 2005). The modafinil was discontinued, and he developed symptoms of sadness, anhedonia, and withdrawal. Modafinil was restarted, and the manic symptoms recurred. He required hospitalization and pharmacological treatment for mania.

An 11-year-old boy with ADHD and a family history of bipolar disorder was treated with atomoxetine (0.8 mg per kg per day; Henderson, 2004). After 3 weeks on atomoxetine treatment, his activity level in the classroom increased substantially, and there was no improvement in his attention. After 4 weeks, he developed marked oppositional and impulsive behavior at school. He threatened to kill a peer, was oppositional toward his teachers, and had a violent anger outburst in school. After 6 weeks, he developed insomnia and became increasingly irritable and violent, both at home and at school. At week 7, he had an angry outburst and brandished a sword at his family. He removed his clothes and covered his body with markings from a pen. Psychiatric hospitalization was necessary, and the atomoxetine was stopped. Within 7 days of atomoxetine discontinuation, the boy's behavior returned to his baseline functioning.

In the case histories of 9 children with mania, it was reported that stimulant treatment for ADHD worsened mania in those children who had family histories of bipolar disorder (Mota-Castillo et al., 2001).

Case Series

Henderson and Hartman (2004) pooled the data of 153 consecutive children (mean age 10.5 years old) treated with atomoxetine in outpatient settings. They reported that 51 (33%) children developed extreme irritability, aggression, mania, or hypomania. Of those individuals, 80% had a personal history of mood symptoms, and 61% had a positive family history for mood disorders. Ten of these patients met diagnostic criteria for mania, and three of them were hospitalized. The onset of mood symptoms and/or aggression began at a mean of 6.4 weeks after starting treatment with atomoxetine. There was no difference in the time of onset of mood symptoms between those patients who were also treated with mood stabilizers or atypical antipsychotics. Some of the patients were treated with stimulant augmentation, which reduced hyperactivity but not the irritability or aggression.

Bhangoo et al. (2003) screened 111 youths by parent phone interview for potential inclusion in a study of bipolar disorder. Of these patients, 89 (80%) had a diagnosis of bipolar disorder, and 56 (63%) also met criteria for ADHD. Seventy-six (68%) of the children had a trial of a stimulant. The reported stimulant side effects and percentages were as follows: hyperactivity (14%), irritability (9%), aggression (8%), decreased sleep (4%), and psychosis (1%). Eighty-seven (78%) of the youths had a trial of an SSRI. The reported SSRI side effects and percentages were as follows: hyperactivity (9%), irritability (9%), aggression (9%), decreased sleep (3%), and psychosis (3%).

Chart Review

The medical records of 267 individuals (83 children and adolescents, 184 adults) with bipolar I disorder in a state mental health system were reviewed (Jerrell & Shugart, 2004b). Compared with the adult patients, the child and adolescent patients were found to be more irritable, to have more functional impairment, to have made more suicide attempts, and to be more likely to be treated with stimulant medication and to meet criteria for major depression. There was no significant difference in treatment with mood stabilizers between children and adults. Given these age-related findings, the investigators postulated that treatment with stimulants may unmask or trigger affective symptoms in youths.

The medical records of 82 children with bipolar disorder were evaluated to assess treatment-emergent mania or increased mood cycling after pharmacological treatment (Faedda, Baldessarini, Glovinsky, & Austin, 2004). Treatment-emergent mania was found in 35 of 69 (50.7%) children who had been treated with a psychoactive agent. Of these cases, treatment-emergent mania was associated with use of a stimulant (24.2%) or an antidepressant (75.7%). With regard to specific agents, the percentages of patients with treatment-emergent mania were as follows: SSRIs, 48.7%; tricyclic antidepressant, 40.0%; other antidepressants, 30.7%; methylphenidate, 21.4%; amphetamines, 16.7%.

The severity of bipolar disorder in hospitalized adolescents with a history of stimulant or antidepressant treatment was assessed by Soutullo et al. (2002). In a retrospective chart review of 80 hospitalized adolescents with bipolar I disorder, manic or mixed, it was found that the lifetime rate of ADHD was 49%. Thirty-five percent of youths had been exposed to stimulants, and 44% had been exposed to antidepressants. The adolescents who had a history of stimulant exposure were younger than those who had no history of stimulant exposure (mean age = 13.7 years vs. 15.1 years). Adolescents with bipolar disorder who had histories of stimulant exposure had a more severe hospital course, defined by length of hospital stay, use of medication as needed, and need for seclusion and restraint. There was no difference in the hospital course between adolescents with or without ADHD. These investigators concluded that adolescents with bipolar disorder who had prior treatment with stimulants may have a more severe course of illness that is not fully accounted for by comorbid ADHD.

A comparison of the clinical characteristics of adolescents with bipolar disorder with and without a history of stimulant treatment was conducted by DelBello et al. (2001). The sample consisted of 34 adolescents who were hospitalized for mania. Of these adolescents, 21 (62%) had histories of stimulant treatment. All of the adolescents who had prior stimulant exposure were initially treated with a stimulant before the onset of the affective episode. Eighty-two percent of the adolescents who were treated with stimulants were prescribed methylphenidate. The mean duration of stimulant exposure was 48 months. It was found that adolescents who had prior stimulant exposure had an earlier age of onset of bipolar disorder than those adolescents with no history of stimulant exposure (mean age = 10.7 years vs. 13.9 years). Furthermore, adolescents who had been treated with at least two stimulant medications in the past had a younger age of onset of bipolar disorder than those adolescents who had been treated with only one stimulant (mean age = 8.9 years vs. 12.7 years old). No significant correlation was found between the duration of stimulant treatment and the age of onset of bipolar disorder. There was no difference in the age of onset of bipolar disorder between those with and without ADHD. These investigators concluded that stimulant treatment, independent of ADHD, is associated with younger age of onset of bipolar disorder. These authors suggest that behavioral sensitization may account for their findings. They hypothesize that children with a predisposition for developing bipolar disorder will experience increased frequency, severity, and duration of their affective symptoms when treated with stimulants.

MEDICATION TREATMENT FOR COMORBID ADHD DOES NOT WORSEN MANIA: EVIDENCE BASE

Case Reports

A 12-year-old boy with ADHD and bipolar II disorder was treated with gabapentin, 200 mg per day, added to methylphenidate, 30 mg per day (Hamrin & Bailey, 2001). Mood stabilization was apparent within 3 weeks and continued at 6-month follow-up.

A 14-year-old brain-injured adolescent with mania was successfully treated with dextroamphetamine after having failed prior trials of mood stabilizers (Max, Richards, & Hamden-Allen, 1995).

Chart Review

A chart review of pharmacological treatment was conducted for 38 children with bipolar disorder and comorbid ADHD (Biederman et al., 1999). It was found that improvement in ADHD required prior mood stabilization in these patients. The probability of improvement in ADHD symptoms was 7.5 times higher following initial improvement in manic symptoms than was the probability of ADHD improvement prior to initial manic improvement. Treatment with tricyclic antidepressants, in the absence of mood stabilization, resulted in a relapse rate of 76% in the visits in which a tricyclic was taken compared with a 42% relapse rate in visits in which a tricyclic was not taken.

A chart review was conducted of 42 hospitalized adolescents with bipolar disorder who were treated with lithium or divalproex (State et al., 2004). Three of the 14 adolescents with bipolar disorder and comorbid ADHD were discharged on stimulant treatment concurrent with a mood stabilizer. Two of these adolescents were much or very much improved at discharge, and the third adolescent was minimally improved. The combination of stimulant plus mood stabilizer did not worsen the clinical course of the bipolar illness in these 3 adolescents.

Thirty-one preschoolers, ages 2–5 years old, with bipolar disorder were identified by chart review (Scheffer & Niskala Apps, 2004). Eighty percent of the children had comorbid ADHD. Twenty-one (68%) had had prior treatment with a stimulant or antidepressant, and, of these, 13 (62%) had worsening of mood symptoms. These children had not been on a mood stabilizer at the time of stimulant or antidepressant treatment. Twenty-six of the preschoolers were treated openly with a mood stabilizer, primarily valproic acid, over a 2-month to 2-year period, with a significant reduction in manic symptoms. Ten children received stimulant treatment for comorbid ADHD. None of these preschoolers experienced a worsening of mood symptoms when a mood stabilizer was administered concurrently with the stimulant.

Open Studies

Kowatch et al. (2000) conducted a 6- to 8-week acute treatment study in which 42 children and adolescents with bipolar I or II disorder were randomized to lithium, divalproex, or carbamazepine. Thirty-five of these youths participated in a 16-week open extension study (Kowatch, Sethuraman, Hume, Kromelis, & Weinberg, 2003). During the extension phase, the treatment options for nonresponders were to switch mood stabilizer or augment mood stabilizer with another mood stabilizer, stimulant, antidepressant, or antipsychotic. Thirteen of these youths were treated with a mood stabilizer and a stimulant during the extension phase. Twelve (92%) showed clinical improvement (much or very much improved) of ADHD symptoms with the added stimulant. Importantly, there was no exacerbation of mood symptoms when the stimulant was added.

A 1-month methylphenidate titration trial was conducted as part of a multimodal treatment study of children with ADHD. Of this sample, a subset of 61 children with ADHD and some manic symptoms were identified (Galanter et al., 2003). Children received methylphenidate over the course of a 1-month trial. There was no difference in outcome measures between children with and without manic symptoms on measures of attention, impulsivity, and aggression. Importantly, there was no difference in adverse events such as irritability for children who received stimulants compared with those who did not receive stimulants.

Acute Controlled Trials

The effects of methylphenidate and lithium on attention and activity level were assessed by Carlson, Rapport, Kelly, and Pataki (1992). Seven hospitalized children with both disruptive behavior disorders and bipolar disorder or major depression were included in this study. Patients were crossed over with placebo, methylphenidate, lithium, and methylphenidate plus lithium. The lithium–methylphenidate combined-treatment group showed improved attention. Neither methylphenidate nor lithium exacerbated hyperactivity. Methylphenidate, if used alone, worsened depression and irritability in some children.

The largest controlled study to date to assess whether adjunctive use of a stimulant is safe and efficacious for treating comorbid ADHD in children with bipolar disorder was conducted by Scheffer, Kowatch, Carmody, and Rush (2005). Forty children and adolescents, ages 6 to 17 years old, with bipolar I or II disorder and comorbid ADHD received 8-week open-label treatment with divalproex sodium. Thirty-two (80%) of the youths had a $\geq$ 50% reduction in Young Mania Rating Scale (YMRS) scores from baseline to end point. Only three youths (.08%) showed significant improvement in ADHD symptoms. Thirty of the youths who were stabilized on divalproex entered a 2-week double-blind crossover trial of mixed amphetamine salts or placebo. It was found that the mixed amphetamine salts were significantly more effective for ADHD symptoms than placebo. Importantly, there was no worsening of manic symptoms for children with bipolar disorder who received mixed amphetamine salts. The investigators concluded that mixed amphetamine salts are safe and effective when added to divalproex sodium for the treatment of comorbid ADHD in pediatric bipolar disorder.

Longitudinal Studies

A longitudinal study of stimulant treatment for children at risk for bipolar disorder was conducted by Carlson, Loney, Salisbury, Kramer, and Arthur (2000). Seventy-five boys, ages 6 to 12 years old, were diagnosed with hyperkinetic reaction and treated with methylphenidate. These boys were presumably at risk for bipolar disorder and were followed up into young adulthood. At ages 21–23 years old, those individuals with bipolar diagnoses did not differ from those without bipolar diagnoses with regard to early methylphenidate treatment history. These investigators concluded that there was no evidence that methylphenidate precipitates young adult bipolar disorder in at-risk individuals.

A 2-year follow-up study was conducted of 89 children and adolescents (mean age = 10.9 years) with a diagnosis of bipolar I disorder (Geller et al., 2002). Comorbid ADHD was present for 77 (86.5%) of these children with bipolar disorder. It was found that neither stimulant medication (administered to 53 participants; 59.6%) nor antidepressant medication (administered to 26 participants; 29.2%) with or without concurrent mood-stabilizing agents predicted recovery or relapse during the 2-year follow-up period.

CONCLUSION

Further controlled data are necessary to resolve with confidence the controversy of whether medications used to treat comorbid ADHD in children with bipolar disorder worsen mania. Given the available data, it appears that stimulants do not worsen mania if the child is currently receiving a mood-stabilizing agent. Those cases in which stimulants induced mania primarily occurred in the absence of a concurrent mood-stabilizing agent. Reassuringly, in an acute 2-week controlled trial, there was no worsening of manic symptoms for children who received stimulants compared with placebo after mood stabilization with an antimanic agent.

Because children with bipolar disorder often have comorbid ADHD, separate treatment is required for each of these disorders. With regard to pharmacological treatment, the clinician should initiate treatment with a mood stabilizer. When adequate mood stabilization is achieved, then introduction of a stimulant for treatment of comorbid ADHD would be a reasonable strategy.

There has been some clinical concern that long-term treatment with stimulants may worsen the course of bipolar illness in children. However, the available evidence to date, based on a 2-year follow-up study, did not find that stimulant or antidepressant treatment predicted recovery or relapse of mood symptoms in youths with bipolar disorder.

An area that requires further research is whether use of a stimulant is associated with an earlier age of onset of bipolar disorder, particularly in those individuals at genetic risk for the development of bipolar disorder. Some retrospective studies support this hypothesis, but controlled longitudinal studies are necessary to determine whether or not stimulant use affects the age of onset of bipolar illness in children.

DISCLOSURE

This research was supported by the National Institute of Mental Health. Karen Dineen Wagner has acted as a consultant to and on the advisory board for Abbott Laboratories, AstraZeneca, Bristol-Myers Squibb, Eli Lilly, Forest Laboratories, Glaxo-Smith Kline, Janssen, Jazz Pharmaceuticals, Johnson & Johnson, Novartis, Ortho-McNeil, Otsuka, Pfizer, Solvay, Wyeth.

REFERENCES

Bhangoo, R. K., Lowe, C. H., Myers, F. S., Treland, J., Curran, J., Towbin, K. E., et al. (2003, Winter). Medication use in children and adolescents treated in the community for bipolar disorder. *Journal of Child and Adolescent Psychopharmacology, 13*(4), 515–522.

Biederman, J., Mick, E., Prince, J., Bostic, J. Q., Wilens, T. E., Spencer, T., et al. (1999). Systematic chart review of the pharmacologic treatment of comorbid attention deficit hyperactivity disorder in youth with bipolar disorder. *Journal of Child and Adolescent Psychopharmacology, 9*(4), 247–256.

Carlson, G. A., Loney, J., Salisbury, H., Kramer, J. R., & Arthur, C. (2000, Fall). Stimulant treatment in young boys with symptoms suggesting childhood mania: A report from a longitudinal study. *Journal of Child and Adolescent Psychopharmacology, 10*(3), 175–184.

Carlson, G. A., Rapport, M. D., Kelly, K. L., & Pataki, C. S. (1992, March). The effects of methylphenidate and lithium on attention and activity level. *Journal of the American Academy of Child and Adolescent Psychiatry, 31*(2), 262–270.

DelBello, M. P., Soutullo, C. A., Hendricks, W., Niemeier, R. T., McElroy, S. L., & Strakowski, S. M. (2001). Prior stimulant treatment in adolescents with bipolar disorder: association with age at onset. *Bipolar Disorders, 3*, 53–57.

Faedda, G. L., Baldessarini, R. J., Glovinsky, I. P., & Austin, N. B. (2004, October 1). Treatment-emergent mania in pediatric bipolar disorder: A retrospective case review. *Journal of Affective Disorders, 82*(1), 149–158.

Galanter, C. A., Carlson, G. A., Jensen, P. S., Greenhill, L. L., Davies, M., Li, W., et al. (2003, Summer). Response to methylphenidate in children with attention deficit hyperactivity disorder and manic symptoms in the multimodal treatment study of children with attention deficit hyperactivity disorder titration trial. *Journal of Child and Adolescent Psychopharmacology, 13*(2), 123–136.

Geller, B., Craney, J. L., Bolhofner, K., Nickelsburg, M. J., Williams, M., & Zimerman, B. (2002). Two-year prospective follow-up of children with a prepubertal and early adolescent bipolar disorder phenotype. *American Journal of Psychiatry, 159*, 927–933.

Hamrin, V., & Bailey, K. (2001). Gabapentin and methylphenidate treatment of a preadolescent with attention deficit hyperactivity disorder and bipolar disorder. *Journal of Child and Adolescent Psychopharmacology, 11*, 301–309.

Henderson, T. A. (2004, October). Mania induction associated with atomoxetine. *Journal of Clinical Psychopharmacology, 24*(5), 567–568.

Henderson, T. A., & Hartman, K. (2004). Aggression, mania and hypomania induction associated with atomoxetine. *Pediatrics, 114*(3), 895–896.

Jerrell, J. M., & Shugart, M. A. (2004a, August). Community-based care for youths with early and very early onset bipolar I disorder. *Bipolar Disorder, 6*(4), 299–304.

Jerrell, J. M., & Shugart, M. A. (2004b, May). A comparison of the phenomenology and treatment of youths and adults with bipolar I disorder in a state mental health system. *Journal of Affective Disorders, 80*(1), 29–35.

Koehler-Troy, C., Strober, M., & Malenbaum, R. (1986). Methylphenidate-induced mania in a prepubertal child. *Journal of Clinical Psychiatry, 47,* 566–567.

Kowatch, R. A., Sethuraman, G., Hume, J. H., Kromelis, M., & Weinberg, W. A. (2003, June 1). Combination pharmacotherapy in children and adolescents with bipolar disorder. *Biological Psychiatry, 53*(11), 978–84.

Kowatch, R. A., Suppes, T., Carmody, T. L., Bucci, J. P., Hume, J. H., Kromelis, M., et al. (2000). Effect size of lithium, divalproex sodium, and carbamazepine in children and adolescents with bipolar disorder. *Journal of the American Academy of Child and Adolescent Psychiatry, 39,* 713–720.

Kowatch, R. A., Suppes, T., Carmody, T. J., Bucci, J. P., Hume, J. H., Kromelis, M., et al. (1995). Case study: Antimanic effectiveness of dextroamphetamine in a brain-injured adolescent. *Journal of American Academy of Child and Adolescent Psychiatry, 34,* 472–476.

Mota-Castillo, M., Torruella, A., Angels, B., Perez, J., Dedrick, C., & Gluckman, M. (2001). Valproate in very young children: An open case series with a brief follow-up. *Journal of Affective Disorders, 67,* 193–197.

Sarampote, C. S., Efron, L. A., Robb, A. S., Pearl, P. L., & Stein, M. A. (2002). Can stimulant rebound mimic pediatric bipolar disorder? *Journal of Child and Adolescent Psychopharmacology, 12,* 63–67.

Scheffer, R. E., Kowatch, R. A., Carmody, T., & Rush, A. J. (2005). Randomized, placebo-controlled trial of mixed amphetamine salts for symptoms of comorbid ADHD in pediatric bipolar disorder after mood stabilization with divalproex sodium. *American Journal of Psychiatry, 162,* 58–64.

Scheffer, R. E., & Niskala Apps, J. A. (2004, October). The diagnosis of preschool bipolar disorder presenting with mania: Open pharmacological treatment. *Journal of Affective Disorders, 82*(Suppl. 1), S25–S34.

Schmidt, K., Delaney, M. A., Jensen, M., Levinson, D. F., & Lewitt, M. (1986). Methylphenidate challenge in a manic boy. *Biological Psychiatry, 21*(11), 1107–1109.

Soutullo, C. A., DelBello, M. P., Ochsner, J. E., McElroy, S. L., Taylor, S. A., Strakowski, S. M., et al. (2002, August). Severity of bipolarity in hospitalized manic adolescents with history of stimulant or antidepressant treatment. *Journal of Affective Disorders, 70*(3), 323–327.

State, R. C., Frye, M. A., Altshuler, L. L., Strober, M., DeAntonio, M., Hwang, S., et al. (2004, August). Chart review of the impact of attention-deficit/hyperactivity disorder comorbidity on response to lithium or divalproex sodium in adolescent mania. *Journal of Clinical Psychiatry, 65*(8), 1057–1063.

Tillman, R., Geller, B., Bolhofner, K., Craney, J. L., Williams, M., & Zimerman, B. (2003, December). Ages of onset and rates of syndromal and subsyndromal comorbid DSM-IV diagnoses in a prepubertal and early adolescent bipolar disorder phenotype. *Journal of the American Academy of Child and Adolescent Psychiatry, 42*(12), 1486–1493.

Vorspan, F., Warot, D., Consoli, A., Cohen, D., & Mazet, P. (2005). Mania in a boy treated with modafinil for narcolepsy. *American Journal of Psychiatry, 162*(4), 813–814.

Weller, E., Weller, R. A., & Dogin, J. W. (1998). A rose is a rose is a rose. *Journal of Affective Disorders, 51,* 189–193.

Wilens, T. E., Biederman, J., Forkner, P., Ditterline, J., Morris, M., Moore, H., et al. (2003). Patterns of comorbidity and dysfunction in clinically referred preschool and school-age children with bipolar disorder. *Journal of Child and Adolescent Psychopharmacology, 13*(4), 495–505.

Wozniak, J., Biederman, J., Kiely, K., Ablon, J. S., Faraone, S. V., Mundy, E., et al. (1995). Mania-like symptoms suggestive of childhood-onset bipolar disorder in clinically referred children. *Journal of the American Academy of Child and Adolescent Psychiatry, 34*(7), 867–876.

CHAPTER 12

Pediatric Bipolar Disorder and Substance Use Disorders

The Nature of the Relationship, Subtypes at Risk, and Treatment Issues

TIMOTHY E. WILENS *and* MARTIN GIGNAC

Bipolar disorder is an increasingly recognized serious psychopathological condition affecting children and adolescents. Whereas prepubescent youths often have pervasive and severe mood dysregulation, irritability, and aggressiveness, adolescents may begin to manifest more typical symptoms of adult bipolarity, including grandiosity, depression, mania, psychosis, risk-taking behaviors, and poor judgment. Although initially conceptualized as including many abject symptoms, bipolar disorder in youths has been reconceptualized to include high rates of both internalizing and externalizing comorbid psychopathology (Biederman, Faraone, Wozniak, & Monuteaux, 2000).

SUBSTANCE USE DISORDERS AND BIPOLAR DISORDER

In recent years, a focus on mood disorders in youths with substance use disorders (SUDs; abuse or dependence of drugs or alcohol) has emerged as a major clinical and public health concern, particularly given the implications of reduction of SUDs, delinquency, and mood symptoms with treatment (Riggs, Mikulich, Coffman, & Crowley, 1997). In addition to non-SUD psychiatric comorbidity, data suggest an excessive overlap and bidirectional overrepresentation between bipolar disorder and SUDs in youths (Biederman et al., 1997; Dunner & Feinman, 1995; West et al., 1996; Wilens, Biederman, Mick, Faraone, & Spencer, 1997; Brady & Sonne, 1995; Himmelhoch, 1979; Reich, Davies, & Himmelhoch, 1974; Strakowski et al., 1998; Winokur et al., 1995; McElroy et al., 2001; Wilens et al., 2004). In epidemiological and clinically based studies, SUD is one of the most common comorbidities found in bipolar disorder (McElroy et al., 1995; Regier et al., 1990; Winokur et al., 1995; Strakowski et al., 1998; Reich et al., 1974). McElroy et al. (1995) reported that drug and alcohol use disorders were found in 39% and 32% of adults with bipolar disorder, respectively. These clinically derived data are similar to Epidemiologic Catchment Area (ECA) data in which the lifetime prevalence of co-occurring SUD exceeds 60% (Regier et al., 1990). In terms of linking SUD to early-onset adult bipolar disorder, Dunner and Feinman (1995) showed that bipolar disorder onset prior to adulthood was strongly and specifically related to SUD development in young adults. Similarly, McElroy and colleagues showed a retrospective association between early-onset bipolar disorder, mixed symptoms and comorbidity, and SUD (McElroy et al., 2001).

A smaller literature suggests that juvenile-onset bipolar disorder is a risk factor for SUD. An excess of SUD has been reported in the literature in adolescents with bipolar disorder or prominent mood lability and dyscontrol (Biederman et al., 1997; West et al., 1996; Wilens, Biederman, Abrantes, & Spencer, 1997; Young et al., 1995), and bipolar disorder is overrepresented in youths with SUD (Biederman et al., 1997; West et al., 1996; Wilens, Biederman, Abrantes, & Spencer, 1997). West et al. (1996) reported that 40% of inpatient adolescents with bipolar disorder suffered from SUD. Strober et al. (1995) reported on the 5-year follow-up of 54 adolescent inpatients with bipolar disorder and described a mixed, highly relapsing picture associated with impairment and comorbidity. At baseline (mean age = 16 years) 10% had SUD, and at follow-up 22% had current substance use issues. No controls or further description of the SUD were available. In contrast, Geller and colleagues (Geller, Bolhofner, et al., 2000; Geller et al., 2000a, 2000b), despite reporting a highly relapsing condition (bipolar disorder) associated with chronic impairment, reported no SUD at 2-year follow-up, but the participants at 2-year follow-up were only 12.9 (SD = 2.7) years old (Geller et al., 2000a, 2000b).

We previously found that psychiatrically referred adolescent outpatients with SUD were more likely than those without SUD to have comorbid bipolar disorder (Wilens, Biederman, Abrantes, & Spencer, 1997). Preliminary prospective findings derived from a longitudinal study of youths with ADHD from our group signaled that early-onset bipolar disorder was reported to be a risk for SUD, independent of ADHD (Biederman et al., 1997). Adolescents with bipolar disorder in this sample were also found to be at higher risk for early initiation of and higher rates of cigarette smoking (Wilens et al., 2000). We further evaluated a separate group of 86 clinically referred adolescents with bipolar disorder and compared them with psychiatric controls without bipolar disorder, all diagnosed by structured interviews (Wilens et al., 1999). We found that adolescents with bipolar disorder were at heightened risk for developing SUD not accounted for by conduct disorder (CD) relative to psychiatric controls.

More recently, we reported the midpoint analysis of a family-based study of SUD in adolescents with bipolar disorder (vs. controls; Wilens et al., 2004; see Figures 12.1A–12.1D). In this study funded by the National Institute on Drug Abuse (MDA), we systematically studied adolescents to age 18 years with bipolar disorder and compared them with a similarly ascertained group of adolescents without any mood disorder history (to ensure that they were at low risk of developing bipolar disorder). Structured psychiatric interviews and subjective measures of SUD were collected. We evaluated specifically the relationship between SUD and the age at onset of bipolar disorder (child vs. adolescent onset) and the presence of comorbid CD. Our youths were a mean age of 13.5 (± 2.4) years and did not differ by group (bipolar disorder vs. controls) for any clinical characteristics or demographics. SUD was found in 32% of youths with bipolar disorder compared with 7% of controls ($Z = 2.9$, $p = .004$). Youths with bipolar disor-

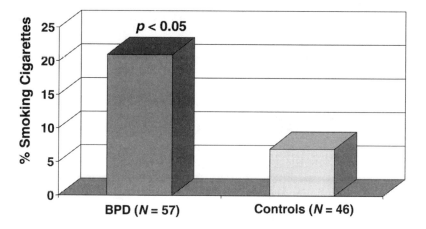

FIGURE 12.1.A. Cigarette smoking in juvenile bipolar disorder. Adapted from Wilens et al. (2004). Copyright 2004 by Lippincott Williams & Wilkins. Adapted by permission.

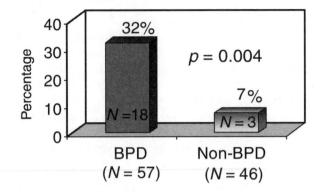

FIGURE 12.1.B. Substance use disorder in juvenile bipolar disorder. Adapted from Wilens et al. (2004). Copyright 2004 by Lippincott Williams & Wilkins. Adapted by permission.

der ubiquitously had higher rates of additional comorbidities and poorer neuropsychological functioning than controls.

We further evaluated whether a developmental effect of bipolar disorder onset was related to SUD onset. We previously found that in a group of adolescents with bipolar disorder, the onset of their bipolar disorder in adolescence was more pernicious in terms of SUD onset than it was when the bipolar disorder began prepubertally (Wilens et al., 1999; see Figure 12.2). Interestingly, we replicated our previous findings in that youths who developed bipolar disorder in adolescence were at higher risk for cigarette smoking and SUD compared with those who developed it prepubertally (for SUD, $\chi^2 = 9.3$, $p = .002$). Comorbidity with CD did not account for bipolar disorder as a risk factor for SUD (odds ratio = 5.4 accounting for conduct).

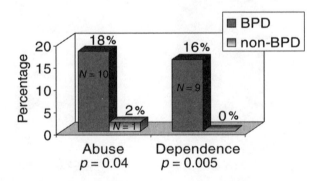

FIGURE 12.1.C. Drug use disorders in juvenile bipolar disorder. Adapted from Wilens et al. (2004). Copyright 2004 by Lippincott Williams & Wilkins. Adapted by permission.

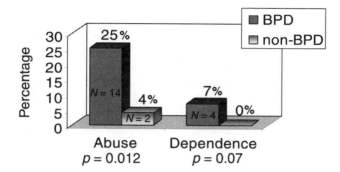

FIGURE 12.1.D. Alcohol use disorders in juvenile bipolar disorder. Adapted from Wilens et al. (2004). Copyright 2004 by Lippincott Williams & Wilkins. Adapted by permission.

We also found that adolescents with bipolar disorder who developed an SUD had a more severe type and course of SUD relative to control participants without mood disorders. We concluded that our findings replicated our previous work, clearly indicating that juvenile bipolar disorder is a risk factor for SUD that was not accounted for by CD, ADHD, or other comorbid psychopathology. Youths who develop bipolar disorder during adolescence were at particularly high risk for SUD. Bipolar disorder attenuated the severity and course of SUD.

Sequence of SUDs and Bipolar Disorder

Having established a link between SUDs and bipolar disorder, a number of important issues remain. Carefully conducted work by Winokur et al.

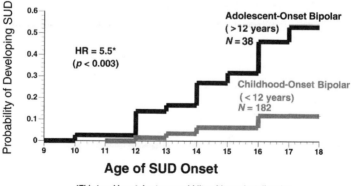

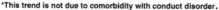

FIGURE 12.2. Development of SUD in juvenile bipolar disorder. Adapted from Wilens et al. (1999). Copyright 1999 by Lippincott Williams & Wilkins. Adapted by permission.

(1995) and Strakowski and colleagues (Strakowski, Tohen, Stoll, Faedda, & Goodwin, 1992; Strakowski, McElroy, Keck, & West, 1995; Strakowski et al., 1998) have helped elucidate the developmental timing of SUD as it pertains to bipolar disorder in adults. These research teams have found that in adults with bipolar disorder, the bipolar disorder preceded SUD in 30–47% of cases (Winokur et al., 1995; Strakowski, et al., 1998). Whereas Winokur has reported that a subgroup with bipolar disorder plus SUD have evidence of alcoholism secondary to bipolar disorder (Winokur et al., 1995), Strakowski has noted that active SUD was associated with unstable bipolar disorder; however, unstable bipolar disorder was not associated with SUD (Strakowski et al., 1998). Although the reasons for the discrepancies in their work are not clear, the influence of the timing of the onset of bipolar disorder as it relates to SUD has not been thoroughly investigated. For example, in contrast to Strakowski's work, we previously reported that in outpatient youths given structured psychiatric interviews, bipolar disorder preceded SUD in 55% of the cases, occurred within 1 year of SUD onset in 9%, and developed after SUD in 36% (Wilens, Biederman, Abrantes, & Spencer, 1997). Similar findings have been reported in adults with bipolar disorder with juvenile onset (Dunner & Feinman, 1995) and in youths with mood disorders (Mezzich, Tarter, Hsieh, & Fuhrman, 1992; Stowell & Estroff, 1992). Hence, in adolescent groups, it appears that the majority of time, bipolar disorder either precedes or occurs simultaneously with the onset of SUD.

Role of CD in SUD Development in Bipolar Disorder

Understanding the risk of SUD in bipolar disorder necessitates a thorough understanding of an important potential confound, namely the role of CD, a common comorbid condition with bipolar disorder (Kovacs & Pollock, 1995; Wozniak, Biederman, Kiely, et al., 1995). Numerous studies have demonstrated that child or adolescent CD predicts early-onset SUD (Robins, 1966; Crowley & Riggs, 1995). Moreover, CD has been consistently overrepresented among adolescents who smoke cigarettes or abuse other substances (West et al., 1996; Wilens, Biederman, Abrantes, & Spencer, 1997; DeMilio, 1989; Hovens, Cantwell, & Kiriakos, 1994). Among many characteristics and needs of delinquent youths with SUD (McKay & Buka, 1994), investigations have highlighted the need for attention to mood symptoms in CD, particularly in SUD (Crowley & Riggs, 1995). Unfortunately, the role and interaction between bipolar disorder and CD in the context of SUD in youths remains relatively understudied.

Studies involving children with bipolar disorder and CD have documented a bidirectional link: a high overlap of CD in youths with bipolar disorder (Kovacs & Pollock, 1995; Wozniak, Biederman, Kiely, et al.,

1995; Faraone et al., 1997) and high rates of bipolar disorder individuals with CD (Kutcher, Marton, & Korenblum, 1989). Epidemiological studies have found similarly high rates of comorbidity between juvenile bipolar disorder and disruptive disorders, including CD (Lewinsohn, Gotlib, & Seeley, 1995). Rates of CD in clinically referred youths with bipolar disorder range from 42% (Kutcher et al., 1989) to 69% (Kovacs & Pollock, 1995). The association between CD and mania is consistent with the comorbidity between CD and major depression (Angold & Costello, 1993) given the link between depression and later bipolar disorder in youths (Geller, Fox, & Clark, 1994; Strober & Carlson, 1982; Geller, Zimerman, Williams, Bolhofner, & Craney, 2001). The reported association between bipolar disorder and CD is not surprising considering that juvenile mania is frequently associated with prolonged and aggressive outbursts (Davis, 1979; Carlson, 1983) that may predispose these youths to developing SUD.

Children with bipolar disorder frequently meet diagnostic criteria for CD and are at risk for SUD. Disentangling the association between bipolar disorder, CD, and SUD is critical in unveiling the role of each disorder independently, or in combination, in mediating SUD. For example, in evaluating the ECA data, Carlson, Bromet, and Jandorf (1998) have reported that adults with bipolar disorder less than 30 years of age with SUD had been significantly overrepresented among youths with CD and suggested that it was the presence of comorbid CD, and not the bipolar disorder, that was the main mediator of the SUD. However, systematic reporting of SUD was not undertaken, and CD in youths was defined, in part, by the presence of SUD, confounding the role of juvenile CD in predicting later SUD. In contrast, our finding of an association between SUD and juvenile bipolar disorder not being mediated by CD is noteworthy (Wilens et al., 1999; Wilens et al., 2004). In our ongoing studies, we have preliminary results replicating the finding that CD, both alone and in association with bipolar disorder, is a risk factor for SUD. However, we have also found that bipolar disorder is a robust risk factor for SUD even controlling for CD. Our findings appeared to support the independence of both CD and bipolar disorder as independent risk factors for adolescent-onset SUD. We are currently investigating the familiality of bipolar disorder, CD, and SUD to further explore their interrelationship.

Given that SUD associated with CD alone is often difficult to treat, the identification of a subset of children with CD and bipolar disorder could permit the development of appropriate intervention strategies with antimanic agents for such children that may have an impact on the onset and course of SUD (Riggs et al., 1997; Geller et al., 1998; Donovan, Susser, & Nunes, 1996). As seen in Figure 12.3, although there is no doubt a major risk for SUD associated with CD, adolescent-onset bipolar disorder poses a similar "stealth" risk for SUD development.

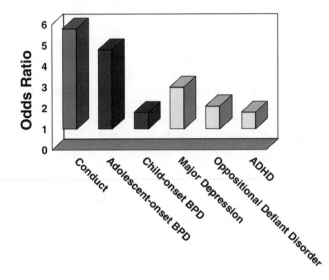

FIGURE 12.3. Risk of SUD in psychiatrically referred adolescent outpatients. Adapted from Wilens et al. (1999). Copyright 1999 by Lippincott Williams & Wilkins. Adapted by permission.

MECHANISM OF SUD RISK IN BIPOLAR DISORDER

The reasons that juvenile bipolar disorder is a risk for SUD in particular and that adolescent-versus child-onset bipolar disorder confers a differential risk for SUD in adolescence in particular remain unclear. Given the prominent genetic influences in both bipolar disorder and ADHD (as individual disorders and perhaps cosegregating), it remains unclear whether SUD in youths with bipolar disorder represent a subtype of bipolar disorder and/or SUD or whether a vulnerability to SUD development exists in these youths. For instance, we previously speculated that the development of bipolar disorder may be particularly predictive of development of SUD during adolescence, considering that adolescence is a time of vulnerability for the development of SUD (Faraone et al., 1997; Wilens et al., 1999; Chambers, Taylor, & Potenza, 2003).

SUDs, Bipolar Disorder, and "Self-Medication"

Among disturbances reported in youths with bipolar disorder, severe affective and self-regulation problems (Wozniak, Biederman, Kiely, et al., 1995; Geller et al., 2000a) may predispose them to seek drugs of abuse. By nature of their intrapsychic distress and behavioral disinhibition, these youths may try to modulate their irritable and labile mood with substances of abuse, such as has been described in adults (Khantzian, 1985, 1997; Pandina, Johnson, & Labouvie, 1992). Three factors interact to make a particular drug especially appealing (Khantzian, 1997): the main action or effect of the drug, the personality organization or characteristics of that individual, and his or her inner states of psychological suffering or disharmony. These affect states, which are developmentally influenced (i.e., somatic, not recognized, nonverbalized), are themselves a risk factor for SUD based on the individual's proneness to act on his or her feelings, such as engaging in substance use (Krystal, 1978). It is notable that the qualitative description and severity of the affective instability referred to in the self-medication theory (Krystal, 1978; Khantzian, 1997) is a key feature in adolescents with bipolar disorder, particularly during chronic mixed, labile mood states.

Self-regulatory mechanisms may additionally operate in the context of SUD and bipolar disorder. Longitudinal data in youths demonstrates that the inability to modulate self-esteem, affect, relationships, or self-care predisposes the individual to later SUD (Shedler & Block, 1990; Newcomb & Bentler, 1988). The connection between SUD and mood disorders has been established in adults (Rounsaville, Weissman, Kleber, & Wilber, 1982). For example, in adults with bipolar disorder, SUD has been shown to occur preferentially during active bipolar disorder symptomatology (Reich et al., 1974; Strakowski et al., 1998), specifically during mania (Reich et al., 1974). Furthermore, in the course of bipolar disorder in adults, not only is SUD connected to an unstable mood (Strakowski et al., 1998) but also SUD and bipolar disorder severity are highly correlated (Winokur et al., 1995). Hence, the marked affective instability and self-regulation deficits seen in juvenile bipolar disorder may be linked to SUD through internal characteristics. Although these findings are compelling, some important issues remain to be elucidated: (1) the existence of such a self-medication phenomenon in juvenile bipolar disorder relative to SUD; (2) the predictive value (e.g., etiological nature) of self-medication on SUD; (3) the apparent risk of only certain youths with bipolar disorder developing SUD; and (4) the effect that treatment of the mood state has on the risk for SUD.

Genes and Adolescent SUDs

There is clearly evidence of genetic influences on adolescent substance use. As reviewed by Hopfer and colleagues (Hopfer, Crowley, & Hewitt, 2003), the literature supports both genetic and shared environmental influences as playing a significant role in the development of substance use and misuse or abuse in adolescence. Moderate heritability has been reported for nicotine dependence and for drug abuse from the Virginia and Minnesota twin studies (Maes et al., 1999; McGue, Elkins, & Iacono, 2000). Moreover, genetic and shared environments are influenced by age, sex, specific substance and contexts, and spirituality (Hopfer et al., 2003). For instance, higher heritability has been noted in older adolescents relative to younger adolescents (Hopfer et al., 2003). There is some evidence for a common genetic influence on substance use, misuse, and abuse across different substances.

Child- and adolescent-onset bipolar disorder may be etiologically distinct, with a variable course and outcome, including the risk for SUD. It may also be that adolescent-onset bipolar disorder and adolescent-onset SUD may represent variable expressivity of a shared risk factor (Comings et al., 1991; Ebstein et al., 1996). In order for us to better understand these competing influences, comprehensive longitudinal assessments of these high-risk youths and family members are necessary (Faraone, Tsuang, & Tsuang, 1999). It may be that substances such as cigarettes and alcohol tend to increase the risk for using illicit drugs (Kandel & Logan, 1984; Yamaguchi & Kandel, 1984), such as has been recently shown for ADHD (Biederman, et al., 2006). This potential pathway to drug use is of significance given that nationwide surveys of high school students reveal that nearly two-thirds of students had tried cigarette smoking in their lifetimes with nearly one-third of students currently smoking (*www.NIDA.nih.gov*). Moreover, 80% had had at least one drink of alcohol during their lifetimes, and nearly one-third had been drunk within the preceding month. The developmental transition from licit to illicit substance use is particularly relevant to bipolar disorder given our findings of a threefold increased risk for smoking (Wilens et al., 2000).

Socialization and SUDs

A rich literature highlights the importance of adequate socialization with peers individually and in groups in the context of the initiation and maintenance of SUD in youths (Glantz & Pickens, 1992; Newcomb, Maddahian, & Bentler, 1986; Brook, Whiteman, & Gordon, 1983). The importance of extremes in socialization has been described and validated independently as social disability (Greene et al., 1996). Determined by using significant discrepancies between social adjustment and expected social functioning (John, Gammon, Prusoff, & Warner, 1987; Greene et al., 1996), social disability has been described in a variety of disturbed youths. Social disability has been shown to be overrepresented in youths with bipolar disorder, oppositional defiant disorder, and CD (Greene, Biederman, Faraone, Sienna, & Garcia-Jetton, 1997). Conversely, participants with marked social dysfunction and disability may be at high risk for later psychopathology and SUD (Ollendick, Weist, Borden, & Greene, 1992). In longitudinal studies, social disability has predicted higher rates of internalizing and externalizing psychopathology, poorer overall outcome, and a higher risk for SUD (Greene et al., 1999). For example, Greene and colleagues (Greene et al., 1997; Greene et al., 1999) have shown that social disability at baseline was a very significant predictor of cigarette smoking and of SUD 4 years later (adjusted odds ratios = 6–17). Unfortunately, no studies to date have examined the longitudinal relationship of social disability in context of bipolar disorder and SUD.

Family Adversity

A variety of research has shown evidence of family risk factors that can also contribute to the development of such disorders. Generally, lower socioeconomic status (SES) has been found to be one of several unitary predictors of substance and alcohol use disorders (Greene et al., 1999), and other research has shown that family stress and siblings' SUD are other significant factors that can lead to the development of SUD (Weinberg, Rahdert, Colliver, & Glantz, 1998; Reinherz, Giaconia, Hauf, Wasserman, & Paradis, 2000). Moreover, for males, being born to younger parents and SUD in parents, primarily the father, lead to an increased risk for SUD (Reinherz et al., 2000). Exposure to parental SUD, especially in adolescence, predicts SUD in offspring (Biederman, Faraone, Monuteaux, & Feighner, 2000). We previously reported (Wilens et al., 2002) that, when controlling for SES and family intactness, SUD was found to be significantly greater in children of parents with alcohol dependence compared with controls. Additionally, other researchers have shown that adolescent and young adult alcohol use problems are directly related to their parents' SUD (Rohde, Lewinsohn, Kahler, Seeley, & Brown, 2001). The interaction of poor parenting abilities and the child's difficult temperament may also lead to early-age onset of SUD.

Academic Underachievement, Neuropsychological Functioning, and SUDs

Bipolar-disorder-related neuropsychological dysfunction and academic failure (Lagace, Kutcher, & Robertson, 2003) may create an additional set of risk factors for SUD. Adults with childhood-onset bipolar disorder (McElroy et al., 1992), as well as youths with bipolar disorder, evidence educational underachievement and neuropsychological disturbances (Wozniak, Biederman, Kiely, et al., 1995; Lagace et al., 2003; Doyle et al., 2005). For instance, Wozniak, Biederman, Kiely, et al. (1995) reported significantly poorer Wechsler Intelligence Scale for Children (WISC-III) subscales, IQ scores, and academic achievement compared with matched psychiatric controls. These youths with bipolar disorder also had higher rates of learning disabilities, repeated grades, need for tutoring, mathematics difficulties, and placement in special classes compared with controls (Wozniak, Biederman, Kiely, et al., 1995). More recently, Shear, DelBello, Lee Rosenberg, and Strakowski (2002) have shown specific executive functioning deficits in adolescents with bipolar disorder. These findings in adolescents with bipolar disorder are of great relevance to the study of SUD given the link between academic and cognitive and neuropsychological dysfunction and later SUD (Kellam, Brown, Rubin, & Ensminger, 1983; Crum, Bucholz, Helzer, & Anthony, 1992; Bry, McKeon, & Pandina, 1982; Labouvie & McGee, 1986). Similarly, we recently reported severe neuropsychological dysfunction in our adolescent sample of youths with bipolar disorder compared with controls (Doyle et al., 2005). In our sample, the massive neuropsychological deficits, including proxies of executive functioning, were substantially more prominent compared with ADHD samples and with our control adolescents without mood disorders.

Longitudinal studies have demonstrated powerful associations between low grade point average, poor academic performance, and a noncommitment to school with later SUD (Bry et al., 1982; Newcomb et al., 1986; Labouvie & McGee, 1986). Cognitive and neuropsychological dysfunction in youths with later SUD has been reported (Hawkins, Catalano, & Miller, 1992). Complicating the picture, SUD has both short- and long-term effects on cognitive and neuropsychological functioning in adults (Block, 1996), although the extent of these findings in youths remains unclear. Given the increasingly growing concern with neuropsychological and executive-function defects in predicting later SUD, children and adolescents with bipolar disorder, by nature of their multiplicity of cognitive deficits, are at independently high risk for SUD.

Novelty Seeking and SUDs

Bardo, Donohew, and Harrington's (1996) review of the literature showed that the bulk of studies support the idea that novelty seekers are at increased risk for SUD relative to those low in novelty seeking. Moreover, the personality dimensions of harm avoidance and reward dependence also are associated with SUD initiation (Cloninger, 1987) and treatment attrition (Kravitz, Fawcett, McGuire, Kravitz, & Whitney, 1999). For example, in a study of 457 adolescents, Wills, Windle, and Cleary (1998) showed that SUD was particularly elevated for persons high in novelty seeking, low in harm avoidance, and low in reward dependence. Masse and Tremblay (1997) examined personality dimensions measured at ages 6 and 10 as predictors of SUD in adolescence. They found that high novelty seeking and low harm avoidance significantly predict early onset of substance use. In contrast, reward dependence was unrelated to any of the outcomes studied. Notably, novelty seekers are impulsive, exploratory, excitable, and quick tempered—clinical features of juvenile bipolar disorder.

DIAGNOSTIC AND TREATMENT CONSIDERATIONS

Evaluation and treatment of comorbid bipolar disorder and SUD should be part of a plan in which consideration is given to all aspects of the child's life. Any intervention should follow a careful evaluation of the patient, including psychiatric, addiction, social, cognitive, educational, and family evaluations. A thorough history of substance use should be obtained, including past and current usage and treatments. Careful attention should be paid to the differential diagnoses, including medical, psychiatric, and neurological conditions whose symptoms may overlap with bipolar disorder (schizophrenia, hyperthyroidism) or be a result of SUD (i.e., protracted withdrawal, intoxication, hyperactivity). Current psychosocial factors contributing to the clinical presentation need to be explored thoroughly. No specific guidelines exist for evaluating the patient with bipolar disorder and active SUD, but at least a few days of abstinence may be useful in assessing for bipolar disorder symptoms. Semistructured psychiatric interviews are invaluable aids for the systematic diagnostic assessment of this group of patients. Heavy, intermittent, binge use of substances is a tip-off to the possible existence of bipolar disorder in youth who are abusing substances.

The first consideration that clinicians should have in mind in the establishment of a specific treatment plan for adolescents with co-occurring mental and substance-related disorders is the determination of the level of care needed. The American Society of Addiction Medicine placement criteria (*www.asam.org/ppc/ppc2.htm*; American Society of Addiction Medicine, 2004) has shed light on the issue of placement, length of stay, and follow-up of adolescents with SUD. Four levels of care should be considered and are defined as the following: level I, outpatient treatments; level II, intensive outpatient/partial hospitalization; level III, residential/inpatient treatment; and level IV, medically managed intensive inpatient treatment. The determination of a level of care relies on the severity of the SUD and associated conditions. Therefore, the assessment of an adolescent with SUD should include the exploration the following six dimensions: (1) intoxication–withdrawal symptoms associated with the substance of abuse; (2) medical evaluation, as the initial treatment period may lead to destabilization of underlying medical problems; (3) psychological evaluation that will ensure safety in regard to suicidality and aggressive behaviors; (4) motivational evaluation, paying careful attention to treatment resistance and expectations; (5) relapse potential, in particular peer influence (one of the most important factors), ambivalence, and drug-seeking behaviors; (6) environmental support, parental attitude, availability of the substances, and quality of the social network. Treatment should begin in the least restrictive setting that ensures personal safety, as it is important to maximize family involvement from the onset. In youths with SUD, family involvement is likely to increase compliance with treatment and may lead to higher rates of sustained abstinence. In all of the different therapies, the social environment, particularly the immediate family, plays a highly influential role in any successful treatment of pediatric SUD, even more so than with adults (Bergmann, Smith, & Hoffmann, 1995). Therefore, education of the individual, family members, and other caregivers is a useful initial step to improve the recognition of the dual diagnosis of SUD and bipolar disorder.

Youths with SUD require frequent visits with the treatment team, especially if they have a comorbid psychiatric condition such as bipolar disorder that is being stabilized. During each visit, the clinician should monitor the patient's SUD, bipolar disorder, and other psychiatric symptoms, his or her social stressors and compliance with medication, and any adverse effects he or she may have experienced. Although random urine "dipstick" testing for substances of abuse, such as the Roche "On Trac" system, can be a useful piece of the treatment plan (provided that the adolescent is aware that such testing may be performed), we previously showed that questionnaires, like structured interviews, are an essential source of information (Gignac et al., 2005). Not only do they provide a better understanding of usage pattern associated with the substance abused, but they have also been shown to be specific and sensitive when compared with urine screen.

When approaching the treatment of a dual diagnosis, such as bipolar disorder and SUD, clinicians should consider a simultaneous approach for individuals. Given limited, albeit important, data on the effects of medication treatment in reducing SUD in bipolar disorder, both psychosocial and medication strategies should be considered in these adolescents with comorbid disorders. It is important to review with the patient and family the fact that medication is one aspect of the treatment plan and is more likely to be effective when used in conjunction with other treatments. The response to treatment may vary according to certain factors related to the relative onsets of SUD and affective symptoms. In a prospective follow-up study of alcohol-use disorders and bipolar disorders, participants with bipolar disorder beginning prior to the SUD had longer affective episodes and alcohol-use symptoms compared with individuals who presented with alcohol-related problems prior to the onset of the bipolar symptoms (Strakowski et al., 2005). It is important to explain that comorbidity is a major clinical concern, as patients with psychiatric disorders and SUD have more complicated treatment courses and higher rates of relapse (Bukstein, Brent, & Kaminer, 1989; Wilens, Biederman, & Mick, 1998).

Psychosocial Treatment

A variety of psychosocial interventions have been implemented successfully in youths with SUD that should also be useful in adolescents with bipolar disorder and SUD, including family therapy, cognitive-behavioral therapy (Kaminer & Slesnick, 2005), multisystemic therapy (Borduin, 1999), and self-help groups (e.g., Alateen) which offer a helpful treatment modality for many teens with SUD. Recently, the large multisite Cannabis Youth Treatment Study (Dennis et al., 2004) compared five psychosocial treatment modalities for youths with cannabis use disorder. Six hundred adolescents (ages 15–16) were randomly assigned to one of the five treatment modalities: five sessions of motivational enhancement therapy (MET) plus cognitive-behavioral therapy (CBT), 12 sessions of MET/CBT, family support network (FSN), adolescent community reinforcement approach (ACRA) and multidimensional family therapy (MDFT). Based on two main outcomes (days of abstinence and percentage of participants in recovery), the most effective interventions were MET/CBT for five or twelve sessions and ACRA. However, the role of these psychosocial interventions for individuals in the context of dual diagnosis, such as SUD and bipolar disorder, has not been studied.

Pharmacotherapy

There is evidence that pharmacological interventions are an effective treatment for youths with SUD and bipolar disorder. Clinicians should review how the medication will work, the possible side effects, and the time frame in which benefit may be expected. An informed and involved family is more likely to encourage compliance from an adolescent than one that has never met their child's treatment team. An adult caretaker and not the patient should store, administer, and monitor all prescription medications to maximize compliance and minimize the inappropriate use of these medications. Unlike other psychiatric disorders in children in which abstinence is often recommended prior to pharmacotherapy (Riggs, 1998; Waxmonsky & Wilens, 2003), based on the trial by Geller et al. (1998), a period of abstinence is not necessary, as medication treatment should be initiated quickly in youths with bipolar disorder and SUD.

Two studies, including one randomized controlled study, have reported that mood stabilizers, specifically lithium and valproic acid, significantly reduced substance use in youths with bipolar disorder (Geller et al., 1998; Donovan & Nunes, 1998). In the one controlled study of youths with SUD and comorbid psychiatric illness, Geller et al. (1998) completed a randomized, placebo-controlled study evaluating the use of lithium in a group of outpatient adolescents with affective dysregulation and substance dependence. All patients were in outpatient treatment for the duration of the study but did not receive any other psychotropic medications besides lithium ($n = 13$) or placebo ($n = 12$). After 6 weeks, the lithium group ($n = 13$) showed a clinically significant decrease in the number of positive urines compared with the placebo-treated group ($n = 12$; $p = .042$), as well as a significant increase in the overall global functioning of this group. However, there was no difference in severity of the affective symptoms between the two groups (measured via K-SADS). No participants discontinued the lithium because of adverse events, although participants receiving lithium did report higher rates of polyuria and polydipsia. (See Figures 12.4A and 12.4B.)

Donovan and Nunes (1998) completed an open study evaluating the use of valproic acid in adolescent outpatients with marijuana abuse/dependence and "explosive mood disorder" (mood symptoms were not classified using the DSM-IV). Eight participants were prescribed 1000 mg of valproic acid for 5 weeks, in addition to regular therapy sessions, but did not receive any other psychotropic medications. All participants showed a significant improvement in their marijuana use ($p < .007$) and their affective symptoms ($p < .001$), although outcomes were measured only by self-report. The most common adverse events were nausea and sedation. No participants discontinued because of these side effects, nor were there any reported interactions between the valproic acid and substances of abuse. The use of atypical neuroleptics as mood-stabilizing agents in comobid SUD–bipolar disorder remains understudied, and further work in this area is needed.

In terms of treating the depressive subphase of bipolar disorder in SUD, relatively little is known, and data are derived from open studies in youths with mood disorders in this age group. An open-label study with fluoxetine 20 mg (> 7 weeks trial) showed that depressive symptoms persisting after SUD stabilization in 8 adolescents (14–18 years) showed 50% improvement on depression scales (Riggs et al., 1997). Preliminary work by Solhkhah and colleagues (2005) has found similar results with bupropion in adolescents with SUD and depression and/or ADHD. There is also very preliminary evidence that treatment of bipolar disorder may *prevent* future cigarette and substance use (Wilens et al., 2000).

More generally for SUD, pharmacological agents may be used to treat SUD in a pediatric population. Kaminer and Slesnick (2005) have proposed categorizing the existing agents by their mechanism of action (aversion, craving reduction, substitution and treatment of comorbid psychiatric disorders). The best known *aversion agent* is disulfiram, which prevents the breakdown of acetaldehyde, a toxic metabolite of alcohol, producing a

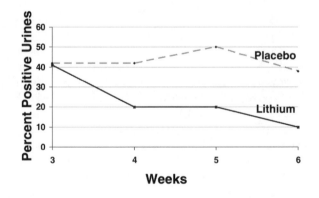

FIGURE 12.4.A. Lithium for bipolar adolescents with substance use disorders: Effect on substance use. Adapted from Geller et al. (1998). Copyright 1998 by Lippincott Williams & Wilkins. Adapted by permission.

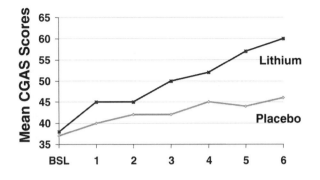

FIGURE 12.4.B. Lithium for bipolar adolescents with substance use disorders: Effect on functioning. Adapted from Geller et al. (1998). Copyright 1998 by Lippincott Williams & Wilkins. Adapted by permission.

noxious reaction when alcohol is consumed. It has not been shown useful in a case report of two teenagers with alcohol abuse disorder (Myers, Donahue, & Goldstein, 1994). The *substitution agents* methadone, levo-alpha acetyl methadol (LAAM), and buprenorphine have been understudied in heroin addiction among adolescents (Hopfer, Mikulich, & Crowley, 2000), and the stimulant replacement strategy for cocaine addiction had no effect on craving for this substance (Grabowski et al., 1997) Naltrexone, the most studied opiate antagonist used as an *anticraving agent*, was used in three adolescents with alcohol dependence, producing a positive response in all three cases with no significant adverse events after 6 months of use (Lifrak, Alterman, O'Brien, & Volpicelli, 1997). However, Hopfer and colleagues reported significant compliance difficulties when using naltrexone in youths with SUD (Hopfer et al., 2000). Other anticraving agents such as nalmefene, acamprosate, and ondansetron have not been studied among adolescents.

In terms of pharmacological treatment of comorbid conditions, a larger literature derived from the ADHD–SUD comorbidity studies exists. As ADHD is often comorbid with bipolar disorders (Wozniak & Biederman, 1996; Wozniak, Biederman, Kiely, et al., 1995; Wozniak, Biederman, Mundy, Mennin, & Faraone, 1995), these data are of great interest to the field. However, clinicians should stabilize mood disorders as a priority and then perhaps use other agents as adjuvant treatment. One should pay careful attention to the risk of inducing mania in individuals with ADHD and bipolar disorder. Agents such as atomoxetine, bupropion, or long-acting stimulants (Schubiner, 2005; Hah & Chang, 2005; Biederman et al., 1998; Ross, 2006) for comorbid ADHD are preferred. Short-acting stimulants should be avoided in this population as they carry a higher risk of abuse and diversion (Wilens, Gignac, Swezey, Monuteaux, & Biederman, 2006).

SUMMARY

In summary, a strong literature supports a relationship between bipolar disorder and SUD. Characterizing the course, outcome, and nature of bipolar disorder and SUD linked to juvenile bipolar disorder is of particular interest because (1) bipolar disorder is an increasingly recognized psychiatric disorder affecting children and adolescents although the course of the disorder is not well mapped out; (2) juvenile bipolar disorder generally has onset prior to SUD; (3) persistent bipolar disorder into adulthood is associated with SUD; (4) bipolar disorder is treatable; (5) bipolar disorder treatment results in reduced SUD in adolescents with active SUD in bipolar disorder; and (6) bipolar disorder treatment over time may reduce the risk or attenuate the course of SUD. Both family–genetic and self-medication influences may be operational in the development and continuation of SUD in adolescents and young adults with bipolar disorder; however, systematic data are lacking. Patients with bipolar disorder and SUD require multimodal interventions incorporating addiction and mental health treatment simultaneously.

Although the existing literature has provided important information on the relationship of bipolar disorder and SUD, it also points to a number of areas in need of further study. The mechanism by which bipolar disorder leads to SUD needs to be better understood. The influence of adequate treatment of bipolar disorder on the onset, course, and remission from SUD needs to be delineated. Given the prevalence and major morbidity and impairment caused by SUD and bipolar disorder, prevention and treatment strategies for these patients need be further developed and evaluated.

ACKNOWLEDGMENTS

This research was supported by the National Institutes of Health (National Institute on Drug Abuse) Grant Nos. RO1 DA12945, K24 DA016264, and 5U10DA015831-0 to Timothy E. Wilens.

REFERENCES

Angold, A., & Costello, E. J. (1993). Depressive comorbidity in children and adolescents: Empirical, theoretical and methodological issues. *American Journal of Psychiatry, 150,* 1779–1791.

Bardo, M. T., Donohew, R. L., & Harrington, N. G. (1996). Psychobiology of novelty seeking and drug seeking behavior. *Behavioural Brain Research, 77,* 23–43.

Bergmann, P. E., Smith, M. B., & Hoffmann, N. G. (1995). Adolescent treatment. Implications for assessment, practice guidelines, and outcome management. *Pediatric Clinics of North America, 42,* 453–472.

Biederman, J., Faraone, S. V., Monuteaux, M. C., & Feighner, J. A. (2000). Patterns of alcohol and drug use in adolescents can be predicted by parental substance use disorders. *Pediatrics, 106,* 792–797.

Biederman, J., Faraone, S. V., Wozniak, J., & Monuteaux, M. C. (2000). Parsing the association between bipolar, conduct, and substance use disorders: A familial risk analysis. *Biological Psychiatry, 48,* 1037–1044.

Biederman, J., Mick, E., Bostic, J., Prince, J., Daly, J., Wilens, T., et al. (1998). The naturalistic course of pharmacologic treatment of children with manic like symptoms: A systematic chart review. *Journal of Clinical Psychiatry, 59,* 628–637.

Biederman, J., Monuteaux, M., Mick, E., Wilens, T., Fontanella, J., Poetzl, K., et al. (2006). Is cigarette smoking a gateway drug to subsequent alcohol and illicit drug use disorders?: A controlled study of youths with and without ADHD. *Biological Psychiatry, 59,* 258–264.

Biederman, J., Wilens, T., Mick, E., Faraone, S., Weber, W., Curtis, S., et al. (1997). Is ADHD a risk for psychoactive substance use disorder?: Findings from a four-year follow-up study. *Journal of the American Academy of Child and Adolescent Psychiatry, 36,* 21–29.

Block, R. I. (1996). Does heavy marijuana use impair human cognition and brain function? *Journal of the American Medical Association, 275,* 560–561.

Borduin, C. (1999). Multisystemic treatment of criminality and violence in adolescents. *Journal of the American Academy of Child and Adolescent Psychiatry, 38,* 242–249.

Brady, K., & Sonne, S. (1995). The relationship between substance abuse and bipolar disorder. *Journal of Clinical Psychiatry, 56*(Suppl. 3), 19–24.

Brook, J. S., Whiteman, M., & Gordon, A. S. (1983). Stages of drug use in adolescence: Personality, peer, and family correlates. *Developmental Psychology, 19,* 269–277.

Bry, B. H., McKeon, P., & Pandina, R. J. (1982). Extent of drug use as a function of number of risk factors. *Journal of Abnormal Psychology, 91,* 273–279.

Bukstein, O. G., Brent, D. A., & Kaminer, Y. (1989). Comorbidity of substance abuse and other psychiatric disorders in adolescents. *American Journal of Psychiatry, 146,* 1131–1141.

Carlson, G. A. (1983). Bipolar affective disorders in childhood and adolescence. In D. P. Cantwell & G. A. Carlson (Eds.), *Affective disorders in childhood and adolescence* (pp. 61–83). New York: Spectrum.

Carlson, G., Bromet, E., & Jandorf, L. (1998). Conduct disorder and mania: What does it mean in adults? *Journal of Affective Disorders, 48,* 199–205.

Chambers, R. A., Taylor, J. R., & Potenza, M. N. (2003). Developmental neurocircuitry of motivation in adolescence: A critical period of addiction vulnerability. *American Journal of Psychiatry, 160,* 1041–1052.

Cloninger, C. R. (1987). Neurogenetic adaptive mechanisms in alcoholism. *Science, 236,* 410–416.

Comings, D., Comings, B., Muhleman, D., Dietz, G., Shahbahrami, B., Tast, D., et al. (1991). The dopamine D2 receptor locus as a modifying gene in neuropsychiatric disorders. *Journal of the American Medical Association, 266,* 1793–1800.

Crowley, T. J., & Riggs, P. D. (1995). Adolescent substance use disorder with conduct disorder and comorbid conditions. *NIDA Research Monographs, 156,* 49–111.

Crum, R. M., Bucholz, K. K., Helzer, J. E., & Anthony, J. C. (1992). The risk of alcohol abuse and dependence in adulthood: The association with educational level. *American Journal of Epidemiology, 135,* 989–999.

Davis, R. E. (1979). Manic-depressive variant syndrome of childhood: A preliminary report. *American Journal of Psychiatry, 136,* 702–706.

DeMilio, L. (1989). Psychiatric syndromes in adolescent substance abusers. *American Journal of Psychiatry, 146,* 1212–1214.

Dennis, M., Godley, S. H., Diamond, G., Tims, F. M., Babor, T., Donaldson, J., et al. (2004). The Cannabis Youth Treatment (CYT) Study: Main findings from two randomized trials. *Journal of Substance Abuse Treatment, 27,* 197–213.

Donovan, S., & Nunes, E. (1998). Treatment of comorbid affective and substance use disorders: Therapeutic potential of anticonvulsants. *American Journal of Addiction, 7*, 210–220.

Donovan, S. J., Susser, E. S., & Nunes, E. V. (1996). Changes in marijuana use in teenagers with temper outbursts and irritable mood after successful treatment with open-label Depakote. In (Eds.) *Fifty-eighth annual meetings of the College on Problems of Drug Dependence,* San Juan, Puerto Rico.

Doyle, A. E., Wilens, T., Kwon, A., Seidman, L. J., Faraone, S. V., Fried, R., et al. (2005). Neuropsychological functioning in youth with bipolar disorder. *Biological Psychiatry, 58*, 540–548.

Dunner, D. L., & Feinman, J. (1995). The effect of substance abuse on the course of bipolar disorder. In (Eds.) *Thirty-fourth annual meeting of the American College of Neuropsychopharmacology,* San Juan, Puerto Rico.

Ebstein, R., Novick, O., Umansky, R., Priel, B., Osher, Y., Blaine, D., et al. (1996). Dopamine D4 receptor exon III polymorphism associated with the human personality trait of novelty seeking. *Nature Genetics, 12*, 78–80.

Faraone, S. V., Biederman, J., Wozniak, J., Mundy, E., Mennin, D., & O'Donnell, D. (1997). Is comorbidity with ADHD a marker for juvenile-onset mania? *Journal of the American Academy of Child and Adolescent Psychiatry, 36*, 1046–1055.

Faraone, S. V., Tsuang, D., & Tsuang, M. T. (1999). *Genetics and mental disorders: A guide for students, clinicians, and researchers.* New York: Guilford Press.

Geller, B., Bolhofner, K., Craney, J. L., Williams, M., DelBello, M. P., & Gundersen, K. (2000). Psychosocial functioning in a prepubertal and early adolescent bipolar disorder phenotype. *Journal of the American Academy of Child and Adolescent Psychiatry, 39*, 1543–1548.

Geller, B., Cooper, T., Sun, K., Zimerman, B., Frazier, J., Williams, M., et al. (1998). Double-blind and placebo controlled study of lithium for adolescent bipolar disorders with secondary substance dependency. *Journal of the American Academy of Child and Adolescent Psychiatry, 37*, 171–178.

Geller, B., Fox, L., & Clark, K. (1994). Rate and predictors of prepubertal bipolarity during follow-up of 6- to 12-year-old depressed children. *Journal of the American Academy of Child and Adolescent Psychiatry, 33*, 461–468.

Geller, B., Zimerman, B., Williams, M., Bolhofner, K., & Craney, J. L. (2001). Adult psychosocial outcome of prepubertal major depressive disorder. *Journal of the American Academy of Child and Adolescent Psychiatry, 40*, 673–677.

Geller, B., Zimerman, B., Williams, M., Bolhofner, K., Craney, J. L., DelBello, M. P., et al. (2000a). Diagnostic characteristics of 93 cases of a prepubertal and early adolescent bipolar disorder phenotype by gender, puberty and comorbid attention deficit hyperactivity disorder. *Journal of Child and Adolescent Psychopharmacology, 10*, 157–164.

Geller, B., Zimerman, B., Williams, M., Bolhofner, K., Craney, J. L., DelBello, M. P., et al. (2000b). Six-month stability and outcome of a prepubertal and early adolescent bipolar disorder phenotype. *Journal of Child and Adolescent Psychopharmacology, 10*, 165–173.

Gignac, M., Wilens, T. E., Biederman, J., Kwon, A., Mick, E., & Swezey, A. (2005). Assessing cannabis use in adolescents and young adults: What do urine screen and parental report tell you? *Journal of Child and Adolescent Psychopharmacology, 15*, 742–750.

Glantz, M., & Pickens, R. (1992). *Vulnerability to drug abuse.* Washington, DC: American Psychological Press.

Grabowski, J., Roache, J. D., Schmitz, J. M., Rhoades, H., Creson, D., & Korszun, A. (1997). Replacement medication for cocaine dependence: Methylphenidate. *Journal of Clinical Psychopharmacology, 17*, 485–488.

Greene, R., Biederman, J., Faraone, S., Ouellette, C., Penn, C., & Griffin, S. (1996). Toward a new psychometric definition of social disability in children with attention-deficit hyperactivity disorder. *Journal of the American Academy of Child and Adolescent Psychiatry, 35*, 571–578.

Greene, R., Biederman, J., Faraone, S., Sienna, M., & Garcia-Jetton, J. (1997). Adolescent outcome of boys with attention-deficit/hyperactivity disorder and social disability: Results from a 4-year longitudinal follow-up study. *Journal of Consulting and Clinical Psychology, 65,* 758–767.

Greene, R. W., Biederman, J., Faraone, S. V., Wilens, T. W., Mick, E., & Blier, H. K. (1999). Further validation of social impairment as a predictor of substance use disorders: Findings from a sample of siblings of boys with and without ADHD. *Journal of Clinical Child Psychology, 28,* 349–354.

Hah, M., & Chang, K. (2005). Atomoxetine for the treatment of attention-deficit/hyperactivity disorder in children and adolescents with bipolar disorders. *Journal of Child and Adolescent Psychopharmacology, 15,* 996–1004.

Hawkins, D., Catalano, R., & Miller, J. (1992). Risk and protective factors for alcohol and other drug problems in adolescence and early adulthood. *Psychological Bulletin, 112,* 64–68.

Himmelhoch, J. M. (1979). Mixed states, manic-depressive illness, and the nature of mood. *Psychiatric Clinics of North America, 2,* 449–459.

Hopfer, C., Crowley, T. J., & Hewitt, J. K. (2003). Review of twin and adoption studies of adolescent substance use. *Journal of the American Academy of Child and Adolescent Psychiatry, 42,* 710–719.

Hopfer, C. J., Mikulich, S. K., & Crowley, T. J. (2000). Heroin use among adolescents in treatment for substance use disorders. *Journal of the American Academy of Child and Adolescent Psychiatry, 39,* 1316–1323.

Hovens, J. G., Cantwell, D. P., & Kiriakos, R. (1994). Psychiatric comorbidity in hospitalized adolescent substance abusers. *Journal of the American Academy of Child and Adolescent Psychiatry, 33,* 476–483.

John, K., Gammon, D., Prusoff, B. A., & Warner, V. (1987). The Social Adjustment Inventory for Children and Adolescents (SAICA): Testing of a new semistructured interview. *Journal of the American Academy of Child and Adolescent Psychiatry, 26,* 898–911.

Kaminer, Y., & Slesnick, N. (2005). Evidence-based cognitive-behavioral and family therapies for adolescent alcohol and other substance use disorders. *Recent Developments in Alcoholism, 17,* 383–405.

Kandel, D. B., & Logan, J. A. (1984). Patterns of drug use from adolescence to young adulthood: I. Periods of risk for initiation, continued use, and discontinuation. *American Journal of Public Health, 74,* 660–666.

Kellam, S., Brown, C., Rubin, B., & Ensminger, M. (1983). Paths leading to teenage psychiatric symptoms and substance use: Developmental epidemiological studies in Woodlawn. In S. Guze, F. Earls, & J. Barrett (Eds.), *Childhood psychopathology and development* (pp. 17–51). New York: Raven Press.

Khantzian, E. J. (1985). The self-medication hypothesis of addictive disorders: Focus on heroin and cocaine dependence. *American Journal of Psychiatry, 142,* 1259–1264.

Khantzian, E. J. (1997). The self-medication hypothesis of substance use disorders: A reconsideration and recent applications. *Harvard Review of Psychiatry, 4,* 231–244.

Kovacs, M., & Pollock, M. (1995). Bipolar disorder and comorbid conduct disorder in childhood and adolescence. *Journal of the American Academy of Child and Adolescent Psychiatry, 34,* 715–723.

Kravitz, H., Fawcett, J., McGuire, M., Kravitz, G., & Whitney, M. (1999). Treatment attrition among alcohol-dependent men: Is it related to novelty seeking personality traits? *Journal of Clinical Psychopharmacology, 19,* 51–56.

Krystal, H. (1978). Self-representation and the capacity for self-care. *Annals of Psychoanalysis, 6,* 209–246.

Kutcher, S., Marton, P., & Korenblum, M. (1989). Relationship between psychiatric illness and conduct disorder in adolescents. *Canadian Journal of Psychiatry, 34,* 526–529.

Labouvie, E. W., & McGee, C. R. (1986). Relation of personality to alcohol and drug use in adolescence. *Journal of Consulting and Clinical Psychology, 54,* 289–293.

Lagace, D. C., Kutcher, S. P., & Robertson, H. A. (2003). Mathematics deficits in adolescents with bipolar I disorder. *American Journal of Psychiatry, 160,* 100–104.

Lewinsohn, P. M., Gotlib, I. H., & Seeley, J. R. (1995). Adolescent psychopathology: IV. Specificity of psychosocial risk factors for depression and substance abuse in older adolescents. *Journal of the American Academy of Child and Adolescent Psychiatry, 34,* 1221–1229.

Lifrak, P. D., Alterman, A. I., O'Brien, C. P., & Volpicelli, J. R. (1997). Naltrexone for alcoholic adolescents. *American Journal of Psychiatry, 154,* 439–441.

Maes, H. H., Woodard, C. E., Murrelle, L., Meyer, J. M., Silberg, J. L., Hewitt, J. K., et al. (1999). Tobacco, alcohol and drug use in eight- to sixteen-year-old twins: The Virginia Twin Study of Adolescent Behavioral Development. *Journal of Studies on Alcohol, 60,* 293–305.

Masse, L. C., & Tremblay, R. E. (1997). Behavior of boys in kindergarten and the onset of substance use during adolescence. *Archives of General Psychiatry, 54,* 62–68.

McElroy, S., Altshuler, L., Suppes, T., Keck, P. E., Frye, M. A., Denicoff, K. D., et al. (2001). Axis I psychiatric comorbidity and its relationship to historical illness variables in 288 patients with bipolar disorder. *American Journal of Psychiatry, 158,* 420–426.

McElroy, S. L., Keck, P. E., Jr., Pope, H. G., Jr., Hudson, J. I., Faedda, G. L, & Swann, A. C. (1992). Clinical and research implications of the diagnosis of dysphoric or mixed mania or hypomania. *American Journal of Psychiatry, 149,* 1633–1644.

McElroy, S. L., Strakowski, S. M., Keck, P. E., Jr., Tugrul, K. L., West, S. A., & Lonczak, H. S. (1995). Differences and similarities in mixed and pure mania. *Comprehensive Psychiatry, 36,* 187–194.

McGue, M., Elkins, I., & Iacono, W. G. (2000). Genetic and environmental influences on adolescent substance use and abuse. *American Journal of Medical Genetics, 96,* 671–677.

McKay, J. R., & Buka, S. L. (1994). Issues in the treatment of antisocial adolescent substance abusers. *Journal of Child and Adolescent Substance Abuse, 3,* 59–81.

Mezzich, A. C., Tarter, R. E., Hsieh, Y., & Fuhrman, A. (1992). Substance abuse severity in female adolescents: Association between age at menarche and chronological age. *American Journal on Addictions, 1,* 217–221.

Myers, W., Donahue, J., & Goldstein, M. (1994). Disulfiram for alcohol use disorders in adolescents. *Journal of American Academy of Child and Adolescent Psychiatry, 33,* 484–489.

Newcomb, M. D., & Bentler, P. M. (1988). Impact of adolescent drug use and social support on problems of young adults: A longitudinal study. *Journal of Abnormal Psychology, 97,* 64–75.

Newcomb, M. D., Maddahian, E., & Bentler, P. M. (1986). Risk factors for drug use among adolescents: Concurrent and longitudinal analyses. *American Journal of Public Health, 76,* 525–531.

Ollendick, T., Weist, M., Borden, M., & Greene, R. (1992). Sociometric status and academic, behavioral, and psychological adjustment: A five-year longitudinal study. *Journal of Consulting and Clinical Psychology, 60,* 80–87.

Pandina, R., Johnson, V., & Labouvie, E. (1992). Affectivity: A central mechanism in the development of drug dependence. In M. Glantz & R. Pickens (Eds.), *Vulnerability to drug abuse* (pp. 179–210). Washington, DC: American Psychological Association Press.

Regier, D. A., Farmer, M. E., Rae, D. S., Zocke, B. Z., Keith, S. J., Judd, L. L., et al. (1990). Comorbidity of mental disorders with alcohol and other drug abuse. *Journal of the American Medical Association, 264,* 2511–2518.

Reich, L. H., Davies, R. K., & Himmelhoch, J. M. (1974). Excessive alcohol use in manic-depressive illness. *American Journal of Psychiatry, 131,* 83–86.

Reinherz, H. Z., Giaconia, R. M., Hauf, A. M., Wasserman, M. S., & Paradis, A. D. (2000). General and specific childhood risk factors for depression and drug disorders by early adulthood. *Journal of American Academy of Child and Adolescent Psychiatry, 39,* 223–231.

Riggs, P. D. (1998). Clinical approach to treatment of ADHD in adolescents with substance use disorders and conduct disorder. *Journal of American Academy of Child and Adolescent Psychiatry, 37,* 331–332.

Riggs, P., Mikulich, S., Coffman, L., & Crowley, T. (1997). Fluoxetine in drug-dependent delinquents with major depression: An open trial. *Journal of Child and Adolescent Psychopharmacology, 7,* 87–95.

Robins, L. N. (1966). *Deviant children grown up.* Baltimore: Williams & Wilkins.

Rohde, P., Lewinsohn, P. M., Kahler, C. W., Seeley, J. R., & Brown, R. A. (2001). Natural course of alcohol use disorders from adolescence to young adulthood. *Journal of the American Academy of Child and Adolescent Psychiatry, 40,* 83–90.

Ross, R. G. (2006). Psychotic and manic-like symptoms during stimulant treatment of attention deficit hyperactivity disorder. *American Journal of Psychiatry, 163,* 1149–1152.

Rounsaville, B. J., Weissman, M. M., Kleber, H., & Wilber, C. (1982). Heterogeneity of psychiatric diagnosis in treated opiate addicts. *Archives of General Psychiatry, 39,* 161–166.

Schubiner, H. (2005). Substance abuse in patients with attention-deficit hyperactivity disorder: Therapeutic implications. *CNS Drugs, 19,* 643–655.

Shear, P. K., DelBello, M. P., Lee Rosenberg, H., & Strakowski, S. M. (2002). Parental reports of executive dysfunction in adolescents with bipolar disorder. *Neuropsychology, Development, and Cognition: Section C. Child Neuropsychology, 8,* 285–295.

Shedler, J., & Block, J. (1990). Adolescent drug use and psychological health: A longitudinal inquiry. *American Psychologist, 45,* 612–630.

Solhkhah, R., Wilens, T. E., Daly, J., Prince, J. B., Patten, S. L., & Biederman, J. (2005). Bupropion SR for the treatment of substance-abusing outpatient adolescents with attention-deficit/hyperactivity disorder and mood disorders. *Journal of Child and Adolescent Psychopharmacology, 15,* 777–786.

Stowell, R., & Estroff, T. W. (1992). Psychiatric disorders in substance-abusing adolescent inpatients: A pilot study. *Journal of the American Academy of Child and Adolescent Psychiatry, 31,* 1036–1040.

Strakowski, S., McElroy, S., Keck, P., Jr., & West, S. (1995). The effects of antecedent substance abuse on the development of first-episode psychotic mania. *Journal of Psychiatric Research, 30,* 59–68.

Strakowski, S. M., DelBello, M. P., Fleck, D. E., Adler, C. M., Anthenelli, R. M., Keck, P. E., Jr., et al. (2005). Effects of co-occurring alcohol abuse on the course of bipolar disorder following a first hospitalization for mania. *Archives of General Psychiatry, 62,* 851–858.

Strakowski, S., Sax, K., McElroy, S., Keck, P., Hawkins, J., & West, S. (1998). Course of psychiatric and substance abuse syndromes co-occurring with bipolar disorder after a first psychiatric hospitalization. *Journal of Clinical Psychiatry, 59,* 465–471.

Strakowski, S., Tohen, M., Stoll, A., Faedda, G., & Goodwin, D. (1992). Comorbidity in mania at first hospitalization. *American Journal of Psychiatry, 149,* 554–556.

Strober, M., & Carlson, G. (1982). Predictors of bipolar illness in adolescents with major depression: A follow-up investigation. *Adolescent Psychiatry, 10,* 299–319.

Strober, M., Schmidt-Lackner, S., Freeman, R., Bower, S., Lampert, C., & DeAntonio, M. (1995). Recovery and relapse in adolescents with bipolar affective illness: A five-year naturalistic, prospective follow-up. *Journal of the American Academy of Child and Adolescent Psychiatry, 34,* 724–731.

Waxmonsky, J., & Wilens, T. (2003). Substance abusing youths. In A. Martin, L. Scahill, D. S. Charney, & J. F. Leckman (Eds.), *Pediatric psychopharmacology: Principles and practice* (pp. 605–616). New York: Oxford University Press.

Weinberg, N., Rahdert, E., Colliver, J., & Glantz, M. (1998). Adolescent substance abuse: A review of the past 10 years. *Journal of the American Academy of Child and Adolescent Psychiatry, 37,* 252–261.

West, S. A., Strakowski, S. M., Sax, K. W., McElroy, S. L., Keck, P. E., & McConville, B. J. (1996). Phenomenology and comorbidity of adolescents hospitalized for the treatment of acute mania. *Biological Psychiatry, 39,* 458–460.

Wilens, T., Biederman, J., Abrantes, A., & Spencer, T. (1997). Clinical characteristics of psychiatrically referred adolescent outpatients with substance use disorders. *Journal of the American Academy of Child and Adolescent Psychiatry, 36,* 941–947.

Wilens, T., Biederman, J., Bredin, E., Hahesy, A., Abrantes, A., Neft, D., et al. (2002). A family study of the high-risk children of opioid- and alcohol-dependent parents. *American Journal on Addictions, 11,* 41–51.

Wilens, T., Biederman, J., Kwon, A., Ditterline, J., Forkner, P., Chase, R., et al. (2004). Risk for substance use disorders in adolescents with bipolar disorder. *Journal of the American Academy Child and Adolescent Psychiatry, 43,* 1380–1386.

Wilens, T., Biederman, J., & Mick, E. (1998). Does ADHD affect the course of substance abuse?: Findings from a sample of adults with and without ADHD. *American Journal on Addictions, 7,* 156–163.

Wilens, T., Biederman, J., Milberger, S., Hahesy, A., Goldman, S., Wozniak, J., et al. (2000). Is bipolar disorder a risk for cigarette smoking in ADHD youth? *American Journal on Addictions, 9,* 187–195.

Wilens, T., Gignac, M., Swezey, A., Monuteaux, M., & Biederman, J. (2006). Characteristics of adolescents and young adults with ADHD who divert or misuse their prescribed medications. *Journal of the American Academy Child and Adolescent Psychiatry, 45,* 408–414.

Wilens, T. E., Biederman, J., Mick, E., Faraone, S. V., & Spencer, T. (1997). Attention deficit hyperactivity disorder (ADHD) is associated with early onset substance use disorders. *Journal of Nervous and Mental Disease, 185,* 475–482.

Wilens, T. E., Biederman, J., Millstein, R., Wozniak, J., Hahesy, A., & Spencer, T. J. (1999). Risk for substance use disorders in youth with child- and adolescent-onset bipolar disorder. *Journal of the American Academy of Child and Adolescent Psychiatry, 38,* 680–685.

Wills, T. A., Windle, M., & Cleary, S. D. (1998, February). Temperament and novelty seeking in adolescent substance use: Convergence of dimensions of temperament with constructs from Cloninger's theory. *Journal of Personality and Social Psychology, 74,* 387–406.

Winokur, G., Coryell, W., Akiskal, H. S., Maser, J. D., Keller, M. B., Endicott, J., et al. (1995). Alcoholism in manic-depressive (bipolar) illness: Familial illness, course of illness, and the primary–secondary distinction. *American Journal of Psychiatry, 152,* 365–372.

Wozniak, J., & Biederman, J. (1996). A pharmacological approach to the quagmire of comorbidity in juvenile mania. *Journal of the American Academy of Child and Adolescent Psychiatry, 35,* 826–828.

Wozniak, J., Biederman, J., Kiely, K., Ablon, S., Faraone, S. V., Mundy, E., et al. (1995). Mania-like symptoms suggestive of childhood-onset bipolar disorder in clinically referred children. *Journal of the American Academy of Child and Adolescent Psychiatry, 34,* 867–876.

Wozniak, J., Biederman, J., Mundy, E., Mennin, D., & Faraone, S. V. (1995). A pilot family study of childhood-onset mania. *Journal of the American Academy of Child and Adolescent Psychiatry, 34,* 1577–1583.

Yamaguchi, K., & Kandel, D. B. (1984). Patterns of drug use from adolescence to young adulthood: II. Sequences of progression. *American Journal of Public Health, 74,* 668–672.

Young, S., Mikulick, S., Goodwin, M., Hardy, J., Martin, C., Zoccolillo, M., et al. (1995). Treated delinquent boys' substance use: Onset, pattern, relationship to conduct and mood disorders. *Drug and Alcohol Dependence, 37,* 149–162.

CHAPTER 13

Pediatric Bipolar Disorder and Comorbid Conditions

Treatment Implications

GAGAN JOSHI *and* JANET WOZNIAK

Pediatric-onset bipolar disorder seldom occurs in the absence of comorbid conditions. The co-occurrence of additional disorders complicates both the accurate diagnosis of bipolar disorder in youth and also its treatment. To date, most pharmacological trials of bipolar disorder in children and adolescents include children with a variety of comorbidities. Thus the mediating effect of the comorbid condition on the treatment of bipolar disorder in children and adolescents is unknown. Treatment trials for anxiety and other conditions routinely exclude participants with bipolar disorder. In addition, treatments for some comorbid conditions, such as antidepressant treatment for anxiety, may make bipolar disorder worse. Thus, when possible, nonmedication treatments, such as interpersonal psychotherapy and cognitive-behavioral therapy, should be used, as these treatments have demonstrated efficacy for conditions such as depression, anxiety disorders, and obsessive–compulsive disorder (OCD), without running the risk of exacerbating mania (Kowatch et al., 2005).

Treatment guidelines for pediatric bipolar disorder indicate that the treatment plan must include treatment for each comorbid disorder, which may become a complex process of trial and error to find the most effective combination of medications (Kowatch et al., 2005). These guidelines further recommend that, in the absence of treatment trials aimed specifically at conditions as they co-occur with bipolar disorder, clinicians use any of the medications and psychosocial treatments that are generally recommended for each comorbid disorder when that disorder occurs as the primary problem. Clinical sense dictates that comorbid conditions are addressed only after the symptoms of bipolar disorder are stabilized (Wozniak & Biederman, 1996).

Comorbid disorders may be hard to diagnose due to overlapping symptoms and complicated patterns of development. Comorbid disorders can manifest simultaneously (concurrent comorbidity) or at different times without overlapping with each other (successive comorbidity). Longitudinally, phenotypic presentation can remain unchanged over time (homotypic continuity) or manifest differently over time (hetrotypic continuity). The comorbid disorders can share nonspecific symptoms, as they may belong to common diagnostic groups (homotypic comorbidity), or they may belong to different diagnostic groups (hetrotypic comorbidity) and not share symptoms that define them. Based on the sequence of onset of comorbid disorders, historically the terms *primary* and *secondary disorders* have sometimes been applied, signifying that the secondary disorder is caused by or is a consequence of the primary disorder, but this hierarchical notion based on sequence of onset is highly debatable and may hinder proper treatment.

Comorbid disorders need further study to delineate in which cases comorbid conditions represent distinct co-occurring conditions, a combined condition that represents a distinct genetic subtype, or the result of methodological bias. *Berkson's bias* refers to the notion that a higher estimate of comorbidity may be apparent in clinically referred cases than would be the case if study were made of nonclinical cases. Nonetheless, current studies based on clinically referred cases likely reflect common clinical experience.

To understand the nature of comorbidity, current and future research focuses on (1) epidemiological studies to document comorbidity rates, (2) systematic examinations of correlates of clinical characteristics, comorbidity profile, course, and treatment outcomes of disorders in the context of comorbidity status (3) family genetic studies to identify familial patterns of comorbidity and to discern distinct genetic subtypes, (4) molecular genetic studies to understand underlying specific neurobiology, and (5) treatment intervention studies to address efficacy and tolerability of psychotropic medication in the context of the comorbidity.

Studies addressing comorbidity generally rely either on cross-sectional data or on recall of disorders over the whole life course. Both of these approaches pose limitations. Long-term longitudinal studies offer the best possibility for observing the developmental progression of the emergence of comorbid conditions.

The presence of comorbid disorders with bipolar disorder results in a more severe clinical condition. Adult studies report that adults with bipolar disorder and additional comorbidity suffer an earlier age of bipolar disorder onset with cycle acceleration and more severe episodes (McElroy et al., 2001). Previous research has suggested that identifying and treating co-occurring psychiatric disorders among individuals with bipolar disorder may help to alleviate the impairment and prolonged course that individuals with bipolar disorder and additional psychiatric disorders often experience.

In addition to attention-deficit/hyperactivity disorder (ADHD), conditions commonly occurring with pediatric-onset bipolar disorder include conduct disorder, multiple anxiety disorders (including panic disorder, posttraumatic stress disorder [PTSD], and OCD), and pervasive developmental disorders. This chapter addresses the co-occurrence and treatment of bipolar disorder in children and adolescents with these additional disorders.

CONDUCT DISORDER

Prevalence and Clinical Characteristics

In a comprehensive literature review, Geller and Luby (1997) concluded that "Available data strongly suggest that prepubertal-onset BPD is a non-episodic, chronic, rapid-cycling, mixed manic state that may be comorbid with attention-deficit/hyperactivity disorder (ADHD) and conduct disorder (CD) or have features of ADHD and/or CD as initial manifestations" (p. 1168). This observation is supported by a body of research documenting a bidirectional overlap between CD and bipolar disorder in children. As both CD and bipolar disorder are highly impairing conditions, their co-occurrence heralds a particularly severe clinical picture and raises important clinical questions. From a diagnostic standpoint, the question remains as to whether antisocial behaviors in a child with bipolar disorder, such as stealing, lying, or vandalizing, should be attributed to the disinhibition of mania with its attendant impulsivity, irritability, and grandiosity or to comorbid CD. From a treatment standpoint in such a child, the question further remains as to whether the symptoms of CD will diminish when the symptoms of bipolar disorder are adequately treated. If this is the case, then some portion of youths in the criminal justice system could be fruitfully diverted to psychiatric treatment.

In addition to improving the treatment of these difficult patients, the delineation of a subtype of CD linked to bipolar disorder may lead to the identification of a more homogeneous subgroup of youths with CD with a distinct pathophysiology and etiology. This, eventually, could lead to a better understanding of the causes of CD and bipolar disorder in this subgroup. If future research finds a relatively homogeneous etiology for comorbid CD and bipolar disorder, that could lead to specialized treatments for these difficult-to-manage patients, which would reduce the burden to the criminal justice system.

The association between CD and mania is consistent with the well-documented comorbidity between CD and major depression (Angold & Costello, 1993) and the frequently bipolar nature of juvenile depression (Geller, Fox, & Clark, 1994; Strober & Carlson, 1982). Moreover, pediatric-onset bipolar disorder is frequently mixed (dysphoric) and commonly associated with "affective storms," with prolonged and aggressive temper outbursts (Davis, 1979; Carlson, 1983, 1984). These irritable outbursts often include threatening or attacking behavior toward family members, children, adults, and teachers, behaviors that overlap with CD. For example, McGlashan (1988) reported that juvenile-onset mania may be particularly explosive and disorganized and that children with mania tended to have more trouble with the law and more "psychotic assaultiveness" (p. 222) than adults with mania. Kovacs and Pollock (1995) reported that some youngsters with mania showed serious acting-out behaviors, including burglary, stealing, vandalism, and a history of school suspensions. Although these aberrant behaviors are consistent with the diagnosis of CD, they may be due to the behavioral disinhibition that characterizes bipolar disorder. Thus it is not surprising that youths with bipolar disorder frequently meet diagnostic criteria for CD.

Kovacs and Pollock (1995) reported a 69% rate of CD in a referred sample of youths with bipolar disorder, and the presence of CD heralded a more complicated course of bipolar disorder. Similarly, Kutcher, Marton, and Korenblum (1989) found that 42% of hospitalized youths with bipolar disorder had comorbid CD, and Wozniak et al. (1995) showed that preadolescent children satisfying structured interview criteria for bipolar disorder very frequently had comorbid CD. A study by Moore, Thompson-Pope, and Whited (1996) suggested that the type of CD associated with mania can be severe. Moreover, data presented by Modestin, Hug, and Ammann (1997) suggest that the antisocial behaviors of youths with bipolar disorder can persist into adulthood. They examined the prevalence of criminal behavior in a population of 261 male inpatients with affective disorders. The full account of conviction records in a criminal register was used as a measure of criminal behavior. Altogether, a higher criminality rate was found in patients with bipolar disorder, whereas no increased criminality rate was found in patients with unipolar major depression.

Carlson and Kashani (1988) examined 150 14- to 16-year-olds randomly selected from a nonreferred population. Among these, 20 endorsed four or more manic symptoms of at least 2 days' duration. Compared with the rest of the sample, these adolescents had significantly higher rates of attention-deficit, conduct, and anxiety disorders and psychotic symptoms. This group was described as dysphoric, impulsive, and emotionally labile. Notably, Lewinsohn, Klein, and Seeley's (1995) epidemiological study found high rates of comorbidity between bipolar and disruptive behavior disorders. Similar findings were reported in the Epidemiologic Catchment Area (ECA) study. In an initial analysis of the ECA data, Robins and Price (1991) showed that the risk for mania increased with the number of CD symptoms. Further work on the ECA data by Carlson, Bromet, and Jandorf (1998) documented a substantial overlap between CD and mania in adults, particularly in those under the age of 30 years. In that study, rates of CD were higher in participants under age 30 with bipolar disorder (32.6%) than in older participants (16.3%). Notably, the younger group of patients with bipolar disorder who also had substance use disorders had CD rates three times those of patients without substance use disorders (52% vs. 14.8%). In comparison, young participants without mania or substance use disorders had CD rates of 7.8%. From these results, the authors concluded that substance abuse in adults with bipolar disorder was more related to childhood CD than to bipolar disorder. The ECA also reported a nearly seven-fold increase in the risk for bipolar disorder among individuals with antisocial personality disorder (Boyd et al., 1984).

In conceptualizing the overlap between bipolar disorder and CD, Kovacs and Pollock (1995) suggested that the high prevalence of comorbid CD in youths with bipolar disorder might confuse the clinical presentation of childhood bipolar disorder and possibly account for some of the documented failure to detect bipolarity in children. Isaac (1992) examined a group of adolescents found to be the most problematic, crisis-prone, and treatment-resistant in a special educational day school and treatment program. These authors found that two-thirds of these youngsters satisfied DSM-III-R criteria for bipolar disorder, which had been misdiagnosed mainly as ADHD and CD. Most of the remaining youngsters showed significant bipolar features but did not fully satisfy DSM-III-R criteria for bipolar disorder. Considering the heterogeneity of bipolar disorder and that of CD, these findings may have important implications in helping to identify a subtype of bipolar disorder with early onset characterized by high levels of comorbid CD (Kovaks & Pollock, 1995) and a subtype of CD with high levels of dysphoria and explosiveness.

Although the reasons for these associations between CD and bipolar disorder remain unknown, a close inspection of the characteristics of juvenile bipolar disorder offers some clues. The literature indicates that juvenile bipolar disorder is frequently mixed (dysphoric), often characterized by irritable mood, with "affective storms," which include threatening or attacking behavior toward others, including family members, children, adults, and teachers. Although these aberrant behaviors are consistent with the diagnosis of CD, they may additionally be exacerbated by the behavioral disinhibition of bipolar disorder. Considering the extreme severity of juvenile bipolar disorder, its emergence in children with CD seriously complicates their already compromised lives, and vice versa.

Thus, in a series of pilot studies, Biederman and colleagues attempted to delineate the relationship between bipolar disorder and CD. These studies relied on systematic evaluation of clinical correlates in affected youths and their relatives. The first study used data from a large, well-characterized, prospective sample of referred children with ADHD (Biederman, Faraone, Hatch, et al., 1997). This study found that probands with CD plus bipolar disorder had a higher familial and personal risk for mood disorders than CD probands without bipolar disorder, whereas these latter probands had a higher personal risk for antisocial personality disorder. These results strongly suggested that the presence of bipolar disorder in some children with CD could be clinically meaningful, at least in the context of ADHD.

Further analysis of structured interview-derived data from a large sample of consecutive, clinic-referred children and adolescents, showed again a large and symmetrical overlap between bipolar disorder and CD (Biederman, Faraone, Chu, & Wozniak, 1999). Examination of the clinical features, patterns of psychiatric comorbidity, and functioning in multiple domains showed that children with CD and bipolar disorder had similar features of each disorder, irrespective of comorbidity with the other disorder. These findings further supported the hypothesis that children who satisfy diagnostic criteria for bipolar disorder and CD suffer from both disorders, rather than it being a case of one disorder misdiagnosed as the other, even outside the context of comorbid ADHD.

In both data sets, there was a similarity in the phenotypic features of both CD and bipolar disorder in children with both diagnoses, irrespective of the comorbidity with the other disorder. CD symptoms were almost identical in children with CD, irrespective of the comorbidity with bipolar disorder, and the same was true for manic symptoms. In both groups, mania presented with a predominantly severe irritable mood, a chronic course, and a mixed presentation, with symptoms of major depression overlapping in time with those of mania.

These authors also documented the fact that psychiatric hospitalizations among probands with CD were almost entirely accounted for by those with comorbid bipolar disorder. This finding is consistent with the notion that probands with CD plus bipolar disorder, along with other symptoms of CD, engage in a disorganized type of aggression associated with bipolar disorder. Because many children in psychiatric hospitals with the diagnosis of CD commonly have a profile of severe aggressiveness, it is likely that these children required psychiatric hospitalizations because of the manic picture and not necessarily because of the CD.

Evidence from Family Genetic Studies

Further evidence that a subtype of CD linked to bipolar disorder could be identified derives from pilot familial-risk analyses (Biederman, Faraone, Wozniak, & Monuteaux, 2000; Wozniak, Biederman, Faraone, Blier, & Monuteaux, 2001). These results showed that relatives of probands with bipolar disorder had an increased risk for bipolar disorder but not CD, whereas relatives of probands with CD had an increased risk for CD but not for bipolar disorder; relatives of probands with CD plus bipolar disorder had an elevated risk for both disorders (Wozniak et al., 2001). Among relatives in this latter group, bipolar disorder and antisocial disorders showed significant cosegregation, that is, relatives with one disorder were highly likely to have the other. As a result of this cosegregation, CD plus bipolar disorder was significantly elevated among relatives of probands with CD plus bipolar disorder but was rare among the relatives of the other proband groups. Probands with the combined condition of CD and bipolar disorder also had high rates of conduct or antisocial disorders without bipolar disorder among the relatives, suggesting a genetic loading with two subtypes of CD: with and without bipolar disorder.

The family study results support the concept of heterogeneity of bipolar disorder and CD. Whereas the rates of bipolar disorder in relatives were identical in both bipolar disorder proband groups, the relatives of probands with CD plus bipolar disorder had almost exclusively the comorbid type of bipolar disorder (CD/antisocial personality disorder plus bipolar disorder) and relatives of the probands with bipolar disorder had higher rates of bipolar disorder without CD/antisocial personality disorder (Wozniak et al., 2001). These results provide compelling evidence that subtypes of CD and of bipolar disorder can be identified based on patterns of comorbidity with the other disorder. Notably, both CD and bipolar disorder show both a within-patient and a familial association with ADHD, suggesting that their co-occurrence may correspond to a distinct familial syndrome (Biederman et al., 2000; Wozniak et al., 2001; Faraone, Biederman, Mennin, Wozniak, & Spencer, 1997; Faraone, Biederman, Mennin, & Russell, 1998; Faraone, Biederman, & Monuteaux, 2001).

Familial-risk analysis also found strong support for the hypothesis that bipolar disorder in probands is a risk factor for substance use disorders (SUDs) in relatives, independently of the comorbidity with CD in probands (Biederman et al., 2000). After accounting for CD in probands, bipolar disorder in probands was a risk factor for SUDs, including both drug and alcohol addiction, in relatives. In contrast, after accounting for bipolar disorder in probands, CD in probands was a risk factor for alcohol dependence in relatives but not for drug dependence, independently of comorbid bipolar disorder in the probands. The effects of bipolar disorder and CD in probands combined additively to predict the risk for SUDs in relatives.

Familial-risk data also showed that regardless of the presence of CD in probands with bipolar disorder, relatives of these probands were at risk for substance dependence onset in their teenage years. In contrast, the risk for alcohol dependence imparted by probands with CD becomes evident only during adulthood. These data suggest that the familial disposition to bipolar disorder—and not CD—is associated with early-onset SUDs, making it especially relevant for prevention programs aimed at adolescents.

Management

Rather than pharmacotherapy, the treatment of CD in youths primarily utilizes psychosocial interventions. A recent report (Tcheremissine & Lieving, 2006) addressing the pharmacological aspects of the treatment of CD in children and adolescents concludes that pharmacological interventions will be most effective when combined with behavioral and psychosocial interventions. These authors write that "a multidisciplinary approach to the treatment of CD, which includes behavioral parent training, interpersonal skills training, family therapy and the use of psychotropic agents targeted at a particular cluster of symptoms, can increase the overall effectiveness of each of the applied interventions" (Tcheremissine & Lieving, 2006, p. 459). The authors go on to suggest that the best targets for psychopharmacological intervention are aggression, hyperactivity, impulsivity, and mood symptoms and that antipsychotics, antidepressants, mood stabilizers, antiepileptics, stimulants, and adrenergic medications should be used for the comorbidity associated with the CD.

Although a small literature addresses the pharmacotherapy of CD, notably these studies generally utilize treatments that are considered mood stabilizers, raising the question of whether responders in these studies suffer additionally from a bipolar spectrum disorder. A review of prevention, treatment, and service configurations for juvenile maladaptive aggression (i.e., conduct problems) indicates, as in the preceding report, that prevention programs and psychosocial treatments are useful in reducing aggression in children and adolescents (Connor et al., 2006). However, in addition, these authors cite the antimanic agents (along with stimulants when ADHD is present) as the pharmacological treatments with the most robust empirical support in the treatment of aggression, suggesting that the aggression could be symptom of mania.

The delineation of a subgroup of children with mania and CD would have important clinical implications. It could lead to improvement in our efforts to ameliorate the guarded outcome of some youths with CD. Because mania may respond to specific pharmacological treatments, correctly identifying those children with mania and CD may afford the opportunity to introduce these medications in the treatment of antisocial and aggressive youths.

Indeed, our preliminary treatment data from extensive chart reviews of children with mania suggest that mood stabilizers and atypical antipsychotics, the very medications most commonly recommended for the treatment of CD, are important for the clinical stabilization of difficult-to-treat patients with bipolar disorder (Wozniak & Biederman, 1996; Biederman et al., 1998). Campbell and Cueva's (1995) review concluded that for children and adolescents, the antimanic agent lithium is useful for reducing a key symptom of CD, aggression. Consistent with this, their double-blind, placebo-controlled study showed lithium to be effective in the treatment of hospitalized aggressive children with CD. In another review, Sheard (1975) noted that lithium had been successfully used to improve aggressive behavior in childhood, and Worrall, Moody, and Naylor (1975) reported that lithium could effectively treat aggressive, nonmanic adolescents.

A small literature suggesting that antipsychotic medications such as haloperidol and molindone were helpful in decreasing aggression in youths with CD (Campbell, Anderson, & Green, 1983) has led to the use of the atypical antipsychotic agents in treating CD with aggressive features. An open-label pharmacokinetic study by Findling et al. (2006) examined quetiapine in 6- to 12-year-olds with the primary diagnosis of CD. The outcome measures included the Rating of Aggression Against People and/or Property Scale (RAAPPS), the Nisonger Child Behavior Rating Form (NCBRF), the Clinical Global Impression Scale of Improvement (CGI-I) and Severity (CGI-S), and the Connors Parent Rating Scale (CPRS-48). Scores on the RAAPPS and the CGI-S improved significantly by week 8 and five of the six problem scales of the NCBRF improved significantly as well. The Conduct, Learning and Hyperactivity scales of the CPRS improved from baseline to week 8, and the Psychosomatic, Impulse, and Anxiety scales improved but not significantly.

Several trials indicate that risperidone can be useful for CD, especially the aggressive features, in both short-term and long-term use (Aman, De Smedt, Derivan, Lyons, & Findling, 2002; Findling, Aman, Eerdekens, Derivan, & Lyons, 2004; Croonenberghs, Fegert, Findling, De Smedt, & Van Dongen, 2005; Findling et al., 2000; Turgay, Binder, Snyder, & Fisman, 2002). These reports, from the Risperidone Disruptive Behavior Study Group, examine the use of risperidone in children with severe disruptive behaviors and below-average IQ in double-blind, placebo-controlled short-term studies and open-label long-term studies. Included children had a clinician-confirmed DSM-IV diagnosis of CD, oppositional defiant disorder, or disruptive behavior disorder not otherwise specified, as well as elevated scores on the Conduct Problem subscale of the NCBRF. In addition, included children had a DSM-IV Axis II diagnosis of mild mental retardation, moderate mental retardation, or borderline intellectual functioning (IQ of 36–84) and a low score on the Vineland Adaptive Behavior Scale. These studies concluded that risperidone was effective in the short- and long-term treatment of disruptive behavior disorders based on statistically significant improvement in the Conduct Problem subscale of the NCBRF.

However, a post-hoc analysis of data from the placebo-controlled 6-week study ($N = 110$) examined 24 candidate affective symptoms extracted from the 64-item NCBRF (Biederman et al., 2006). These symptoms reflected the bipolar symptoms of explosive irritability, agitation, expansiveness, grandiosity, and depression. Risperidone was also effective in treating these putative symptoms of mania. This analysis raises the question of whether studies that examine the effects of antimanic agents on CD may include participants with comorbid bipolar spectrum illness and, further, whether the improvement in CD symptoms is a function in part of the improvement in bipolar disorder symptoms.

Consistent with this notion, an open-label trial of risperidone in children and adolescents with bipolar disorder concluded that risperidone was associated with significant short-term improvement of symptoms of pediatric bipolar disorder but, in addition, reported that 55% of participants with comorbid CD were "much" or "very much" improved on the CGI-S for CD (Biederman, Mick, Wozniak, et al., 2005). Nine of the 30 participants with bipolar disorder (30%) treated with risperidone had impairment at baseline on conduct symptoms. In open-label studies of olanzapine and risperidone in preschool-age participants (4–6 years; Biederman, Mick, Hammerness, et al., 2005) the authors reported rapid reduction of symptoms of mania in preschool children. At baseline, 39% of the 16 participants on risperidone and 57% of the 15 participants on olanzapine had symptoms of CD as indicated by a CGI-S score of 3 or more. At follow-up evaluation 8 weeks later, 50% of the 5 risperidone-treated participants with CD and 38% of the 8 olanzapine-treated participants with CD were "much" or "very much" improved on the CGI-I scale for CD.

OPPOSITIONAL DEFIANT DISORDER

High rates with bidirectional overlap of comorbid oppositional defiant disorder (ODD) and bipolar disorder are reported by various studies. Rates of ODD in the population with bipolar disorder range from 47–88% (Wozniak et al., 1995; Findlay et al., 2001; Geller et al., 2000), and, conversely, 20% of children with ODD are reported to have comorbid bipolar disorder (Greene & Doyle, 1999). A recent meta-analysis reported that among samples of children and adolescents with bipolar disorder, ODD was the second most common comorbidity after ADHD, with weighted rate of 53% (Kowatch et al., 2005).

Diagnosis of ODD in the context of mania is challenging, as, nosologically, ODD shares overlapping symptoms with mania, without any symptom specific to ODD that could diagnostically differentiate it from mania. Because ODD is so frequently comorbid with pediatric bipolar disorder, understanding of ODD's relationship with bipolar disorder ranges from ODD being a secondary disorder as a consequence of bipolar illness or being a prodrome or early manifestation of bipolar disorder to representing a "true independent" comorbid psychopathological phenomenon. However, many children with disruptive behavior disorders do not go on to develop bipolar disorder (Biederman et al., 1996), suggesting that different forms of disruptive behavior disorders may exist—one that could be prodromal to bipolar disorder and another form that is not. More work is needed to further evaluate this issue.

A clinical inquiry summarized eight reviews of ODD treatment in children and found improved behavior, with 20–30% decrease in disruptive or aggressive behaviors with parenting interventions and behavioral therapy, including cognitive-behavioral therapy, social problem-solving skills training, and parent management training involving child and/or parent for 12–25 sessions (Farley et al., 2005). Though treatment for ODD is primarily behavioral in nature, when it is comorbid with other medication-responsive psychiatric conditions (bipolar disorder, ADHD), pharmacological treatment of the comorbid disorder often reduces overall symptoms. A double-blind crossover randomized controlled trial evaluating children with either CD or ODD with explosive temper and mood lability reported significant reduction in aggressive behaviors and anger and hostility following divalproex treatment (Donovan et al., 2000). There are currently no data available on the treatment of ODD in the context of bipolar disorder comorbidity. Further prospective studies addressing course and treatment of ODD when comorbid with bipolar disorder are warranted.

ENURESIS

Significantly higher rates of enuresis have been observed with pediatric bipolar disorder. Epidemiological studies report high prevalence of enuresis in children and adolescents (5–8% of 7- to 17-year-olds) (Bellman, 1966; Costello et al., 1996; Linna, Moilanen, Keistinen, Ernvall, & Karppinen, 1991; Shaffer et al., 1996; Spee-van der Wekke, Hirasing, Meulmeester, & Radder, 1998). Higher than expected rates (21.5%) of enuresis are reported with bipolar disorder (Klages, Geller, Tillman, Bolhofner, & Zimerman, 2005; Henin et al., 2006) and other common childhood-onset disorders such as ADHD (21–32% of 6- to 17-year-olds) (Klages et al., 2005; Biederman et al., 1995; Robson, Jackson, Blackhurst, & Leung, 1997). Genetic factors appear to be important in the pathophysiology of enuresis, as evidenced by family studies reporting that enuretics versus nonenuretics had a significantly higher prevalence of familial aggregation of enuresis. This is evident both in the general population and in populations with bipolar disorder (Klages et al., 2005; Arnell et al., 1997; Loeys et al., 2002). It is unlikely that enuresis is part of the symptom picture of a severe manic episode or due to medication (lithium) side effects, because of this evidence of familial aggregation plus evidence that onset of enuresis tends to occur prior to onset of mania (Klages et al., 2005; Henin et al., 2006).

Medication treatment may play a role in this comorbidity as well. High rates of bipolar disorder occurring in youths with enuresis have been suggested to be a result of hypomania induced by antidepressant treatment for enuresis in youths. Conversely, psychotropic treatment for mania in youths, such as lithium treatment, may result in enuresis as a side effect. The issue of enuresis in youths with bipolar disorder secondary to anti-manic psychotropic treatment has been addressed by Klages et al. (2005), who examined the temporal relationship between onset of enuresis and treatment with lithium in youths with bipolar disorder and reported that no participant with enuresis had received lithium before the onset of enuresis. These authors concluded that enuresis in youths with bipolar disorder is not secondary to treatment with lithium. The risk of antidepressant-induced hypomania should be considered when treating enuresis in children at risk of bipolar disorder with tricyclic antidepressants. Alternative treatment with desmopressin could be the treatment of choice for enuretic children with enuresis with or at risk for bipolar disorder.

ANXIETY DISORDERS

The presence of anxiety disorders in individuals who suffer from bipolar disorder has been underrecognized and understudied. One reason for this lack of recognition could be the notion that it is counterintuitive to suggest that bipolar disorder, which is characterized by high levels of disinhibition, could coexist with anxiety, which is characterized by fear and inhibition. However, in the first study to demonstrate the high frequency (16%) of bipolar disorder in an outpatient pediatric psychopharmacology clinic (Wozniak et al., 1995) 56% of the children with bipolar disorder suffered from two or more lifetime anxiety disorders (multiple anxiety disorders) comorbidly. These findings have been replicated in a larger sample (Biederman et al., 2004). Furthermore, a recent detailed analysis of the comorbidity between pediatric bipolar disorder and anxiety disorders revealed that 75% of youths with bipolar disorder have one or more anxiety disorders comorbid with their bipolar disorder. In a community sample, Lewinsohn et al. (1995) reported that a third of nonreferred adolescents with bipolar disorder had comorbid anxiety disorders, a significantly higher rate than that found in those without a history of mania. Similar findings were reported by Faraone, Biederman, Mennin, et al. (1997), who found that 56% of adolescents with a diagnosis of bipolar disorder had multiple anxiety disorders.

This association is also evident in adults, as demonstrated by Simon and colleagues, who reported in one of the largest studies of bipolar adults to date that over half of their sample had at least one anxiety disorder (Simon et al., 2003; Simon et al., 2005). Anxiety has been found to occur relatively frequently in both the manic and depressive phases of bipolar disorder in adults (Cassidy, Forest, Murry, & Carroll, 1998; Cassidy, Murry, Forest, & Carroll, 1998). Data from both ECA (Chen & Dilsaver, 1995) and the National Comorbidity Survey (NCS) document higher than expected rates of several anxiety disorders in participants with bipolar disorder (OCD, social phobia, panic disorder, PTSD).

Because the anxiety disorders are heterogeneous (eight are included in the DSM-IV; American Psychiatric Association, 1994), uncertainties remain as to which anxiety disorders are associated with bipolar disorder, and most studies lump them together. Various clinical and epidemiological studies in adult and pediatric populations have identified a wide range of anxiety disorders associated with bipolar disorder, including generalized anxiety disorder, panic disorder, agoraphobia, simple phobia, social phobia, separation anxiety disorder, PTSD, and OCD. Rates of comorbid association range between 12.5 and 56% (McElroy et al., 2001; Lewinsohn et al., 1995; Chen & Dilsaver, 1995; Johnson, Cohen, & Brook, 2000; Masi et al., 2001; Faedda, Baldessarini, Glovinsky, & Austin, 2004; Harpold et al., 2005; Tillman et al., 2003; Wozniak, Biederman, Monuteaux, Richards, & Faraone, 2002; Biederman, Faraone, Marrs, et al., 1997; Faraone, Biederman, Wozniak, et al., 1997; Feske et al., 2000; Kessler, Sonnega, Bromet, Hughest, & Nelson, 1995; Kessler, Stang, Wittchen, Stein, & Walters, 1999; Perugi, 1999; Masi et al., 2004; Wozniak et al., 1999; Judd et al., 1002; Perugi, Akiskal, Toni, Simonini, & Gemignani, 2001; Perugi, Frare, Toni, Mata, & Akiskal, 2001). A specific association in youths between separation anxiety disorder and bipolar disorder is suggested by Tillman et al. (2003). However, Harpold et al. (2005) found high rates of anxiety disorders in 297 clinically referred youths with bipolar disorder with no specific link to any particular anxiety disorder over others. Thus more information is needed as to whether the association between bipolar disorder and anxiety disorders in youths is limited to a single anxiety disorder or is more extensive and includes other anxiety disorders as well.

Panic Disorder

A preponderance of investigators have suggested that a particular link exists between bipolar disorder and panic disorder in adults (Chen & Dilsaver, 1995; Goodwin & Hoven, 2002; Goodwin, Hamilton, Milne, & Pine, 2002) and children (Birmaher et al., 2002). Data from adult studies report a lifetime prevalence of panic disorder in 21–33% of individuals with bipolar disorder (Chen & Dilsaver, 1995; Goodwin & Hoven, 2002;

Goodwin et al., 2002; Kessler, Davis, & Kendler, 1997; Kessler et al., 1998) and, conversely, lifetime bipolar disorder in 6–23% of individuals with panic disorder (Perugi, 1999; Rowen, South, & Hawkes, 1994). MacKinnon and colleagues (MacKinnon et al., 1998; MacKinnon et al., 2002) utilize family genetic methodology in 57 families to argue that panic disorder with bipolar disorder is a genetic subtype of bipolar disorder. Savino et al. (1993) systematically explored the intraepisodic and longitudinal comorbidity of 140 adults with panic disorder, and the reported comorbidity with bipolar disorder in 13.5% of the patients with panic disorder. They also note that an additional 34.3% met features of "hyperthymic temperament," a possible bipolar spectrum condition. Likewise, a recent report by Birmaher et al. (2002) suggested a specific association between bipolar disorder and panic disorder in youths, and Biederman, Faraone, Marrs, et al. (1997) reported high rates of panic disorder (52%) among youths with bipolar disorder.

There is growing evidence that anxiety comorbidity is a frequent, albeit a hitherto neglected, precursor for pediatric-onset bipolar disorder (Masi et al., 2001; Bashir, Russell, & Johnson, 1987; Geller, Biederman, Griffin, Jones, & Lefkowitz, 1996). In a longitudinal study, Johnson et al. (2000) found that having an anxiety disorder as an adolescent increased the risk of developing bipolar disorder in early adulthood.

Posttraumatic Stress Disorder

Individuals who work with trauma victims make the clinical observation that mood swings are common in this group. Although a considerable literature implicates psychosocial stresses in the onset and recurrence of bipolar disorder (Kraepelin, 1921; Brown & Harris, 1982; Hlastala et al., 2000), there is paucity of research on the association of PTSD with bipolar disorder. Findings from the National Comorbidity Survey (NCS) estimate the lifetime prevalence of PTSD in the general population as 7.8% (Kessler et al., 1995). By contrast, reported rates of PTSD comorbidity in patients with bipolar disorder have varied widely from 7 to 50%.

Although many studies have looked at possible links between early traumatic events and development of psychopathology over the life span (Breslau et al., 1998; Bryer, Nelson, Miller, & Krol, 1987; Grilo, Sanislow, Fehon, Martino, & McGlashan, 1999; Kaplan et al., 1998; Kessler et al., 1997; Levitan et al., 1998), few studies have examined the potential role of early traumatic life stresses on the development of bipolar disorder and PTSD. Emerging evidence suggests that trauma significantly compromises the course of bipolar disorder. Leverich et al. (2006) evaluated 631 outpatients with bipolar disorder and reported that nearly half of the females (49%) and one-third of the males (36%) reported early sexual and physical abuse. Those who endorsed a history of child or adolescent physical or sexual abuse, compared with those who did not, had significantly higher rates of comorbid PTSD, a history of an earlier onset of bipolar illness, and a higher rate of suicide attempts. On the other hand Geller et al. (2000) reported high rates (43%) of the symptom of hypersexuality (higher in pubertal vs. prepubertal bipolar disorder population) and low rates (< 1%) of history of sexual abuse in their prepubertal and early-adolescent bipolar disorder cohort, suggesting that the symptom of hypersexuality in pediatric bipolar disorder is etiologically unrelated to sexual abuse and more reflective of mania and puberty. Similarly, Garno, Goldberg, Ramirez, and Ritzler (2005) studied 100 adult patients with bipolar disorder, and half (51%) reported a history of abuse, whereas a quarter suffered from comorbid PTSD (24%).

A report by Wozniak et al. (1999) raises the question as to whether a diagnosis of bipolar disorder may pose a risk factor for trauma. Using data from a large longitudinal sample of well-characterized boys with and without ADHD, these authors failed to find meaningful associations between ADHD, trauma, and PTSD. Instead, they identified early bipolar disorder as an important antecedent to later trauma. When traumatized children present with severe irritability and mood lability, clinicians may have a tendency to attribute these symptoms to having experienced a trauma. These longitudinal results, in contrast, suggest the opposite: Mania may be an antecedent risk factor for later trauma (possibly because of the attendant reckless, disinhibited state) rather than representing a reaction to the trauma. If confirmed, these results could help dispel the commonly held notion that mania-like symptoms in youths represent a reaction to trauma and would further suggest that children with bipolar disorder should be monitored closely to prevent trauma.

Obsessive–Compulsive Disorder

Minimal extant literature and no systematic data exist on the challenging clinical dilemma of children and adolescents presenting with comorbid OCD and bipolar disorder. Descriptions of OCD symptoms in patients with bipolar disorder date back to the 19th century (Morel, 1860). Most data on comorbid OCD and bipolar disorder are not based on systematic studies (Goodwin & Jamison, 1990; Rasmussen & Eisen, 1992) but consist of documentation from naturalistic studies. In adults, evidence of a higher-than-expected overlap between OCD and bipolar disorder first came from the ECA study, in which 23% of those with bipolar disorder also met criteria for OCD (Robins & Price, 1991). Subsequent studies have consistently found the overlap between OCD and bipolar disorder to be as high as 15–35% (Chen & Dilsaver, 1995; Perugi et al., 1997; Kruger, Cooke, Hasey, Jorne, & Persad, 1995). When comorbid with bipolar disorder, OCD in adults has a more episodic course, often featuring higher rates of sexual and religious obsessions, lower rates of checking rituals, greater frequency of concurrent major depressive episodes, and panic disorder. These individuals also exhibit increased rates of suicidality, more frequent hospitalizations, and more complex pharmacological interventions than those without bipolar disorder (Chen & Dilsaver, 1995; Perugi et al., 1997; Perugi et al., 2002; Centorrino et al., 2006). A recent survey conducted among the French Association of OCD Patients provides corroborating evidence for this comorbidity in participants who gave retrospective childhood reports. The authors, while reporting a high prevalence of comorbid lifetime bipolarity, also noted that many of these participants had had a juvenile onset of OCD (Hantouche et al., 2002; Kochman et al., 2002).

Until recently, the presence of comorbid OCD and bipolar disorder in children and adolescents had drawn little attention. Recently, several separate studies have reported a bidirectional overlap between bipolar disorder and OCD in children at rates greater than expected. Masi and colleagues in 2001 reported that 44% of their pediatric patients with bipolar disorder had a lifetime diagnosis of OCD, which usually preceded the onset of mood symptoms. In 2005, Masi et al. reported that 24.5% of their pediatric population with OCD had comorbid bipolar disorder. Geller et al. (1996; Geller, 1996) also found high rates of bipolar disorder (27%), as well as disruptive behavior disorders, in a pediatric population with OCD. Similarly, recent findings in a pediatric population with bipolar disorder reveal rates of comorbid OCD in the range of 15–27% (Faedda et al., 2004; Harpold et al., 2005; Tillman et al., 2003). On the other hand, Reddy and colleagues (2000) reported a much lower rate of bipolar disorder (1.9%) in their pediatric population with OCD that was largely treatment naïve and of moderate severity. Inconsistency in the rate of co-occurrence of the two disorders could be attributed to selection and/or referral bias and suggests that a true comorbidity risk may have been overlooked in these patients.

Although the available literature suggests substantial impact on clinical presentation, global functioning, and treatment decisions when bipolar disorder and OCD co-occur in young patients (Masi et al., 2004), the nature of this relationship remains unknown. For example, the agitation, racing thoughts, and feelings of distress that can be associated with severe OCD could mimic a bipolar picture; conversely, the manic symptom of increase in goal-directed activity ("mission mode" behavior) or repetitive, unwanted hypersexual thoughts in a child or adolescent with bipolar disorder could mimic an OCD presentation.

There is a paucity of systematic data addressing the clinical characteristics of the comorbid OCD and bipolar disorder in a pediatric population. One of the two studies that address this comorbid presentation comes from Masi et al. (2004), who conducted a naturalistic prospective 3-year follow-up study of 102 children and adolescents with OCD, bipolar disorder, and bipolar disorder plus OCD; the other study examined 228 youths ascertained to have OCD and bipolar disorder for clinical features, patterns of psychiatric comorbidity, functioning in multiple domains, and treatment history and compared groups based on comorbidity and ascertainment status (Joshi et al., 2005). Barring a few differences, the findings from these two studies are consistent.

Masi et al. (2004) reported that in comparison with youths with OCD, youths with comorbid OCD and bipolar disorder were significantly more impaired, had earlier age of onset of OCD, and had more frequent existential, philosophical, odd and/or superstitious obsessions, indicating that comorbidity with bipolar disorder may have a clinically relevant influence on the symptom expression of the OCD. Half of the comorbid population in this study had type II bipolar disorder, and one-third experienced pharmacological hypomania. This high risk of (hypo)manic switches in pediatric OCD treated with antidepressants is suggestive of a bipolar diathesis which has been reported in some youths with OCD (Go, Malley, Birmaher, & Rosenberg, 1998; Diler & Avci, 1999; King et al., 1991).

Joshi et al. (2005) found a significant and symmetrical bidirectional overlap between bipolar disorder and OCD (18% of the cohort with bipolar disorder and 12% of the cohort with OCD satisfied criteria for both bipolar disorder and OCD). Compared with youths with OCD, those with comorbid OCD and bipolar disorder had more frequent obsessions and compulsions (hoarding/saving), higher rates of comorbidity (ODD, major depressive disorder, and social phobia), worse functioning, and more frequent hospitalization. Compared with youths with bipolar disorder without OCD, those with comorbid OCD and bipolar disorder had more frequent mania symptoms of pressured speech, flight of ideas, and increased sociability. In both groups, mania presented with a predominantly severe irritable mood, a chronic course, and a mixed presentation, with symptoms of major depression overlapping in time with those of mania. Overall, this study concluded that when OCD and bipolar disorder occur together, the clinical picture is complicated by more symptoms, more comorbidity, and worse functioning than when each disorder occurs alone.

Limited family genetic data suggest a genetic linkage between OCD and bipolar disorder. Coryell (1981) reported an equal incidence (2.3%) of mania in families of probands with OCD and in families of probands with bipolar disorder. Similarly, an increased incidence of obsessional traits has been reported in the offspring of probands with bipolar disorder (Klein, Depue, & Slater, 1985).

Treatment Implications

Improving the understanding of the relationship between anxiety disorders and bipolar disorder in youths has important treatment implications. Because bipolar disorder and anxiety disorders respond to different treatments, identification of the comorbid state is essential for proper treatment and for achieving optimal functioning. In addition, children and adolescents with comorbid bipolar disorder and anxiety disorders are likely to suffer from a more severe clinical condition that may be less responsive to antimanic and anti-anxiety agents compared with children without such comorbidity.

Feske et al. (2000) found that adults with bipolar disorder who had histories of panic attacks had significantly higher rates of nonremission, required a greater number of medications, and experienced more severe side effects compared with those without panic attacks. Moreover, high levels of anxiety in bipolar disorder have been found to be associated with greater symptom severity, poor treatment response, alcohol abuse, and a risk factor for suicide (Young, Cooke, Robb, Levitt, & Joffe, 1993; Gaudiano & Miller, 2005). Recently, Otto et al. (2006) prospectively followed 1,000 adult outpatients with bipolar disorder for 1 year to examine the impact of comorbid anxiety disorders and concluded that presence of anxiety disorders with bipolar disorder predicted poor course and functioning. Likewise, Olvera et al. (2005) found that children with bipolar disorder plus multiple anxiety disorders displayed manic symptoms at an earlier age and were more likely to have been hospitalized for their illnesses. Masi et al. (2001) reported high rates of pharmacological hypomania in youths with bipolar disorder with comorbid anxiety disorders, with mean age of onset of anxiety disorders preceding bipolar disorder. This finding suggests caution when considering antidepressant pharmacotherapy in a pediatric population with multiple anxiety disorders.

Though no systematic data to date are available that examine the therapeutic response of bipolar disorder in the context of anxiety disorder comorbidity in youths, Joshi et al. (2006) conducted a secondary data analysis to examine the treatment response of mania to atypical antipsychotics in children and adolescents with comorbid bipolar disorder and anxiety disorders by comparing the antimanic response to olanzapine of youths with bipolar disorder in the context of comorbidity status with OCD and generalized anxiety disorder (GAD) and concluded that the comorbid presence of lifetime OCD, but not GAD, in children and adolescents with bipolar disorder is associated with poor response to antimanic agents. This suggests that certain anxiety disorders in the heterogeneous pool of anxiety disorders, when comorbid with bipolar disorder, may have a larger mediating effect on treatment outcome of bipolar disorder than others.

Conversely, the presence of bipolar disorder with anxiety disorders may have a negative effect on the treatment outcome of the anxiety disorder. For example, compared with youths with without comorbid bipolar disorder, children and adolescents with comorbid OCD and bipolar disorder have been reported to show poorer response to psychotropic medication and are more frequently on a polypharmacy regimen (Maci et al., 2005). To date, only one open-label trial has assessed response of co-occurring panic attacks and GAD in adults with bipolar disorder, reporting significant decrease in or remission of anxiety symptoms with divalproex therapy (Calabrese & Delucchi, 1990).

In the absence of data on the efficacy of mood-stabilizing agents in treating anxiety disorders comorbid with bipolar disorder, corroborative evidence for an antianxiety effect comes from treatment studies of mood stabilizers for anxiety disorders in adults. Valproate has been shown to be effective in treating panic disorder and certain combat-related PTSD symptoms. Consistent with open-label studies (Baetz & Bowen, 1998; Primeau, Fontaine, & Beauclair, 1990; Woodman & Noyes, 1994) and case reports (McElroy, Keck, & Lawrence, 1991; Brady, Sonne, & Lydiard, 1994), the only randomized controlled trial (RCT) of valproate reported significant improvement in symptoms of panic disorder in adults (Lum, Fontaine, Elie, & Ontiveros, 1990). As suggested by open-label trials, valproate is effective in treating combat-related but not non-combat-related PTSD in adults (Fesler, 1991; Clark, Canive, Calais, Qualls, & Tuason, 1999; Petty et al., 2002; Otte, Wiedemann, Yassouridis, & Kellner, 2004). In contrast to open-label trials, RCT of carbamazepine did not show any significant improvement in symptoms of panic disorder in adults (Unde, Stein, & Post, 1988; Tondo et al., 1989). Several open-label studies suggest that carbamazepine may be useful for treating PTSD symptoms of flashbacks, nightmares, and intrusive thoughts (Brodsky, Doerman, Palmer, Slade, & Munasifi, 1990; Lipper et al., 1986; Wolf, Alavi, & Mosnaim, 1988; Looff, Grimley, Kuller, Martin, & Shonfield, 1995; Stewart & Bartucci, 1986). In an open-label study for OCD in adults, carbamazepine failed to exhibit any therapeutic benefit (Joffe & Swinson, 1986). On the other hand, lamotrigine, in a preliminary RCT, exhibited potential efficacy in the treatment of PTSD symptoms of reexperiencing, avoidance, and numbing in adults (Hertzberg et al., 1999).

No systematic data are available that examine treatment of anxiety disorders in the context of bipolar comorbidity. Every single published RCT of pediatric anxiety disorders has excluded children with bipolar disorder by protocol design, and, similarly, children with a bipolar disorder diagnosis are typically excluded from RCTs of treatment for both depression and anxiety. In the absence of systematic data, children with comorbid anxiety disorders and bipolar disorder are frequently treated with a variety of medications with unclear efficacy and safety data. Recent concerns regarding increased suicidality in youths taking selective serotonin reuptake inhibitors (SSRIs) may especially be relevant in youths with bipolar disorder, which further complicates the treatment. Because comorbidity with anxiety disorder puts these already compromised children and adolescents suffering from bipolar disorder at additional risk for further impairment, there is a pressing need to address the unique therapeutic needs of youths suffering from the combination of bipolar disorder and comorbid anxiety disorders.

Considering that treatments for bipolar disorder with traditional mood stabilizers do not generally treat anxiety disorders, and that treatment of anxiety disorders with SSRIs can aggravate the bipolar disorder, the pharmacological approach to children with bipolar disorder and comorbid anxiety disorders needs to be defined. Nonpharmacological treatments such as cognitive-behavioral therapy (CBT) have been found to be useful and should be instituted when possible, as should any of the pharmacological alternatives to SSRIs. Also, because the various anxiety disorders have unique therapeutic needs, a better understanding of what type of anxiety disorder is associated with pediatric bipolar disorder may lead to improved therapeutic approaches for youths with bipolar disorder plus anxiety comorbidity.

PERVASIVE DEVELOPMENTAL DISORDERS

Pervasive developmental disorders (PDDs) are estimated to affect 7 in 1,000 children and adolescents, and, with improved understanding of their presentation, a recent ten-fold increase in the rates has been reported (Centers for Disease Control, 2006; Fombonne, 2003). These neurodevelopmental disorders are a group of disorders that share common deficits characterized by communication, socialization, and behavioral problems that can develop in the absence or presence of adequate intellectual and language skills. PDD encompasses autistic disorder, Asperger syndrome, pervasive developmental disorder not otherwise specified (PDD-NOS)—together also referred to as autism spectrum disorders—and Rett syndrome and childhood disintegrative disorder.

Literature is limited, and no systematic data exist on the diagnosis and treatment of comorbid bipolar disorder and PDD in children and adolescents. In the absence of systematic research on comorbid bipolar disorder and PDD, indirect evidence suggestive of comorbid bipolar disorder in pediatric populations with PDD comes from high rates of aggressive behaviors documented in children with PDD, from a high incidence of bipolar disorder in family members of children with PDD, and from case reports.

Case reports of periodic and phasic severe mood disturbances highly suggestive of mania have been described in individuals with autism (Kerbeshian & Burd, 1996; Komoto, Seigo, & Hirata, 1984; Sovner & Hurley, 1983) with good response to lithium treatment (Steingard & Biederman, 1987; Shafey, 1986). Campbell et al. (1972) reported treating 10 severely disturbed children (at least one child with early infantile autism) with hyperactivity and mood symptoms with lithium and chlorpromazine and concluded that "lithium may prove of some value in treatment of severe psychiatric disorders in childhood involving aggressiveness, explosive affect and hyperactivity" (p. 234). Similarly, Duggal (2001) reported bipolar disorder in an adult with Asperger syndrome with good response to lithium and valproate. In a case series study of children with PDD with and without family histories of bipolar disorder, clear differences in symptom profile suggestive of bipolar disorder were seen. Children with PDD with family histories of bipolar disorder had more severe cycling patterns, agitation, and aggression, with neurovegetative disturbances, and had higher functioning compared with the children without family histories of bipolar disorder (DeLong, 1994). In a study of a group of patients with Asperger syndrome who were followed into adolescence, Wing (1981) found that nearly one-half of the patients developed affective disorders.

Conversely, high rates of PDD or PDD traits are reported in children and adolescents with bipolar disorder. Presence of PDD symptoms is reported to be as high as 62% in pediatric populations with mood and anxiety disorders (Towbin, Pradella, Gorrindo, Pine, & Leibenluft, 2005). In the first study to use accepted operationalized criteria to assess the bidirectional overlap between PDD and bipolar disorder in youths, Wozniak et al. (1997) reported comorbid bipolar disorder and PDD in 21% of the participants with PDD and 11% of the participants with mania. They also observed striking homology in the phenotypic features of PDD irrespective of comorbidity with bipolar disorder, and, similarly, phenotypic features of mania were analogous in youths with bipolar disorder with and without PDD comorbidity, suggesting that bipolar disorder and PDD are bona fide disorders when comorbidly present.

An accumulating body of literature suggests that PDD may be associated with high rates of family history of bipolar disorder. A high incidence of affective disorders, especially bipolar disorder, has been reported in families of about one-third of individuals with PDD (DeLong, 1994; DeLong & Nohria, 1994; Herzberg, 1976; DeLong & Dwyer, 1988). Several of the studies indicate that there is a greater risk of bipolar disorder in family members of individuals with Asperger syndrome in particular. On the other hand, Piven et al. (1991) did not observe any difference in the prevalence of bipolar disorder in the parents of probands with PDD when compared with the general population.

Despite direct or indirect evidence of higher than expected rates of PDD comorbidity with bipolar disorder, most of the literature on mood symptoms and disorder associated with PDD is focused on symptoms of "irritability" and "aggression," and pharmacotherapy is limited to management of these target symptoms. If children with PDD are not identified appropriately with comorbid bipolar disorder, irritability and aggression related to bipolar mania may be inappropriately attributed to the PDD itself, to depression, or to ADHD (Mick, Spencer, Wozniak, & Biederman, 2005). On the other hand, if PDD is not correctly diagnosed in a child with bipolar disorder, the PDD symptoms of limited abstract thinking, odd and restricted expression of emotions, and limited capacity to understand the mental states could be misjudged for psychotic process. If this comorbid state is not identified correctly, it may lead to inappropriate treatment, unnecessary exposure to neuroleptics, worsening of symptoms, delayed diagnosis, and misuse of mental health resources. Furthermore, compared with a population without PDD, PDD treatment studies consistently report different efficacy and tolerability profiles, with increased susceptibility to adverse responses, suggesting that participants with PDD respond differently to psychotropic agents than those without PDD (Campbell, Adams, Perry, Spencer, & Overall, 1988). This calls for systematic research aimed at improving our understanding of PDD and bipolar disorder when present comorbidly.

REFERENCES

Aman, M. G., De Smedt, G., Derivan, A., Lyons, B., & Findling, R. L. (2002). Double-blind, placebo-controlled study of risperidone for the treatment of disruptive behaviors in children with subaverage intelligence. *American Journal of Psychiatry, 159*(8), 1337–1346.

American Psychiatric Association. (1994). *Diagnostic and statistical manual of mental disorders* (4th ed.). Washington, DC: Author.

Angold, A., & Costello, E. J. (1993). Depressive comorbidity in children and adolescents: Empirical, theoretical and methodological issues. *American Journal of Psychiatry, 150*(12), 1779–1791.

Arnell, H., Hjalmas, K., Jagervall, M., Lackgren, G., Stenberg, A., Bengtsson, B., et al. (1997). The genetics of primary nocturnal enuresis: Inheritance and suggestion of a second major gene on chromosome 12q. *Journal of Medical Genetics, 34*(5), 360–365.

Baetz, M., & Bowen, R. C. (1998). Efficacy of divalproex sodium in patients with panic disorder and mood instability who have not responded to conventional therapy. *Canadian Journal of Psychiatry, 43*(1), 73–77.

Bashir, M., Russell, J., & Johnson, G. (1987). Bipolar affective disorder in adolescence: A 10-year study. *Australian and New Zealand Journal of Psychiatry, 21*(1), 36–43.

Bellman, M. (1966). Studies on encopresis. *Acta Paediatrica Scandinavica, 170*(Suppl.), 1–151.

Biederman, J., Faraone, S. V., Chu, M. P., & Wozniak, J. (1999). Further evidence of a bidirectional overlap between juvenile mania and conduct disorder in children. *Journal of the American Academy of Child and Adolescent Psychiatry, 38*(4), 468–476.

Biederman, J., Faraone, S., Hatch, M., Mennin, D., Taylor, A., & George, P. (1997). Conduct disorder with and without mania in a referred sample of ADHD children. *Journal of Affective Disorders, 44*(2–3), 177–188.

Biederman, J., Faraone, S. V., Marrs, A., Moore, P., Garcia, J., Ablon, J. S., et al. (1997). Panic disorder and agoraphobia in consecutively referred children and adolescents. *Journal of the American Academy of Child and Adolescent Psychiatry, 36*(2), 214–223.

Biederman, J., Faraone, S. V., Mick, E., Wozniak, J., Chen, L., Ouellette, C., et al. (1996). Attention deficit hyperactivity disorder and juvenile mania: An overlooked comorbidity? *Journal of the American Academy of Child and Adolescent Psychiatry, 35*(8), 997–1008.

Biederman, J., Faraone, S. V., Wozniak, J., & Monuteaux, M. C. (2000). Parsing the association between bipolar, conduct, and substance use disorders: A familial risk analysis. *Biological Psychiatry, 48*(11), 1037–1044.

Biederman, J., Mick, E., Bostic, J., Prince, J., Daly, J., Wilens, T., et al. (1998). The naturalistic course of pharmacologic treatment of children with manic-like symptoms: A systematic chart review. *Journal of Clinical Psychiatry, 59*(11), 628–638.

Biederman, J., Mick, E., Faraone, S. V., Wozniak, J., Spencer, T., & Pandina, G. (2006).

Risperidone in the treatment of affective symptoms: A secondary analysis of a randomized clinical trial in children with disruptive behavior disorder. *Clinical Therapeutics, 28*(5), 794–800.

Biederman, J., Mick, E., Hammerness, P., Harpold, T., Aleardi, M., Dougherty, M., et al. (2005). Open-label, 8-week trial of olanzapine and risperidone for the treatment of bipolar disorder in preschool-aged children. *Biological Psychiatry, 58*(7), 589–594.

Biederman, J., Mick, E., Wozniak, J., Aleardi, M., Spencer, T., & Faraone, S. V. (2005). An open-label trial of risperidone in children and adolescents with bipolar disorder. *Journal of Child and Adolescent Psychopharmacology, 15*(2), 311–317.

Biederman, J., Petty, C., Faraone, S. V., Hirshfeld-Becker, D. R., Henin, A., Gilbert, J., et al. (2004). Moderating effects of major depression on patterns of comorbidity in referred adults with panic disorder: A controlled study. *Psychiatry Research, 126*(2), 143–149.

Biederman, J., Santangelo, S., Faraone, S., Kiely, K., Guite, J., Mick, E., et al. (1995). Clinical correlates of enuresis in ADHD and non-ADHD children. *Journal of Child Psychology and Psychiatry, 36*(5), 865–877.

Birmaher, B., Kennah, A., Brent, D., Ehmann, M., Bridge, J., & Axelson, D. (2002). Is bipolar disorder specifically associated with panic disorder in youths? *Journal of Clinical Psychiatry, 63*(5), 414–419.

Bowen, R., South, M., & Hawkes, J. (1994, March). Mood swings in patients with panic disorder. *Canadian Journal of Psychiatry, 39*(2), 91–94.

Boyd, J. H., Burke, J. D., Gruenberg, E., Holzer, C. E., Rae, D. S., George, L. K., et al. (1984). Exclusion criteria of DSM-III: A study of co-occurrence of hierarchy-free syndromes. *Archives of General Psychiatry, 41*, 983–989.

Brady, K. T., Sonne, S., & Lydiard, R. B. (1994). Valproate treatment of comorbid panic disorder and affective disorders in two alcoholic patients. *Journal of Clinical Psychopharmacology, 14*(1), 81–82.

Breslau, N., Kessler, R. C., Chilcoat, H. D., Schultz, L. R., Davis, G. C., & Andreski, P. (1998). Trauma and posttraumatic stress disorder in the community: The 1996 Detroit Area Survey of Trauma. *Archives of General Psychiatry, 55*(7), 626–632.

Brodsky, L., Doerman, A. L., Palmer, L. S., Slade, G. F., & Munasifi, F. A. (1990). Posttraumatic stress disorder: An eclectic approach. *International Journal of Psychosomatics, 37*(1–4), 89–95.

Brown, G. W., & Harris, T. (1982). Disease, distress and depression. A comment. *Journal of Affective Disorders, 4*(1), 1–8.

Bryer, J. B., Nelson, B. A., Miller, J. B., & Krol, P. A. (1987). Childhood sexual and physical abuse as factors in adult psychiatric illness. *American Journal of Psychiatry, 144*(11), 1426–1430.

Calabrese, J., & Delucchi, G. (1990). Spectrum of efficacy of valproate in 55 patients with rapid-cycling bipolar disorder. *American Journal of Psychiatry, 147*(4), 431–434.

Campbell, M., Adams, P., Perry, R., Spencer, E. K., & Overall, J. E. (1988). Tardive and withdrawal dyskinesia in autistic children: A prospective study. *Psychopharmacology Bulletin, 24*(2), 251–255.

Campbell, M., Anderson, L. T., & Green, W. H. (1983). Behavior-disordered and aggressive children: New advances in pharmacotherapy. *Journal of Developmental and Behavioral Pediatrics, 4*(4), 265–271.

Campbell, M., & Cueva, J. E. (1995). Psychopharmacology in child and adolescent psychiatry: A review of the past seven years: Part II. *Journal of the American Academy of Child and Adolescent Psychiatry, 34*(10), 1262–1272.

Campbell, M., Fish, B., Korein, J., Shapiro, T., Collins, P., & Koh, C. (1972). Lithium and chlorpromazine: A controlled crossover study of hyperactive severely disturbed young children. *Journal of Autism and Developmental Disorders, 2*(3), 234–263.

Carlson, G. A. (1983). Bipolar affective disorders in childhood and adolescence. In D. P.

Cantwell & G. A. Carlson (Eds.), *Affective disorders in childhood and adolescence: An update* (pp. 61–83). New York: Spectrum.

Carlson, G. A. (1984). Classification issues of bipolar disorders in childhood. *Psychiatric Developments, 2*(4), 273–285.

Carlson, G. A., Bromet, E. J., & Jandorf, L. (1998). Conduct disorder and mania: What does it mean in adults? *Journal of Affective Disorders, 48*(2–3). 199–205.

Carlson, G. A., & Kashani, J. H. (1988). Manic symptoms in a non-referred adolescent population. *Journal of Affective Disorders, 15*(3), 219–226.

Cassidy, F., Forest, K., Murry, E., & Carroll, B. J. (1998). A factor analysis of the signs and symptoms of mania. *Archives of General Psychiatry, 55*(1), 27–32.

Cassidy, F., Murry, E., Forest, K., & Carroll, B. J. (1998). Signs and symptoms of mania in pure and mixed episodes. *Journal of Affective Disorders, 50*, 187–201.

Centers for Disease Control. (2006). Parental report of diagnosed autism in children aged 4–17 years. *Morbidity and Mortality Weekly Report, 55*, 481–486.

Centorrino, F., Hennen, J., Mallya, G., Egli, S., Clark, T., & Baldessarini, R. J. (2006). Clinical outcome in patients with bipolar I disorder, obsessive compulsive disorder or both. *Human Psychopharmacology, 21*(3), 189–193.

Chen, Y., & Dilsaver, S. (1995). Comorbidity of panic disorder in bipolar illness: Evidence from the Epidemiologic Catchment Area survey. *American Journal of Psychiatry, 152*(2), 280–283.

Clark, R. D., Canive, J. M., Calais, L. A., Qualls, C. R., & Tuason, V. B. (1999). Divalproex in posttraumatic stress disorder: An open-label clinical trial. *Journal of Traumatic Stress, 12*(2), 395–401.

Connor, D. F., Carlson, G. A., Chang, K. D., Daniolos, P. T., Ferziger, R., Findling, R. L., et al. (2006). Juvenile maladaptive aggression: A review of prevention, treatment, and service configuration and a proposed research agenda. *Journal of Clinical Psychiatry, 67*(5), 808–820.

Coryell, W. (1981). Obsessive-compulsive disorder and primary unipolar depression: Comparisons of background, family history, course, and mortality. *Journal of Nervous and Mental Disorders, 169*(4), 220–224.

Costello, J., Angold, A., Burns, B. J., Stangl, D., Tweed, D., Erkanli, A., et al. (1996, December). The Great Smoky Mountains study of youth: Goals, design, methods, and the prevalence of DSM-III-R disorders. *Archives of General Psychiatry, 53*, 1129–1136.

Croonenberghs, J., Fegert, J. M., Findling, R. L., De Smedt, G., & Van Dongen, S. (2005). Risperidone in children with disruptive behavior disorders and subaverage intelligence: A 1-year, open-label study of 504 patients. *Journal of the American Academy of Child and Adolescent Psychiatry, 44*(1), 64–72.

Davis, R. E. (1979). Manic-depressive variant syndrome of childhood: A preliminary report. *American Journal of Psychiatry, 136*(5), 702–706.

DeLong, G. R. (1994). Children with autistic spectrum disorder and a family history of affective disorder. *Developmental Medicine and Child Neurology, 36*, 674–688.

DeLong, G. R., & Dwyer, J. T. (1988). Correlation of family history with specific autistic subgroups: Asperger's syndrome and bipolar affective disease. *Journal of Autism and Developmental Disorders, 18*(4), 593–600.

DeLong, G. R., & Nohria, C. (1994). Psychiatric family history and neurological disease in autistic spectrum disorders. *Developmental Medicine and Child Neurology, 36*, 441–448.

Diler, R. S., & Avci, A. (1999). SSRI-induced mania in obsessive-compulsive disorder. *Journal of the American Academy of Child and Adolescent Psychiatry, 38*(1), 6–7.

Donovan, S. J., Stewart, J. W., Nunes, E. V., Quitkin, F. M., Parides, M., Daniel, W., et al. (2000). Divalproex treatment for youth with explosive temper and mood lability: A double-blind, placebo-controlled crossover design. *American Journal of Psychiatry, 157*(5), 818–820.

Duggal, H. S. (2001). Mood stabilizers in Asperger's syndrome. *Australian and New Zealand Journal of Psychiatry, 35*(3), 390–391.

Faedda, G. L., Baldessarini, R. G., Glovinsky, I. P., & Austin, N. B. (2004). Pediatric bipolar disorder: Phenomenology and course of illness. *Bipolar Disorders, 6*, 305–313.

Faraone, S. V., Biederman, J., Mennin, D., & Russell, R. L. (1998). Bipolar and antisocial disorders among relatives of ADHD children: Parsing familial subtypes of illness. *American Journal of Medical Genetics, 81*(1), 108–116.

Faraone, S. V., Biederman, J., Mennin, D., Wozniak, J., & Spencer, T. (1997). Attention-deficit hyperactivity disorder with bipolar disorder: A familial subtype? *Journal of the American Academy of Child and Adolescent Psychiatry, 36*(10), 1378–1390.

Faraone, S. V., Biederman, J., & Monuteaux, M. C. (2001). Attention deficit hyperactivity disorder with bipolar disorder in girls: Further evidence for a familial subtype? *Journal of Affective Disorders, 64*(1), 19–26.

Faraone, S. V., Biederman, J., Wozniak, J., Mundy, E., Mennin, D., & O'Donnell, D. (1997). Is comorbidity with ADHD a marker for juvenile onset mania? *Journal of the American Academy of Child and Adolescent Psychiatry, 36*(8), 1046–1055.

Farley, S. E., Adams, J. S., Lutton, M. E., Scoville, C., Fulkerson, R. C., & Webb, A. R. (2005). Clinical inquiries. What are effective treatments for oppositional and defiant behaviors in preadolescents? *Journal of Family Practice, 54*(2), 162, 164–165.

Feske, U., Frank, E., Mallinger, A. G., Houck, P. R., Fagiolini, A., Shear, M. K., et al. (2000). Anxiety as a correlate of response to the acute treatment of bipolar I disorder. *American Journal of Psychiatry, 157*(6), 956–962.

Fesler, F. A. (1991). Valproate in combat-related posttraumatic stress disorder. *Journal of Clinical Psychiatry, 52*(9), 361–364.

Findling, R. L., Aman, M. G., Eerdekens, M., Derivan, A., & Lyons, B. (2004). Long-term, open-label study of risperidone in children with severe disruptive behaviors and below-average IQ. *American Journal of Psychiatry, 161*(4), 677–684.

Findling, R. L., Gracious, B. L., McNamara, N. K., Youngstrom, E. A., Demeter, C. A., Branicky, L. A., et al. (2001). Rapid, continuous cycling and psychiatric co-morbidity in pediatric bipolar I disorder. *Bipolar Disorders, 3*(4), 202–210.

Findling, R. L., McNamara, N. K., Branicky, L. A., Schluchter, M. D., Lemon, E., & Blumer, J. L. (2000). A double-blind pilot study of risperidone in the treatment of conduct disorder. *Journal of the American Academy of Child and Adolescent Psychiatry, 39*(4), 509–516.

Findling, R. L., Reed, M. D., O'Riordan, M. A., Demeter, C. A., Stansbrey, R. J., & McNamara, N. K. (2006). Effectiveness, safety, and pharmacokinetics of quetiapine in aggressive children with conduct disorder. *Journal of the American Academy of Child and Adolescent Psychiatry, 45*(7), 792–800.

Fombonne, E. (2003). The prevalence of autism. *Journal of the American Medical Association, 289*(1), 87–89.

Garno, J. L., Goldberg, J. F., Ramirez, P. M., & Ritzler, B. A. (2005). Impact of childhood abuse on the clinical course of bipolar disorder. *British Journal of Psychiatry, 186*, 121–125.

Gaudiano, B. A., & Miller, I. W. (2005). Anxiety disorder comobidity in bipolar I disorder: Relationship to depression severity and treatment outcome. *Depression and Anxiety, 21*(2), 71–77.

Geller, B. (1996). The high prevalence of bipolar parents among prepubertal mood-disordered children necessitates appropriate questions to establish bipolarity. *Current Opinion in Psychiatry, 9*, 239–240.

Geller, B., Fox, L., & Clark, K. (1994). Rate and predictors of prepubertal bipolarity during follow-up of 6- to 12-year-old depressed children. *Journal of the American Academy of Child and Adolescent Psychiatry, 33*(4), 461–468.

Geller, B., & Luby, J. (1997, September). Child and adolescent bipolar disorder: A review of the past 10 years. *Journal of the American Academy of Child and Adolescent Psychiatry, 36*, 1168–1176.

Geller, B., Zimerman, B., Williams, M., Bolhofner, K., Craney, J. L., DelBello, M. P., et al. (2000). Diagnostic characteristics of 93 cases of a prepubertal and early adolescent bipolar disorder phenotype by gender, puberty and comorbid attention deficit hyperactivity disorder. *Journal of Child and Adolescent Psychopharmacology, 10*(3), 157–164.

Geller, D. A., Biederman, J., Griffin, S., Jones, J., & Lefkowitz, T. R. (1996). Comorbidity of juvenile obsessive-compulsive disorder with disruptive behavior disorders: A review and a report. *Journal of the American Academy of Child and Adolescent Psychiatry, 35*(12), 1637–1646.

Go, F. S., Malley, E. E., Birmaher, B., & Rosenberg, D. R. (1998). Manic behaviors associated with fluoxetine in three 12- to 18-year-olds with obsessive-compulsive disorder. *Journal of Child and Adolescent Psychopharmacology, 8*(1), 73–80.

Goodwin, F., & Jamison, K. (1990). *Manic-depressive illness.* New York: Oxford University Press.

Goodwin, R., Hamilton, S., Milne, B., & Pine, D. (2002). Generalizability and correlates of clinically derived panic subtypes in the population. *Depression and Anxiety, 15*(2), 69–74.

Goodwin, R. D., & Hoven, C. W. (2002). Bipolar-panic comorbidity in the general population: prevalence and associated morbidity. *Journal of Affective Disorders, 70*(1), 27–33.

Greene, R. W., & Doyle, A. E. (1999). Toward a transactional conceptualization of oppositional defiant disorder: Implications for assessment and treatment. *Clinical Child and Family Psychology Review, 2*(3), 129–148.

Grilo, C. M., Sanislow, C., Fehon, D. C., Martino, S., & McGlashan, T. H. (1999). Psychological and behavioral functioning in adolescent psychiatric inpatients who report histories of childhood abuse. *American Journal of Psychiatry, 156*(4), 538–543.

Hantouche, E. G., Demonfaucon, C., Angst, J., Perugi, G., Allilaire, J. F., & Akiskal, H. S. (2002). Trouble obsessionnel compulsif cyclothymique. Caractéristiques cliniques d'une entité négligee et non reconnue. [Cyclothymic obsessive-compulsive disorder. Clinical characteristics of a neglected and underrecognized entity]. *Presse Medicale, 31*(14), 644–648.

Harpold, T., Wozniak, J., Kwon, A., Gilbert, J., Wood, J., Smith, L., et al. (2005). Examining the association between pediatric bipolar disorder and anxiety disorders in psychiatrically referred children and adolescents. *Journal of Affective Disorders, 88*(1), 19–26.

Henin, A., Biederman, J., Mick, E., Hirshfeld-Becker, D. R., Sachs, G. S., Wu, Y., et al. (2006). Childhood antecedent disorders to bipolar disorder in adults: A controlled study. *Journal of Affective Disorders, 99*(1–3), 51–57.

Hertzberg, M. A., Butterfield, M. I., Feldman, M. E., Beckham, J. C., Sutherland, S. M., Connor, K. M., et al. (1999). A preliminary study of lamotrigine for the treatment of posttraumatic stress disorder. *Biological Psychiatry, 45*(9), 1226–1229.

Herzberg, B. (1976). The families of autistic children. In M. Coleman (Ed.), *The autistic syndromes* (pp. 151–172). Amsterdam: North Holland.

Hlastala, S. A., Frank, E., Kowalski, J., Sherrill, J. T., Tu, X. M., Anderson, B., et al. (2000). Stressful life events, bipolar disorder, and the "kindling model". *Journal of Abnormal Psychology, 109*(4), 777–786.

Isaac, G. (1992). Misdiagnosed bipolar disorder in adolescents in a special educational school and treatment program. *Journal of Clinical Psychiatry, 53*(4), 133–136.

Joffe, R. T., & Swinson, R. P. (1987). Carbamazepine in obsessive-compulsive disorder. *Biological Psychiatry, 22*(9), 1169–1171.

Johnson, J. G., Cohen, P., & Brook, J. S. (2000). Associations between bipolar disorder and other psychiatric disorders during adolescence and early adulthood: A community-based longitudinal investigation. *American Journal of Psychiatry, 157*(10), 1679–1681.

Joshi, G., Mick, E., Wozniak, J., Geller, D., Park, J., & Biederman, J. (2006). *Impact of obsessive–compulsive disorder on antimanic response of pediatric bipolar disorder to second generation atypical antipsychotics.* Paper presented at the 53rd annual meeting of the American Academy of Child and Adolescent Psychiatry, San Diego, CA.

Joshi, G., Wozniak, J., Geller, D., Petty, C., Vivas, F., & Biederman, J. (2005, October). *Clinical characteristics of comorbid obsessive–compulsive disorder and bipolar disorder in chil-*

dren and adolescents. Paper presented at the 52nd annual meeting of American Academy of Child and Adolescent Psychiatry, Toronto, Ontario, Canada.

Judd, L. L., Akiskal, H. S., Schettler, P. J., Coryell, W., Maser, J., Rice, J. A., et al. (2003). The comparative clinical phenotype and long term longitudinal episode course of bipolar I and II: A clinical spectrum or distinct disorders? *Journal of Affective Disorders, 73*(1–2), 19–32.

Kaplan, S. J., Pelcovitz, D., Salzinger, S., Weiner, M., Mandel, F. S., Lesser, M. L., et al. (1998). Adolescent physical abuse: Risk for adolescent psychiatric disorders. *American Journal of Psychiatry, 155*(7), 954–959.

Kerbeshian, J., & Burd, L. (1996). Case study: Comorbidity among Tourette's syndrome, autistic disorder, and bipolar disorder. *Journal of the American Academy of Child and Adolescent Psychiatry, 35*(5), 681–685.

Kessler, R., Sonnega, A., Bromet, E., Hughes, M., & Nelson, C. (1995). Posttraumatic stress disorder in the National Comorbidity Survey. *Archives of General Psychiatry, 52,* 1048–1060.

Kessler, R. C., Davis, C. G., & Kendler, K. S. (1997). Childhood adversity and adult psychiatric disorder in the U.S. National Comorbidity Survey. *Psychological Medicine, 27*(5), 1101–1119.

Kessler, R. C., Stang, P., Wittchen, H. U., Stein, M., & Walters, E. E. (1999). Lifetime co-morbidities between social phobia and mood disorders in the U.S. National Comorbidity Survey. *Psychological Medicine, 29*(3), 555–567.

Kessler, R., Stang, P., Wittchen, H., Ustun, B., Roy-Byrne, P., & Walters, E. (1998). Lifetime panic-depression comorbidity in the National Comorbidity Survey. *Archives of General Psychiatry, 55,* 801–808.

King, R. A., Riddle, M. A., Chappel, P. B., Hardin, M. T., Anderson, G. M., Lombroso, P., et al. (1991). Case study: Emergence of self-destructive phenomena in children and adolescents during fluoxetine treatment. *Journal of the American Academy of Child and Adolescent Psychiatry, 30*(2), 179–186.

Klages, T., Geller, B., Tillman, R., Bolhofner, K., & Zimerman, B. (2005). Controlled study of encopresis and enuresis in children with a prepubertal and early adolescent bipolar-I disorder phenotype. *Journal of the American Academy of Child and Adolescent Psychiatry, 44*(10), 1050–1057.

Klein, D., Depue, R., & Slater, J. (1985). Cyclothymia in the adolescent offspring of parents with bipolar affective disorder. *Journal of Abnormal Psychology, 94*(2), 115–127.

Kochman, F. J., Hantouche, E. G., Millet, B., Lancrenon, S., Demonfaucon, C., Barrot, I., et al. (2002). Trouble obsessionnel compulsif et bipolarite attenuee chez l'enfant et l'adolescent: Resultants de l'enquete 'ABC-TOC'. *Neuropsychiatrie de l'Enfance et de l'Adolescence, 50,* 1–7.

Komoto, J., Seigo, U., & Hirata, J. (1984). Infantile autism and affective disorder. *Journal of Autism and Developmental Disorders, 14*(1), 81–84.

Kovacs, M., & Pollock, M. (1995). Bipolar disorder and comorbid conduct disorder in childhood and adolescence. *Journal of the American Academy of Child and Adolescent Psychiatry, 34*(6), 715–723.

Kowatch, R. A., Fristad, M., Birmaher, B., Wagner, K. D., Findling, R. L., & Hellander, M. (2005). Treatment guidelines for children and adolescents with bipolar disorder. *Journal of the American Academy of Child and Adolescent Psychiatry, 44*(3), 213–235.

Kraepelin, E. (1921). *Manic-depressive insanity and paranoia.* Edinburgh, UK: E. & S. Livingstone.

Kruger, S., Cooke, R. G., Hasey, G. M., Jorna, T., & Persad, E. (1995). Comorbidity of obsessive compulsive disorder in bipolar disorder. *Journal of Affective Disorders, 34*(2), 117–120.

Kutcher, S. P., Marton, P., & Korenblum, M. (1989). Relationship between psychiatric illness and conduct disorder in adolescents. *Canadian Journal of Psychiatry, 34*(6), 526–529.

Leverich, G. S., Altshuler, L. L., Frye, M. A., Suppes, T., McElroy, S. L., Keck, P. E., Jr., et al.

(2006). Risk of switch in mood polarity to hypomania or mania in patients with bipolar depression during acute and continuation trials of venlafaxine, sertraline, and bupropion as adjuncts to mood stabilizers. *American Journal of Psychiatry, 163*(2), 232–239.

Levitan, R. D., Parikh, S. V., Lesage, A. D., Hegadoren, K. M., Adams, M., Kennedy, S. H., et al. (1998). Major depression in individuals with a history of childhood physical or sexual abuse: Relationship to neurovegetative features, mania, and gender. *American Journal of Psychiatry, 155*(12), 1746–1752.

Lewinsohn, P., Klein, D., & Seeley, J. (1995). Bipolar disorders in a community sample of older adolescents: Prevalence, phenomenology, comorbidity, and course. *Journal of the American Academy of Child and Adolescent Psychiatry, 34*(4), 454–463.

Linna, S. L., Moilanen, I., Keistinen, H., Ernvall, M. L., & Karppinen, M. M. (1991). Prevalence of psychosomatic symptoms in children. *Psychotherapy and Psychosomatics, 56*(1–2), 85–87.

Lipper, S., Davidson, J. R., Grady, T. A., Edinger, J. D., Hammett, E. B., Mahorney, S. L., et al. (1986). Preliminary study of carbamazepine in post-traumatic stress disorder. *Psychosomatics, 27*(12), 849–854.

Loeys, B., Hoebeke, P., Raes, A., Messiaen, L., De Paepe, A., & Vande Walle, J. (2002). Does monosymptomatic enuresis exist? A molecular genetic exploration of 32 families with enuresis/incontinence. *British Journal of Urology International, 90*(1), 76–83.

Looff, D., Grimley, P., Kuller, F., Martin, A., & Shonfield, L. (1995). Carbamazepine for PTSD. *Journal of the American Academy of Child and Adolescent Psychiatry, 34*(6), 703–704.

Lum, M., Fontaine, R., Elie, R., & Ontiveros, A. (1990). Divalproex sodium's anti-panic effect in panic disorder: A placebo-controlled study. *Biological Psychiatry, 27,* 164A–165A.

MacKinnon, D., Xu, J., McMahon, F., Simpson, S., Stine, O., McInnis, M., et al. (1998). Bipolar disorder and panic disorder in families: An analysis of chromosome 18 data. *American Journal of Psychiatry, 155*(6), 829–831.

MacKinnon, D. F., Zandi, P. P., Cooper, J., Potash, J. B., Simpson, S. G., Gershon, E., et al. (2002). Comorbid bipolar disorder and panic disorder in families with a high prevalence of bipolar disorder. *American Journal of Psychiatry, 159*(1), 30–35.

Masi, G., Millepiedi, S., Mucci, M., Bertini, N., Milantoni, L., & Arcangeli, F. (2005). A naturalistic study of referred children and adolescents with obsessive-compulsive disorder. *Journal of the American Academy of Child and Adolescent Psychiatry, 44*(7), 673–681.

Masi, G., Perugi, G., Toni, C., Millepiedi, S., Mucci, M., Bertini, N., et al. (2004). Obsessive-compulsive bipolar comorbidity: Focus on children and adolescents. *Journal of Affective Disorders, 78,* 175–183.

Masi, G., Toni, C., Perugi, G., Mucci, M., Millepiedi, S., & Akiskal, H. S. (2001). Anxiety disorders in children and adolescents with bipolar disorder: A neglected comorbidity. *Canadian Journal of Psychiatry, 46*(9), 797–802.

McElroy, S. L., Altshuler, L. L., Suppes, T., Keck, P. E., Jr., Frye, M. A., Denicoff, K. D., et al. (2001). Axis I psychiatric comorbidity and its relationship to historical illness variables in 288 patients with bipolar disorder. *American Journal of Psychiatry, 158*(3), 420–426.

McElroy, S. L., Keck, P. E., Jr., & Lawrence, J. M. (1991). Treatment of panic disorder and benzodiazepine withdrawal with valproate. *Journal of Neuropsychiatry and Clinical Neurosciences, 3*(2), 232–233.

McGlashan, T. (1988). Adolescent versus adult onset of mania. *American Journal of Psychiatry, 145*(2), 221–223.

Mick, E., Spencer, T., Wozniak, J., & Biederman, J. (2005). Heterogeneity of irritability in ADHD subjects with and without mood disorders. *Biological Psychiatry, 58*(7), 576–582.

Modestin, J., Hug, A., & Ammann, R. (1997). Criminal behavior in males with affective disorders. *Journal of Affective Disorders, 42*(1), 29–38.

Moore, J. M., Jr., Thompson-Pope, S. K., & Whited, R. M. (1996). MMPI-A profiles of adolescent boys with a history of firesetting. *Journal of Personality Assessment, 67*(1), 116–126.

Morel, B. A. (1860). *Traite de maladies metales.* Paris: Librairie Victor Masson.

Olvera, R. L., Hunter, K., Fonseca, M., Caetano, S. C., Bowden, C. L., Soares, J. C., et al. (2005, October). Juvenile onset bipolar disorder and comorbid anxiety. In *Proceedings of the 52nd annual meeting of American Academy of Child and Adolescent Psychiatry*, Toronto, Ontario, Canada.

Otte, C., Wiedemann, K., Yassouridis, A., & Kellner, M. (2004). Valproate monotherapy in the treatment of civilian patients with non-combat-related posttraumatic stress disorder: An open-label study. *Journal of Clinical Psychopharmacology, 24*(1), 106–108.

Otto, M. W., Simon, N. M., Wisniewski, S. R., Miklowitz, D. J., Kogan, J. N., Reilly-Harrington, N. A., et al. (2006). Prospective 12-month course of bipolar disorder in out-patients with and without comorbid anxiety disorders. *British Journal of Psychiatry, 189*, 20–25.

Perugi, G. (1999). Depressive comorbidity of panic, social phobic, and obsessive compulsive disorders re-examined: Is there a bipolar II connection? *Journal of Psychiatric Research, 33*, 53–61.

Perugi, G., Akiskal, H. S., Pfanner, C., Presta, S., Gemignani, A., Milanfranchi, A., et al. (1997). The clinical impact of bipolar and unipolar affective comorbidity on obsessive-compulsive disorder. *Journal of Affective Disorders, 46*(1), 15–23.

Perugi, G., Akiskal, H. S., Toni, C., Simonini, E., & Gemignani, A. (2001). The temporal relationship between anxiety disorders and (hypo)mania: A retrospective examination of 63 panic, social phobic and obsessive-compulsive patients with comorbid bipolar disorder. *Journal of Affective Disorders, 67*(1–3), 199–206.

Perugi, G., Frare, F., Toni, C., Mata, B., & Akiskal, H. S. (2001). Bipolar II and unipolar comorbidity in 153 outpatients with social phobia. *Comprehensive Psychiatry, 42*(5), 375–381.

Perugi, G., Toni, C., Frare, F., Travierso, M. C., Hantouche, E., & Akiskal, H. S. (2002). Obsessive-compulsive-bipolar comorbidity: A systematic exploration of clinical features and treatment outcome. *Journal of Clinical Psychiatry, 63*(12), 1129–1134.

Petty, F., Davis, L. L., Nugent, A. L., Kramer, G. L., Teten, A., Schmitt, A., et al. (2002). Valproate therapy for chronic, combat-induced posttraumatic stress disorder. *Journal of Clinical Psychopharmacology, 22*(1), 100–101.

Piven, J., Chase, G. A., Landa, R., Wzorek, M., Gayle, J., Cloud, D., et al. (1991). Psychiatric disorders in the parents of autistic individuals. *Journal of the American Academy of Child and Adolescent Psychiatry, 30*(3), 471–478.

Primeau, F., Fontaine, R., & Beauclair, L. (1990). Valproic acid and panic disorder. *Canadian Journal of Psychiatry, 35*(3), 248–250.

Rasmussen, S., & Eisen, J. (1992, April). The epidemiology and differential diagnosis of obsessive compulsive disorder. *Journal of Clinical Psychiatry, 53*(Suppl.), 4–10.

Reddy, Y. C., Reddy, P. S., Srinath, S., Khanna, S., Sheshadri, S. P., & Girimaji, S. C. (2000). Comorbidity in juvenile obsessive-compulsive disorder: A report from India. *Canadian Journal of Psychiatry, 45*(3), 274–278.

Robins, L., & Price, R. (1991). Adult disorders predicted by childhood conduct problems: Results from the NIMH Epidemiologic Catchment Area project. *Psychiatry, 54*(2), 116–132.

Robson, W. L., Jackson, H. P., Blackhurst, D., & Leung, A. K. (1997). Enuresis in children with attention-deficit hyperactivity disorder. *Southern Medical Journal, 90*(5), 503–505.

Savino, M., Perugi, G., Simonini, E., Soriani, A., Cassano, G., & Akiskal, H. (1993). Affective comorbidity in panic disorder: Is there a bipolar connection? *Journal of Affective Disorders, 28*(3), 155–163.

Shafey, H. (1986). Use of lithium and flupenthixol in a patient with pervasive developmental disorder [Letter to the editor]. *American Journal of Psychiatry, 143*(5), 681.

Shaffer, D., Fisher, P., Dulcan, M., Davies, M., Piacentini, J., Schwab-Stone, M., et al. (1996). The NIMH Diagnostic Interview Schedule for Children, version 2.3 (DISC-2.3): Description, acceptability, prevalence rates, and performance in the MECA study. *Journal of the American Academy of Child and Adolescent Psychiatry, 35*(7), 865–877.

Sheard, M. H. (1975). Lithium in the treatment of aggression. *Journal of Nervous and Mental Disorders*, 160(2–1), 108–118.

Simon, N. M., Otto, M. W., Fischmann, D., Racette, S., Nierenberg, A. A., Pollack, M. H., et al. (2005). Panic disorder and bipolar disorder: Anxiety sensitivity as a potential mediator of panic during manic states. *Journal of Affective Disorders*, 87(1), 101–105.

Simon, N. M., Smoller, J. W., Fava, M., Sachs, G., Racette, S. R., Perlis, R., et al. (2003). Comparing anxiety disorders and anxiety-related traits in bipolar disorder and unipolar depression. *Journal of Psychiatric Research*, 37(3), 187–192.

Sovner, R., & Hurley, A. D. (1983). Do the mentally retarded suffer from affective illness? *Archives of General Psychiatry*, 40, 61–67.

Spee-van der Wekke, J., Hirasing, R. A., Meulmeester, J. F., & Radder, J. J. (1998). Childhood nocturnal enuresis in The Netherlands. *Urology*, 51(6), 1022–1026.

Steingard, R., & Biederman, J. (1987). Lithium responsive manic-like symptoms in two individuals with autism and mental retardation. *Journal of American Academy of Child and Adolescent Psychiatry*, 26(6), 932–935.

Stewart, J. T., & Bartucci, R. J. (1986). Posttraumatic stress disorder and partial complex seizures. *American Journal of Psychiatry*, 143(1), 113–114.

Strober, M., & Carlson, G. (1982). Bipolar illness in adolescents with major depression: Clinical, genetic, and psychopharmacologic predictors in a three- to four-year prospective follow-up investigation. *Archives of General Psychiatry*, 39, 549–555.

Tcheremissine, O. V., & Lieving, L. M. (2006). Pharmacological aspects of the treatment of conduct disorder in children and adolescents. *CNS Drugs*, 20(7), 549–565.

Tillman, R., Geller, B., Bolhofner, K., Craney, J. L., Williams, M., & Zimerman, B. (2003). Ages of onset and rates of syndromal and subsyndromal comorbid DSM-IV diagnoses in a prepubertal and early adolescent bipolar disorder phenotype. *Journal of the American Academy of Child and Adolescent Psychiatry*, 42(12), 1486–1493.

Tondo, L., Burrai, C., Scamonatti, L., Toccafondi, F., Poddighe, A., Minnai, G., et al. (1989). Carbamazepine in panic disorder. *American Journal of Psychiatry*, 146(4), 558–559.

Towbin, K. E., Pradella, A., Gorrindo, T., Pine, D. S., & Leibenluft, E. (2005). Autism spectrum traits in children with mood and anxiety disorders. *Journal of Child and Adolescent Psychopharmacology*, 15(3), 452–464.

Turgay, A., Binder, C., Snyder, R., & Fisman, S. (2002). Long-term safety and efficacy of risperidone for the treatment of disruptive behavior disorders in children with subaverage IQs. *Pediatrics*, 110(3), e34.

Uhde, T. W., Stein, M. B., & Post, R. M. (1988). Lack of efficacy of carbamazepine in the treatment of panic disorder. *American Journal of Psychiatry*, 145(9), 1104–1109.

Wing, L. (1981). Asperger's syndrome: A clinical account. *Psychological Medicine*, 11(1), 115–129.

Wolf, M. E., Alavi, A., & Mosnaim, A. D. (1988). Posttraumatic stress disorder in Vietnam veterans clinical and EEG findings: Possible therapeutic effects of carbamazepine. *Biological Psychiatry*, 23(6), 642–644.

Woodman, C. L., & Noyes, R., Jr. (1994). Panic disorder: Treatment with valproate. *Journal of Clinical Psychiatry*, 55(4), 134–136.

Worrall, E. P., Moody, J. P., & Naylor, G. J. (1975). Lithium in non-manic-depressives: Antiaggressive effect and red blood cell lithium values. *British Journal of Psychiatry*, 126, 464–468.

Wozniak, J., & Biederman, J. (1996). A pharmacological approach to the quagmire of comorbidity in juvenile mania. *Journal of the American Academy of Child and Adolescent Psychiatry*, 35(6), 826–828.

Wozniak, J., Biederman, J., Faraone, S. V., Blier, H., & Monuteaux, M. C. (2001). Heterogeneity of childhood conduct disorder: Further evidence of a subtype of conduct disorder linked to bipolar disorder. *Journal of Affective Disorders*, 64(2–3), 121–131.

Wozniak, J., Biederman, J., Faraone, S., Frazier, J., Kim, J. Millstein, R., et al. (1997). Mania in children with pervasive developmental disorder revisited. *Journal of the American Academy of Child and Adolescent Psychiatry, 36*(11), 1552–1560.

Wozniak, J., Biederman, J., Kiely, K., Ablon, S., Faraone, S., Mundy, E., et al. (1995). Mania-like symptoms suggestive of childhood onset bipolar disorder in clinically referred children. *Journal of the American Academy of Child and Adolescent Psychiatry, 34*(7), 867–876.

Wozniak, J., Biederman, J., Monuteaux, M. C., Richards, J., & Faraone, S. V. (2002). Parsing the comorbidity between bipolar disorder and anxiety disorders: A familial risk analysis. *Journal of Child and Adolescent Psychopharmacology, 12*(2), 101–111.

Wozniak, J., Crawford, M. H., Biederman, J., Faraone, S. V., Spencer, T. J., Taylor, A., et al. (1999). Antecedents and complications of trauma in boys with ADHD: Findings from a longitudinal study. *Journal of the American Academy of Child and Adolescent Psychiatry, 38*(1), 48–55.

Young, L., Cooke, R., Robb, J., Levitt, A., & Joffe, R. (1993). Anxious and non-anxious bipolar disorder. *Journal of Affective Disorders, 29*(1), 49–52.

CHAPTER 14

Treatment of Preschool Bipolar Disorder

A Novel Parent–Child Interaction Therapy and Review of Data on Psychopharmacology

JOAN L. LUBY, MELISSA MEADE STALETS,
SAMANTHA BLANKENSHIP, JENNIFER PAUTSCH,
and MOLLY MCGRATH

Converging data from numerous research groups have established the construct validity of bipolar disorder arising in children 6 years of age and older (e.g., Biederman et al., 2004; Birmaher et al., 2006; Geller, Tillman, Craney, & Bolhofner, 2004). However, to date there have been very few systematic investigations of whether preschool-age children can manifest formal DSM-IV criteria for bipolar disorder or whether mania symptoms can even arise at this early stage of development. Several compelling published case studies have described the clinical characteristics of putative mania in preschool children (Mota-Castillo et al., 2001; Pavuluri, Janicak, & Carbray, 2002; Tuzun, Zoroglu, & Savas, 2002). Retrospective chart reviews have also suggested that clinical mania can present during the preschool period (Tumuluru, Weller, Fristad, & Weller, 2003). Although these data are compelling and suggestive, the lack of standardized diagnostic measures, appropriate comparison groups, and blind raters used in the assessments limits the scientific conclusions that can be drawn.

However, objective evidence of early alterations in the behavior of the preschool-age offspring of parents with bipolar disorder has been provided (Hirshfeld-Becker et al., 2006). In a study of the young children of adults with bipolar disorder, higher rates of observed behavioral disinhibition were found in preschoolers who had a parent with bipolar disorder compared with low-risk controls. These findings demonstrate that behaviors suggestive of the kind of emotional dysregulation that might be expected to be associated with a prodrome of later mania are evident in preschoolers at high risk for the disorder by virtue of having an affected parent. These findings are strengthened by the use of observational data scored by raters blind to the diagnostic status of the caregivers, thus providing objective evidence that is not affected by potential parental distortion.

An exploratory investigation of mania symptoms in a large, community-based preschool sample oversampled for mood disorders has provided the first systematic evidence that DSM-IV bipolar I disorder can be identified in preschool children ages 3–6 when age-adjusted symptom manifestations are assessed (Luby & Belden, 2006b). Based on parent report data from a reliable and age-appropriate preschool mania module, evidence for a specific symptom constellation that distinguished preschoolers with bipolar disorder from those who were healthy and those with major depressive disorder (MDD) and DSM-IV disruptive disorders (attention-deficit/hyperactivity disorder, oppositional defiant disorder, conduct disorder) was found (Luby & Belden, 2006b). This preschool group also displayed significantly higher levels of functional impairment and delays in adaptive functioning relative to preschoolers without psychiatric disorders. Highly notable was the finding that this preschool group with bipolar disorder demonstrated significantly higher levels of impairment, even when compared with preschoolers with other DSM-IV Axis I disorders. Highlighting the clinical severity of this symptom constellation, depressed preschoolers with bipolar disorder were found to have higher depression severity than even the most severely depressed melancholic subgroup without bipolar disorder (Luby et al., 2007). Preschoolers with bipolar disorder also displayed high levels of comorbidity with attention-deficit/hyperactivity disorder (ADHD) and oppositional defiant disorder (ODD), similar to the pattern established in older school-age children with bipolar disorder (Luby & Belden, 2006b; Geller et al., 2000). These findings suggest that a highly impairing and comorbid bipolar syndrome can be identified in the preschool period, underscoring the clinical significance of this early-onset syndrome.

Based on the findings of a preschool bipolar disorder that shows discriminant validity from other Axis I disruptive disorders and that is associated with high levels of functional impairment, depression severity, and comorbidity, the design of age-appropriate treatment strategies for early intervention is now warranted. Although treatment of this severe mood disorder in older children has required psychopharmacological interventions to control cycling and elevations of mood, psychosocial and family therapy interventions have also served as effective adjuncts to medication management (Miklowitz et al., 2004; Fristad, Goldberg-Arnold, & Gavazzi, 2002). Early intervention holds particular promise due to the rapid neurobiological change known to occur during this stage of development, potentially providing a unique opportunity to minimize deviation from the normative developmental trajectory. Given the very young age of the participants targeted, initial treatment investigations must focus first on strategies that pose the least risk to the rapidly developing child. Several psychotherapy models for the treatment of other preschool-onset disorders have been empirically tested and have demonstrated efficacy (e.g., Eyberg, 1988; Webster-Stratton, 2005), suggesting that psychotherapy may be considered a promising and logical first step in the treatment of preschool-onset bipolar disorder.

Given the young child's inextricable reliance on the caregiver, psychotherapeutic interventions for preschool-age children in general are most successful if conducted with the child and primary caregiver together. In keeping with this principle, most empirically supported treatments for preschool-age disorders target the parent–child dyad. The importance of the quality of the parent–child relationship in social and emotional outcomes in young children, as well as in negative behaviors associated with early-onset preschool mood disorders, has been well established (Eisenberg et al., 2001; Belden & Luby, 2006). Relational factors such as maternal warmth have also been associated with outcome in older children with bipolar disorder (Geller et al., 2004). Thus treatment aimed toward parent–child interaction would seem to be particularly well suited to the treatment of preschool bipolar disorder.

In addition to the treatment of the cardinal symptoms of preschool bipolar disorder, the nonspecific disruptive symptoms of bipolar disorder must also be targeted. Further, as high rates of comorbidity with disruptive behavioral disorders, in particular ADHD and ODD, have been demonstrated in childhood and preschool bipolar disorder (Geller, Williams, et al., 1998; Biederman et al., 2004; Luby & Belden, 2006b), symptoms of these disorders must be addressed. Management of disruptive symptoms is believed to be a crucial first step in the treatment of preschool bipolar disorder for several reasons. First, disruptive behaviors may stand as an impediment to treatment aimed specifically at cardinal bipolar disorder symptoms. Second, parents may be overwhelmed by their child's disruptive behaviors to the extent that their motivation for addressing their child's mood disorder is diminished (Weiss, Jackson, & Susser, 1997). Finally, given the success of treatments designed to target disruptive behaviors in preschoolers, parents likely will meet with success in their attempts to better manage externalizing behaviors, providing a sense of mastery and control that may be beneficial to treatment of mood symptoms.

Given the necessity to treat the caregiver and child together as a dyad and the need to address disruptive behaviors in preschool bipolar disorder, an available empirically supported treatment designed for early-age disruptive behavior provides a useful base for a planned psychotherapeutic intervention for preschool bipolar disorder. Parent–child interaction therapy (PCIT; Eyberg, 1988), a treatment for disruptive behaviors in young children, was selected because of its focus on the parent–child dyad in session and due to the relatively large database supporting its efficacy. Statistically and clinically significant reductions in children's disruptive behaviors following treatment with PCIT have been reported (see Brinkmeyer & Eyberg, 2003, for a review). Notably, several long-term follow-up studies have demonstrated gains that were sustained even after treatment was completed. These findings were based on both parent report and independent observations of child behavior (Nixon, Sweeney, Erickson, & Touyz, 2004; Boggs et al., 2004). Remarkably, one study demonstrated treatment gains evident as late as 6 years posttreatment without interim follow-up visits (Hood & Eyberg, 2003). Among other gains, parents have reported an increased internal locus of control and decreased stress following treatment (Timmer, Urquiza, Zebell, & McGrath, 2005; Boggs et al., 2004; Hood & Eyberg, 2003; Schuhmann, Foote, Eyberg, Boggs, & Algina, 1998). Studies have demonstrated positive changes in parental interaction with the child, including increased praise and reflective listening as well as decreased negative talk (Eisenstadt, Eyberg, McNeil, Newcomb, & Funderburk, 1993; Schuhmann et al., 1998; Eyberg, Boggs, & Algina, 1995). Recently, a pilot study has demonstrated the effectiveness of PCIT in the treatment of separation anxiety disorder (Choate, Pincus, Eyberg, & Barlow, 2005), suggesting that PCIT may be effective for internalizing, as well as externalizing, disorders. This body of evidence supports the feasibility and potential utility of adaptation of PCIT for the treatment of preschool bipolar disorder.

PCIT—EMOTION DEVELOPMENT

Given the importance of managing disruptive behavior and of improving parent–child dyadic interaction, the proposed treatment model utilizes PCIT as a foundation for additional treatment components designed specifically to address emotional dysregulation, a core feature of bipolar disorder. Based on this, we have named this proposed intervention PCIT—Emotion Development (ED). PCIT has two primary components: (1) child-directed interaction (CDI), aimed toward improving the parent–child relationship and increasing child self-esteem and (2) parent-directed interaction (PDI), in which parents are taught to give appropriate commands and to effectively manage the child's misbehavior. Treatment involves weekly sessions in which parents are coached in specific skills by the therapist through a "bug-in-the-ear" device from which the parent receives direct and "on the spot" feedback and direction from the observing therapist. Parents are instructed to practice CDI at home on a daily basis in order to maintain and enhance gains in the quality of the parent–child relationship. They are also instructed to use skills learned in the PDI portion of treatment at home to address problem behaviors as they arise, noting particular areas of difficulty. Sessions can be used to work through these trouble points and enhance parents' ability to manage their child's behavior and improve their own sense of parenting efficacy. Duration of treatment is not specified, but instead treatment is terminated once parents demonstrate mastery of the skills and the child's behavior is near normal limits.

Our proposed PCIT-ED treatment of preschool-age bipolar disorder begins with PCIT in a largely unmodified format, with the exception that the number of sessions allocated to PCIT is fixed and limited to 14, such that parental mastery of skills is not required to move forward to other treatment components. Skills targeted during PCIT are monitored throughout, however. This modification is believed to be necessary in order to maintain the feasibility of our proposed treatment for the families of children with bipolar disorder who face multiple psychosocial stressors and may be unable to sustain participation in psychotherapy beyond several months. Following the abbreviated PCIT, psychoeducation on bipolar disorder is provided, as well as a parent–child session aimed at improving identification of feelings and development of relaxation techniques. In addition, a parent-only session is included, in which the parents' personal experience regarding expression of emotion (e.g., how emotion expression was handled in the family of origin), as well as the parents' feelings and thoughts about their child's behavior and expression of emotion, are addressed. The content of these sessions is believed to be important in positioning the parents to more effectively assist the child in maintaining stable mood states by enhancing their awareness and understanding of the process of dysregulation.

Treatment targeted specifically to the emotional dysregulation that is a central feature of bipolar disorder departs from Eyberg's program and is based on a novel model of conceptualizing mood disorders in young children posited by Luby and Belden (2006a). This model integrates Thompson's (1994) emotional dynamic model of emotional reactivity and regulation with Saarni's (1999) cogent model of the development of emotional competence. Briefly, Thompson (1994) has outlined key features of emotional response to incentive events, including: (1) latency to respond, (2) time from initial arousal to peak arousal intensity, (3) peak of emotional intensity, (4) total duration of response, and (5) duration and rate of return to euthymic baseline. Saarni (1999) described a model in which emotional competence is characterized by, among other features, the ability to experience a broad range of emotions at sufficient intensity and reasonable duration.

The model of "optimal emotional reactivity curves" posited by Luby and Belden (2006a) can be represented graphically (see Figure 14.1), with time represented on the X axis and emotional intensity represented on the Y axis. This graphic representation helps to characterize and quantify individual differences in this domain. An "optimal" reactivity curve thought to represent adaptive functioning encompasses spontaneous reaction to an emotionally evocative event in a timely manner, sufficient intensity of emotional peak, and reasonable duration to return to euthymic baseline. The features of an optimal or adaptive emotional reactivity curve are proposed to vary depending on the specific emotion expressed, as well as contextual factors, including cultural or familial norms for emotional expression. Using this model, Luby and Belden (2006a) propose that emotional disorders may be characterized by significant deviations from the optimal emotional reactivity curve. For example, a child experiencing mania may demonstrate sustained positive emotion and inability to return to a baseline euthymic state (see Figure 14.1).

The ED component of PCIT-ED is designed to focus on improving the child's developing capacity for effective emotion regulation by enhancing the primary caregiver's ability to guide the child in this domain. PCIT-ED

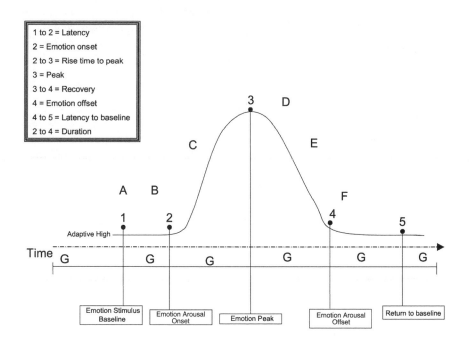

FIGURE 14.1. Emotion reactivity: Time course of response and recovery.

focuses on enhancing the quality of the caregiver–child relationship and aims to help the caregiver serve as a more effective emotion regulator for the young child by focusing on the specific aspects (e.g., very short duration between event and emotional response, very high intensity of response) of an individual child's emotional responses that differ significantly from features of the response curve thought to represent optimal or adaptive emotional competence (see Figure 14.1).

Using the emotional reactivity curve model, it is possible to identify both opportunities (e.g., circumstances and/or points in time) for the parent to intervene using particular skills and desired goals (i.e., increasing or decreasing duration and/or intensity of emotion) of treatment. In this vein, we used the emotional reactivity curve model to guide selection of skills determined to be necessary for parents to learn in order to assist their child in regulating emotions in a more competent and adaptive fashion. These skills and the corresponding points/portion of the reactivity curve (see Figure 14.1) are described next.

Recognize the Triggers of the Child's Emotional Reaction (A, Figure 14.1)

Recognizing triggers allows the parents to be aware of when their child needs their help in managing emotions. The therapist assists the parents in generating a list of their child's triggers and thereby improves parental capacity to detect these triggers in advance. In addition, treatment aims to help parents appreciate and empathize with the child's experience of these triggers.

Align with the Child (B, Figure 14.1)

In order to successfully assist their child in managing difficult emotions, the parents need to be aligned with the child. That is, parents must shift their view of themselves as people who need to suppress expression of emotion or who are irritated or frustrated by emotional expression to people who are able to help the child manage the emotion. Ideally, the parents are aligned with their child on a continuous basis or as much as possible. To the extent that this is not achievable, the parents are encouraged to align with the child immediately after recognizing a trigger.

Label Trigger/Emotion/Behavior (C, Figure 14.1)

Parents are taught how to give clear and developmentally appropriate labels to their child's triggers, emotions, and behaviors with the goal that the child later will be able to provide appropriate labels independently. In addition, by labeling these sequentially (e.g., "You didn't get the snack you want so you're feeling angry and you're stomping"), the parent and child may better understand the relation among the trigger, emotion, and behavior. Furthermore, parental labeling of the child's triggers, emotions, and behaviors acknowledges the child's experience instead of minimizing it. Labeling may result in decreased intensity of emotion as the child learns to use labels in place of disruptive displays of emotion.

Assist the Child in Utilizing Calming Techniques (D, Figure 14.1)

The parents help the child use previously learned calming techniques, such as deep breathing and visualization, which have been used in treatment of preschool-age children with other disruptive psychiatric disorders. In addition to these techniques, parents are coached to use touch to calm the child. The use of calming touch is believed to be especially important given the young age of the child, who may require physical support to regulate physiological reaction to triggers. These strategies may reduce peak emotional intensity and decrease time to return to euthymic baseline.

Assist the Child in Utilizing Alternative Calming Techniques (E, Figure 14.1)

Some children may refuse to engage in the self-calming techniques. In these situations, parents are coached to verbally reflect their child's emotional experience and assist the child by modeling and providing suggestions. If the child remains upset and engages in undesirable behavior for which time out is not appropriate, the parent will utilize a "calming space." The "calming space" is a physical spot that the child finds comforting. If the child refuses to utilize the calming space or gets out of the calming space before he or she is calm, the parent suggests returning to the calming space one time only. The goal of this technique is to encourage the child in calming while minimizing opportunities for the parent and child to engage in conflict. This technique may shorten the duration between peak emotional intensity and return to euthymic baseline.

Mark a New Beginning and Express Confidence in the Child (F, Figure 14.1)

The parents are instructed to mark a new start once the child is calm. This is important as it serves (1) as a reminder to the parents to attempt to "let go" of negative feelings that may have arisen during their interaction with the child and (2) to prevent the parents and child from allowing the negative interaction to continue indefinitely. In addition, the parents are instructed to express confidence in the child in order to reaffirm the parents' alignment with the child and to prevent the child and parents from becoming mired in hopeless thinking.

The following set of skills should be utilized by the parent for the duration of the emotional reactivity curve.

Monitor Personal Reaction (G, Figure 14.1)

Parents are encouraged to monitor their reactions to their child's emotional expression and to consider how their reactions may contribute to escalating or sustaining the child's expression of emotion. By monitoring their reactions, the parents may learn to better tolerate their child's emotional expression, instead of trying to distract from the emotion, minimize it, or alleviate it immediately, thereby providing a supportive environment in which their child may experience and express emotions. Parents will be coached to remain calm, to use a soothing voice, and to avoid power struggles while trying to help the child. Parental monitoring of personal reactions may result in decreased peak intensity of emotion and quicker return to euthymic baseline.

Praise Specific Behavior (G, Figure 14.1)

Parents are encouraged to praise specific desirable behaviors (e.g., attempts to label feeling, to appropriately seek comfort, etc.) throughout in order to increase those adaptive behaviors.

Set Firm Limits on Harmful Behavior (G, Figure 14.1)

Parents are taught to use previously learned time-out behaviors when the child demonstrates any behavior that warrants such intervention, such as harming him- or herself or someone else.

Once the child has calmed down, the parents are taught to do some "emotion work" with the child. This involves again identifying the trigger, then processing thoughts and feelings, gently correcting maladaptive thoughts, and generating more appropriate behavioral alternatives. While parents do much of the "work" with very young children, the framework is in place so that the child will eventually internalize the skills the parents display during this external modulation.

Similar to Eyberg's PCIT, in PCIT-ED parents practice these specific skills in session with the support of an observing therapist coaching via the bug-in-the-ear device (a device the parent wears in the ear by which the therapist, who is observing through a one-way mirror, can verbally coach the parent) or *in vivo*. In order to create opportunities to learn and practice these skills, two strategies are employed to elicit emotional reactions in the child. In one strategy, the parent reminds the child of an emotionally evocative event from the child's life (e.g., a favorite toy breaking) and guides the child through a discussion of the event, emotions related to the event, and related behaviors. The intent is that discussing the event will itself elicit the relevant emotion. If it does not, then the discussion is used as an opportunity for the parent to assist the child in recognizing triggers, labeling emotions, recognizing the behaviors related to the emotion, and generating alternative strategies for coping with the emotion.

The other strategy for eliciting the relevant emotion during the treatment session is the use of various therapist-created scenarios designed specifically to generate emotional responses. For example, the child may be given an undesirable toy after being told that he or she would receive a toy he or she found desirable, or the parent and child may be asked to engage in an activity in which the child is likely to become too excited or elated, such as an electric bubble game. Once parents demonstrate competency and comfort with these skills, the skills are utilized at home between sessions as relevant situations arise. Parents complete a daily log for homework during this period of treatment, in which they record episodes of emotional upset in their child and their use of the skills in assisting their child in regulating his or her emotions.

This proposed treatment model for preschool-onset mania syndrome builds on PCIT, an empirically supported treatment known to be effective in improving the parent–child relationship and minimizing disruptive behavior. Addressing these areas is critical for the treatment of preschool bipolar disorder, as they often are the most functionally impairing and have the most negative impact on family functioning. The first portion of treatment in PCIT focuses on creating positive experiences in a relationship that likely is strained. Treatment next focuses on strategies important to minimizing disruptive behavior. This is valuable in its own right, but it also improves parents' confidence in their ability to effectively manage their child's extreme behaviors. Both aspects of the PCIT set the stage for the additional treatment component that targets emotional dysregulation, believed to be a key feature of early-onset mania. PCIT allows the development of new skills and improved confidence that may prove beneficial as parents learn to assist their child in developing the capacity for effective emotion regulation by focusing on the maladaptive aspects of the child's emotional responses and guiding them toward more optimal adaptive expressions. Given the known rapid development during the preschool period, intervention during this time offers a unique opportunity to minimize disruption from the normal developmental trajectory, potentially minimizing the long-term negative impact of preschool bipolar disorder. This novel treatment model has been successfully piloted in several preschoolers to date with observed gains. A controlled preliminary study of these methods, funded by the National Institute of Mental Health, is now under way.

PSYCHOPHARMACOLOGICAL TREATMENTS FOR PRESCHOOL BIPOLAR DISORDER: EXPLORATORY STUDIES AND CASE REPORTS

The paucity of data on the question of whether mania can arise during the preschool period has stood as an impediment to the conduct of investigations of early intervention. Despite the absence of these necessary data to guide treatment decisions, psychotropic medications are being prescribed to treat irritability and mood instability in preschool children at alarmingly high rates in the community (Rushton & Whitmire, 2001; Zito et al., 2000). To date, few studies have examined pharmacological approaches to treating mental disorders in preschoolers in general, and an even smaller number of these address the specific treatment of bipolar disorder in this young age group. In this section, we attempt to summarize those studies addressing pharmacological treatments for presumptive preschool bipolar disorder and to outline future research directions in this area.

Lithium

It is well established that mood stabilizers in general, and lithium in particular, are effective in treating bipolar symptoms in adult patients (Muzina & Calabrese, 2005). Their efficacy in children, particularly adolescents, has been explored in several open-label studies and only one placebo-controlled study to date, although other studies are currently in progress. Geller, Cooper, et al. (1998) conducted a double-blind and placebo-controlled study of lithium for adolescents with bipolar disorders and secondary substance dependency ($N = 25$) and found that lithium was an efficacious treatment for both disorders. A detailed review of the literature on the use of lithium in older children with bipolar disorder is contained in other chapters in this volume.

In a retrospective chart review exploring the efficacy of mood stabilizers such as valproate and atypical antipsychotics in a preschool sample ($n = 31$) of children 2–5 years old clinically diagnosed as bipolar, mood stabilizers appeared to be well tolerated and clinically effective (Scheffer & Niskala Apps, 2004). Significant developmental benefits, such as improved mastery of social and emotional skills and the ability to engage in cognitive tasks, were also observed in this very young sample. Tumuluru et al. (2003) have provided clinical case reports of 6 preschoolers with bipolar disorder for whom lithium carbonate was recommended. Five of the 6 participants "responded positively"; the sixth child's mother refused treatment. In a retrospective chart review of 3- to 19-year-olds ($n = 46$), 11 of whom were preschool age (3–6 years old), Youngerman and Canino (1978) report that there were 30 positive responses to lithium. Of the 11 preschoolers participating, 6 reported an improvement, 4 reported no change, and 1 reported a worsening of symptoms (Youngerman & Canino, 1978). It is noteworthy that higher doses of lithium carbonate and, accordingly, levels at the higher end of the therapeutic window were associated with greater decreases in manic symptoms in a childhood sample ranging in age from 3 to 17 (Biederman et al., 1998).

Valproate

Clinical case reports of children 18 months to 5 years of age (N = 9) suggest that when lithium is not tolerated or proves ineffective, valproate may be given safely and effectively as a next choice once baseline labs establish normal liver, thyroid, and bone marrow function (Mota-Castillo et al., 2001). A retrospective chart review of preschoolers (N = 31) who were initially treated clinically with a mood stabilizer, mainly valproate, substantiates the claim that mood stabilizers can significantly decrease manic symptoms, evidenced by 84% of patients "responding favorably" on initial treatment and with improvement from baseline based on clinical assessment (Scheffer & Niskala Apps, 2004). Notably, unlike lithium carbonate, no association between dose and response for valproate was evident in the sample studied by Biederman and colleagues (1998).

These findings suggest that controlled treatment trials of mood-stabilizing agents in samples of preschool participants with operationally defined bipolar disorder are now needed. Studies of the efficacy of these medications in the treatment of preschool bipolar disorder must pay special attention to tolerance for side effects and the requirements of appropriate medication management for compounds with narrow therapeutic windows. That is, due to their more complex management, such as the need for frequent blood draws due to the risk of toxicity, the use of mood-stabilizing agents such as lithium carbonate or valproate may be more problematic in young children. In addition, side effects may be an impediment to the use of these medications in this young age group. In particular, enuresis, a common side effect of lithium, can be particularly problematic during the developmental period in which toilet training is being mastered and may cause regression in this area. Further, lithium and valproate can have an imposing side-effect profile of persistent gastrointestinal disturbances, which can be difficult for a preschooler to tolerate. These issues must be carefully addressed in future treatment studies to determine the place of these medications in a comprehensive treatment plan for preschool bipolar disorder.

Atypical Antipsychotics

In addition to studies investigating mood stabilizers, an open-label study comparing the efficacy of risperidone and olanzapine for the treatment of mania in preschool children has been conducted. In this 8-week, open-label trial of 31 preschoolers with symptoms of mania, no differences in the rate of response were found when comparing risperidone to olanzapine (Biederman et al., 2005). Findings demonstrated statistically significant improvement in preschoolers' manic symptoms in response to both medications (Biederman et al., 2005). However, of note was that treatment with risperidone was associated with statistically greater improvement of depressive symptoms compared with treatment with olanzapine. The most common side effects for both medications were increased appetite, headache and sedation, and weight gain, whereas risperidone was associated with increased prolactin (Biederman et al., 2005).

Combinations and Other Agents

A clinical case report of a 4.5-year-old on risperidone, lithium, and topiramate reported that the child became stable on a combination of topiramate and risperidone. In the same patient, risperidone as a monotherapy and in combination with lithium resulted in reduced irritability and rage and worsening of depressive symptoms after 1 week (Pavuluri et al., 2002). Despite the clinical improvement in irritability, side effects such as weight gain, polyuria, cognitive dulling, and parasthesia were observed (Pavuluri et al., 2002).

One case report has illustrated that the use of carbamazepine was effective and safe in treating the manic symptoms of a 5-year-old without major side effects. The patient response was reportedly "gradual though considerable," with remission of manic symptoms within 2 weeks (Tuzun et al., 2002). One key advantage of carbamazepine is that due to its long history of use for the treatment of seizures in very young children, its effects on growth and development during this early period have been tested, and thus this medication is proven safe and well tolerated.

The newer anticonvulsant lamotrigine, which has been used as an effective mood stabilizer in adults with bipolar disorder, has a similar advantage in having been tested for its effects on growth and development, safety, and tolerability in young child patients (Messenheimer, 2002). In a summary of the available data on the efficacy and safety of lamotrigine in pediatric seizure patients, the authors conclude that lamotrigine is well tolerated in very young pediatric patients, with a side-effect profile comparable to that found in adults (Messenheimer, 2002). Lamotrigine is associated with a low incidence of neurological adverse events such as asthenia, dizziness, and somnolence, with no apparent negative impact on cognition, an issue of particular importance in child populations (Messenheimer, 2002). Importantly, it was noted that children appear to be at a greater risk for developing life-threatening rashes than adults; however, the authors indicate that this risk can be minimized by not exceeding current dosing guidelines and by titrating the dose very slowly (Messenheimer, 2002).

Use of Stimulants

There is clear evidence that the rates of prescribing stimulants to preschoolers between the ages of 3 and 6 have been increasing (Zito et al., 2000). Whether these medications are being prescribed for the treatment of inattention or for more nonspecific disruptive symptoms, some of which could be symptoms of mania that are mistaken for symptoms of ADHD, remains unclear. This issue is complicated by the fact that ADHD is very commonly comorbid with bipolar disorder and may be the more readily clinically identifiable disorder (Geller, Williams, et al., 1998; Luby & Belden, 2006b). Along these lines, Scheffer and Niskala Apps (2004) reported that 21 out of 31 patients with bipolar disorder had a history of prior treatment with either a stimulant or an antidepressant without the protective benefit of a mood stabilizer; of these, 13 (62%) reported a worsening of mood symptoms in response to this treatment. Based on 9 clinical case reports of children 18 months of age to 5 years, Mota-Castillo and colleagues (2001) propose one rationale or algorithm for the use of mood stabilizers rather than stimulants in this population, suggesting the use of a mood stabilizer for patients when initial symptom presentation appeared clearly distinct from ADHD as well as for patients whose symptoms were exacerbated when treated with a stimulant (Mota-Castillo et al., 2001).

CONCLUSIONS AND FUTURE DIRECTIONS

Despite these promising and suggestive findings, clinicians' reluctance to prescribe mood-stabilizing medications to preschoolers because of their off-label status and the related lack of sufficient safety and efficacy data is well founded. Zito et al. (2000) underscore the ongoing need for caution in prescribing mood-stabilizing agents to preschoolers based on the fact that there is little or no proven efficacy for this indication and due to the related lack of product package insert labeling information approved by the U.S. Food and Drug Administration (FDA). Along these lines, in those circumstances in which the clinical indication appears highly compelling, specific care should be taken to provide families with the most up-to-date information regarding side effects and a clear explanation that the FDA has not approved the medication for use in the treatment of bipolar disorder or for use in the preschool age group.

Although the current literature is informative and suggests directions for future research, it falls far short of providing the needed empirical data to direct treatment in preschool patients with bipolar disorder. This paucity of data is particularly notable in light of the dramatic increase of psychotropic medications, including mood-stabilizing agents, being prescribed to preschool children in the community (Zito et al., 2000). The absence of necessary available data regarding the safety and efficacy of pharmacological treatments for preschoolers, taken together with new evidence suggesting that a DSM-IV bipolar disorder can arise in preschool children, suggests that controlled investigations of appropriate medications are now needed.

Based on the severity of this syndrome in younger children, if PCIT-ED proves insufficient, psychotherapy and medication combinations may be warranted. Studies of this kind in young children must now use operationalized criteria to identify the participants who meet DSM-IV criteria and have sufficient severity to warrant participation. Further, the need for careful weekly monitoring of growth, drug response, and side effects is particularly important for such young study participants. Given the limited ability of preschool children to provide reliable self-reports, observational measures of play behavior in such a young sample should also be a part of the assessment battery to more accurately assess treatment response. Adaptive strategy designs in which titration of the medication is based on the individual child's response, such as those employed in the ongoing treatment of early-age mania study, are particularly well suited for use in such young samples (Tillman & Geller, 2007).

REFERENCES

Belden, A. C., & Luby, J. L. (2006). Preschoolers' depression severity and behaviors during dyadic interactions: The mediating role of parental support. *Journal of the American Academy of Child and Adolescent Psychiatry, 45*(2), 213–222.

Biederman, J., Faraone, S. V., Wozniak, J., Mick, E., Kwon, A., & Aleardi, M. (2004). Further evidence of unique developmental phenotypic correlates of pediatric bipolar disorder: Findings from a large sample of clinically referred preadolescent children assessed over the last 7 years. *Journal of Affective Disorders, 82*(Suppl. 1), S45–S58.

Biederman, J., Mick, E., Bostic, J. Q., Prince, J., Daly, J., Wilens, T. E., et al. (1998). The naturalistic course of pharmacologic treatment of children with maniclike symptoms: A systematic chart review. *Journal of Clinical Psychiatry, 59*(11), 628–637.

Biederman, J., Mick, E., Hammerness, P., Harpold, T., Aleardi, M., Dougherty, M., et al. (2005). Open-label, 8-week trial of olanzapine and risperidone for the treatment of bipolar disorder in preschool-age children. *Biological Psychiatry, 58*(7), 589–594.

Birmaher, B., Axelson, D., Strober, M., Gill, M. K., Valeri, S., Chiappetta, L., et al. (2006). Clinical course of children and adolescents with bipolar spectrum disorders. *Archives of General Psychiatry, 63*(2), 175–183.

Boggs, S. R., Eyberg, S. M., Edwards, D. L., Rayfield, A., Jacobs, J., Bagner, D., et al. (2004). Outcomes of parent–child interaction therapy: A comparison of treatment completers and study dropouts one to three years later. *Child and Family Behavior Therapy, 26*(4), 1–22.

Brinkmeyer, M. Y., & Eyberg, S. M. (2003). Parent–child interaction therapy for oppositional children. In A. E. Kazdin & J. R. Weisz (Eds.), *Evidence-based psychotherapies for children and adolescents* (pp. 204–223). New York: Guilford Press.

Choate, M. L., Pincus, D. B., Eyberg, S. M., & Barlow, D. H. (2005). Parent–child interaction therapy for treatment of separation anxiety disorder in young children: A pilot study. *Cognitive and Behavioral Practice, 12*(1), 126–135.

Eisenberg, N., Losoya, S., Fabes, R. A., Guthrie, I. K., Reiser, M., Murphy, B., et al. (2001). Parental socialization of children's dysregulated expression of emotion and externalizing problems. *Journal of Family Psychology, 15*(2), 183–205.

Eisenstadt, T. H., Eyberg, S. M., McNeil, C., Newcomb, K., & Funderburk, B. (1993). Parent–child interaction therapy with behavior problem children: Relative effectiveness of two stages and overall treatment outcome. *Journal of Clinical Child Psychology, 22*(1), 42–51.

Eyberg, S. M. (1988). Parent–child interaction therapy: Integration of traditional and behavioral concerns. *Child and Family Behavior Therapy, 10,* 33–46.

Eyberg, S. M., Boggs, S. R., & Algina, J. (1995). Parent–child interaction therapy: A psychosocial model for the treatment of young children with conduct problem behavior and their families. *Psychopharmacology Bulletin, 31*(1), 83–91.

Fristad, M. A., Goldberg-Arnold, J. S., & Gavazzi, S. M. (2002). Multifamily psychoeducation groups (MFPG) for families of children with bipolar disorder. *Bipolar Disorders, 4*(4), 254–262.

Geller, B., Cooper, T. B., Sun, K., Zimerman, B., Frazier, J., Williams, M., et al. (1998). Double-blind and placebo-controlled study of lithium for adolescent bipolar disorders with secondary substance dependency. *Journal of the American Academy of Child and Adolescent Psychiatry, 37*(2), 171–178.

Geller, B., Tillman, R., Craney, J. L., & Bolhofner, K. (2004). Four-year prospective outcome and natural history of mania in children with a prepubertal and early adolescent bipolar disorder phenotype. *Archives of General Psychiatry, 61*(5), 459–467.

Geller, B., Williams, M., Zimerman, B., Frazier, J., Beringer, L., & Warner, K. (1998). Prepubertal and early adolescent bipolarity differentiate from ADHD by manic symptoms, grandiose delusions, ultra-rapid or ultradian cycling. *Journal of Affective Disorders, 51*(2), 81–91.

Geller, B., Zimerman, B., Williams, M., Bolhofner, K., Craney, J., DelBello, M., et al. (2000). Diagnostic characteristics of 93 cases of a prepubertal and early adolescent bipolar disorder phenotype by gender, puberty and comorbid attention deficit hyperactivity disorder. *Journal of Child and Adolescent Psychopharmacology, 10,* 157–164.

Hirshfeld-Becker, D. R., Biederman, J., Henin, A., Faraone, S. V., Cayton, G. A., & Rosenbaum, J. F. (2006). Laboratory-observed behavioral disinhibition in the young offspring of parents with bipolar disorder: A high-risk pilot study. *American Journal of Psychiatry, 163*(2), 265–271.

Hood, K., & Eyberg, S. M. (2003). Outcomes of parent–child interaction therapy: Mothers' reports of maintenance three to six years after treatment. *Journal of Clinical Child and Adolescent Psychology, 32*(3), 419–429.

Luby, J., & Belden, A. (2006a). Mood disorders in the preschool period: Phenomenology and a developmental emotion reactivity model. In J. Luby (Ed.), *Preschool mental health: Development, disorders and treatment* (pp. 209–230). New York: Guilford Press.

Luby, J., & Belden, A. (2006b). Validating and defining bipolar disorder in the preschool period. *Development and Psychopathology, 18,* 971–988.

Messenheimer, J. (2002). Efficacy and safety of lamotrigine in pediatric patients. *Journal of Child Neurology, 17*(Suppl. 2), 2S34–32S42.

Miklowitz, D. J., George, E. L., Axelson, D. A., Kim, E. Y., Birmaher, B., Schneck, C., et al. (2004). Family-focused treatment for adolescents with bipolar disorder. *Journal of Affective Disorders, 82*(Suppl. 1), S113–S128.

Mota-Castillo, M., Torruella, A., Engels, B., Perez, J., Dedrick, C., & Gluckman, M. (2001). Valproate in very young children: An open case series with a brief follow-up. *Journal of Affective Disorders, 67*(1–3), 193–197.

Muzina, D. J., & Calabrese, J. R. (2005). Maintenance therapies in bipolar disorder: Focus on randomized controlled trials. *Australian and New Zealand Journal of Psychiatry, 39*(8), 652–661.

Nixon, R. D., Sweeney, L., Erickson, D. B., & Touyz, S. W. (2004). Parent–child interaction

therapy: One- and two-year follow-up of standard and abbreviated treatments for oppositional preschoolers. *Journal of Abnormal Child Psychology, 32*(3), 263–271.

Pavuluri, M. N., Janicak, P. G., & Carbray, J. (2002). Topiramate plus risperidone for controlling weight gain and symptoms in preschool mania. *Journal of Child and Adolescent
Psychopharmacology, 12*(3), 271–273.

Rushton, J. L., & Whitmire, J. T. (2001). Pediatric stimulant and selective serotonin reuptake inhibitor prescription trends: 1992 to 1998. *Archives of Pediatric and Adolescent Medicine,
155*(5), 560–565.

Saarni, C. (1999). *The development of emotional competence.* New York: Guilford Press.

Scheffer, R. E., & Niskala Apps, J. A. (2004). The diagnosis of preschool bipolar disorder presenting with mania: Open pharmacological treatment. *Journal of Affective Disorders,
82*(1001), S25–S34.

Schuhmann, E. M., Foote, R. C., Eyberg, S. M., Boggs, S. R., & Algina, J. (1998). Efficacy of parent–child interaction therapy: Interim report of a randomized trial with short-term maintenance. *Journal of Clinical Child Psychology, 27*(1), 34–45.

Thompson, R. A. (1994). Emotion regulation: A theme in search of definition. *Monographs of
the Society for Research in Child Development, 59*(2–3), 25–52, 250–283.

Tillman, R., & Geller, B. (2007). Diagnostic characteristics of child bipolar I disorder: Does the
"Treatment of Early Age Mania (TEAM)" sample generalize? *Journal of Clinical Psychiatry, 68,* 307–314.

Timmer, S. G., Urquiza, A. J., Zebell, N. M., & McGrath, J. M. (2005). Parent–child interaction
therapy: Application to maltreating parent–child dyads. *Child Abuse and Neglect, 29*(7),
825–842.

Tumuluru, R. V., Weller, E. B., Fristad, M. A., & Weller, R. A. (2003). Mania in six preschool
children. *Journal of Child and Adolescent Psychopharmacology, 13*(4), 489–494.

Tuzun, U., Zoroglu, S. S., & Savas, H. A. (2002). A 5-year-old boy with recurrent mania successfully treated with carbamazepine. *Psychiatry and Clinical Neuroscience, 56*(5), 589–591.

Webster-Stratton, C. (2005). The incredible years: A training series for the prevention and treatment of conduct problems in young children. In E. Hibbs & P. Jensen (Eds.), *Psychosocial
treatments for child and adolescent disorders: Empirically based strategies for clinical
practice* (Vol. 15, pp. 839). Washington, DC: American Psychological Association.

Weiss, B., Jackson, E. W., & Susser, K. (1997). Effect of co-occurrence on the referability of internalizing and externalizing problem behaviors in adolescents. *Journal of Clinical Child Psychology, 26,* 198–204.

Youngerman, J., & Canino, I. A. (1978). Lithium carbonate use in children and adolescents. A
survey of the literature. *Archives of General Psychiatry, 35*(2), 216–224.

Zito, J., Safer, D., dosReis, S., Gardner, J., Boles, M., & Lynch, F. (2000). Trends in the prescribing of psychotropic medications to preschoolers. *Journal of the American Medical Association, 283*(8), 1025–1030.

CHAPTER 15

Treatment of Children and Adolescents at High Risk for Bipolar Disorder

Kiki D. Chang

Bipolar disorder remains a significant public health issue, with high levels of morbidity and mortality and great cost to the United States (Kessler, Chiu, Demler, Merikangas, & Walters, 2005; Kleinman et al., 2003). Despite ongoing research designed to discover better treatments for bipolar disorder, patients remain treatment-resistant, and suicide attempts and completions remain frequent (Raja & Azzoni, 2004). Clearly, early intervention designed to prevent or at least ameliorate the course of bipolar disorder deserves intense study. Yet the field of prevention of psychiatric disorders is still in its infancy. Other fields, including schizophrenia and depression, have had more activity. For example, much progress has been made in identifying individuals at risk for mild to severe psychosis and implementing early intervention pharmacotherapy (Cannon et al., 2002; McGorry et al., 2002). A similar approach to bipolar disorder would have the potential to reduce enormous suffering and save millions of lives. Yet inherent in this area of study are ethical land mines. How do we know with certainty who will develop bipolar disorder without such intervention? Do the risks of using psychotropic agents in young children outweigh the benefits? Is there anything that we as a society lose by preventing individuals from having manic episodes? With these questions unanswered, many may feel that "it is too early" to discuss preventative intervention, especially when the phenomenological presentation and course of childhood bipolar disorder is still unclear and in debate (Carlson, 2005). The ultimate responsibility for a child, however, remains with the parent, and parents who themselves suffer from bipolar disorder have repeatedly told me that they do not want their child to go through what they did.

POPULATIONS AT HIGH RISK FOR BIPOLAR DISORDER

The population that has received the most scrutiny as being at high risk for bipolar disorder development has been offspring of parents with bipolar disorder ("bipolar offspring"). These children are naturally at risk due to the highly heritable nature of bipolar disorder. Contemporary cross-sectional studies of such offspring in the United States reveal that approximately 50% have some psychiatric disorder, with 14–50% already having bipolar spectrum disorders (Chang & Steiner, 2003; DelBello & Geller, 2001). Of greater interest are the approximately 25% with attention-deficit/hyperactivity disorder (ADHD) and 20% with unipolar depression (Chang, Steiner, & Ketter, 2000; Henin et al., 2005). Why are these rates five times greater than expected in the general population? It is likely that a subset of these children will go on to develop bipolar disorder. For example, prospective studies have found the risk of developing bipolar disorder to be 30% in a prepubertal child with major depressive disorder (MDD; Geller, Fox, & Clark, 1994). The risk would appear to be greater if that child has a first-degree relative with bipolar disorder, but this quantification has not yet been done. Similarly, ADHD is now recognized as the earliest sign of bipolar disorder in an early-onset subtype of bipolar disorder (Faraone, Biederman, Mennin, Wozniak, & Spencer, 1997; Sachs, Baldassano, Truman, & Guille, 2000), and up to 28% of children with ADHD may eventually develop bipolar disorder (Tillman & Geller, 2006). Yet the majority of children with MDD and ADHD do *not* progress to bipolar disorder. Even those with strong family histories of bipolar disorder may not progress, and so other means at identifying bipolar disorder risk are necessary.

Certain temperamental traits have been postulated to be predictive of bipolar outcome in children, including cyclothymic temperament (Kochman et al., 2005), cognitive biases toward threat and negativity (Gotlib, Traill, Montoya, Joorman, & Chang, 2005), and decreased task orientation and flexibility (Chang, Blasey, Ketter, & Steiner, 2003). However, these theorized traits have largely not been validated through longitudinal follow-up and may be somewhat nonspecific.

Biological markers appear to be a better bet for improving the specificity of an early detection process. Melatonin suppression by bright light was found to be greater in bipolar offspring, particularly when both parents have bipolar disorder, compared with healthy controls (Nurnberger et al., 1988). These results are intriguing, as 91% of a cohort of euthymic adults with bipolar disorder experienced the same increased melatonin suppression (Lewy et al., 1985), suggesting that this may be an endophenotype of bipolar disorder that might be used for early detection. However, no follow-up studies in this arena have been conducted. Impaired prefrontal executive function, as measured by the Wisconsin Card Sorting Task (WCST) in bipolar and unipolar offspring was found to be predictive of bipolar disorder development in young adulthood (Meyer et al., 2004). Neuroimaging studies may prove to be the most sensitive test for revealing brain abnormalities in at-risk offspring. The most consistent brain abnormality seen in magnetic resonance imaging (MRI) studies in pediatric participants with fully developed bipolar disorder has been a decreased amygdalar volume (Blumberg, Kaufman, et al., 2003; Chang et al., 2005; Chen et al., 2004; DelBello, Zimmerman, Mills, Getz, & Strakowski, 2004; Dickstein et al., 2005; Frazier et al., 2005; Wilke, Kowatch, DelBello, Mills, & Holland, 2004). Bipolar offspring with early symptoms of bipolar disorder have also been found to have a similarly decreased volume (Karchemskiy et al., 2006), so it is possible that relatively small amygdalae may be one predictor of bipolar disorder development. Functional brain anomalies in children with bipolar disorder have been reported in prefrontal, orbitofrontal, medial frontal cortex, and in striatum and amygdala (Adler et al., 2005; Blumberg, Martin, et al., 2003; Chang et al., 2004; Rich et al., 2006). Similar abnormalities have been reported in bipolar offspring with putative prodromal bipolar disorder (Chang, Wagner, et al., 2006). Longitudinal follow-ups of these putatively prodromal offspring are under way to determine those who develop full bipolar disorder and then to characterize brain morphometry and function in those offspring that may have predicted bipolar disorder development.

Genetic markers also have great promise in identifying bipolar risk. It currently appears that the val66 polymorphism of the BDNF gene is associated with early-onset bipolar disorder (Geller et al., 2004). The serotonin transporter gene (SERT) also holds great interest, as the s-allele has already been associated with the development of depression in conjunction with psychosocial trauma (Caspi et al., 2003). Very preliminary findings indicate that the s-allele may also increase risk for progression toward bipolar disorder in offspring of parents with bipolar disorder (Howe et al., 2006).

It has been found that 30.6% of children and adolescents with bipolar disorder not otherwise specified (BD NOS) and a family history of bipolar disorder develop full bipolar disorder I or II within 2 years (Birmaher et al., 2006). Thus one could wait until the development of BD NOS to intervene, but by then the child would likely be already experiencing functional difficulties and may have already received psychiatric treatment. Earlier intervention appears necessary to stave off dysfunction, but how early? Some might consider the appearance of depression or ADHD as too late, already the first sign of a developing bipolar disorder.

RATIONALE FOR EARLY INTERVENTION

What is the rationale for early intervention? First, intervening during childhood catches brains while they are still developing. Children are still able to change radically, as they are both biologically and behaviorally responsive to environmental stimuli and thus to changes in those stimuli. Shaping of circuits, especially those in the prefrontal cortex, continues rapidly through early adulthood. Thus these changes can occur for the better or for the worse. The kindling hypothesis of affective disorder development holds that significant external stress interacts with genetic predisposition to slowly develop mood episodes. Each such episode creates neurobiological change that results in facilitation of the next episode. Eventually, fewer stressors are needed, episodes become spontaneous, and rapid cycling and treatment resistance develop (Post, 1992). These are changes for the worse. Early intervention may halt or reverse this course, leading to changes for the better. These interventions may do several things, but foremost they either decrease stress, improve the response to stress, or provide direct neuroprotection of brain areas sensitive to "changes for the worse."

MEDICATION ISSUES

Stimulants

There has been some concern that treatment with stimulants might hasten the development of mania in at-risk children (Chang, 2003). Stimulants have been reported to cause *de novo* manic episodes in children with ADHD (Koehler-Troy, Strober, & Malenbaum, 1986). It has been suggested that perhaps childhood bipolar disorder is rarer in Europe than in the United States (Soutullo et al., 2005; Post et al., 2006) because of the relatively widespread use of stimulants in the United States (Reichart & Nolen, 2004). DelBello et al. (2001) found prior stimulant exposure to be predictive of earlier age at onset (AAO) of bipolar disorder in a cohort of adolescents with mania. In this study, retrospective medication histories from 34 adolescents with bipolar disorder were obtained. In the 21 adolescents with past stimulant exposure (at least 1 week of treatment), the mean AAO was 10.7 years, compared with 13.9 years in those participants who were never treated with stimulants. However, although the percentage of participants in each group having ADHD was not different, severity of ADHD was not controlled for. Thus those adolescents with more severe symptoms of ADHD might have been more likely to receive stimulant therapy, and those same adolescents may already therefore have been showing early signs of bipolar disorder. A follow-up analysis of these adolescents did find that those with stimulant exposure had a worse course of illness (Soutullo et al., 2002), which may have been present even before mania onset. Furthermore, multiple studies have now reported earlier-onset bipolar disorder to be more severe than later-onset bipolar disorder (Carter et al., 2003; Perlis et al., 2004).

More recent data suggest that stimulants may not be associated with an earlier AAO of mania. In a cohort of children with ADHD and moderate mood symptoms followed longitudinally, stimulant treatment was not found to predict a bipolar outcome (Carlson, Loney, Salisbury, Kramer, & Arthur, 2000; Galanter et al., 2003). Furthermore, the phenomenon of stimulant rebound also may not be associated with bipolar disorder in children (Carlson & Kelly, 2003). Finally, a prospective study of children with only ADHD found that *decreased* stimulant use was associated with later development of bipolar disorder (Tillman & Geller, 2006). Certainly, on a case-by-case basis, it is possible that some children may develop mania secondary to stimulant treatment, leading to spontaneous episodes of mania that occur earlier than they otherwise would have. However, overall it is unclear whether stimulant exposure in at-risk children leads to an earlier AAO of bipolar disorder.

Case 1

An 8-year-old boy with ADHD presents for medication evaluation. His father has bipolar I disorder, early onset (at age 14), and a history of ADHD himself. There is a more remote family history of mood disorder and ADHD. The boy has irritable periods, usually triggered when he does not get his way, lasting up to 1 hour, but there is no physical aggression associated with them. There is significant oppositionality. Family environment is unremarkable. The boy does *not* have significant symptoms of euphoria, grandiosity, decreased need for sleep, hypersexuality, or increased goal-directed behavior.

In Favor of Stimulants. They are first-line medication options for ADHD, with a long track record of safety and efficacy (Hechtman & Greenfield, 2003). Even long-acting stimulants are cleared fairly rapidly from the system, so that they can be stopped rapidly if the patient's mood worsens or manic symptoms appear. Efficacy is also quick, and the clinician would know fairly soon whether the stimulant is effective in treating the target symptoms.

Against Stimulants. Up to 1 in 4 children with ADHD may go onto develop bipolar disorder (Biederman et al., 1996; Tillman & Geller, 2006). This child has a first-degree relative with bipolar disorder who also had ADHD as a child, presenting 6 years before his first manic episode. Therefore, the boy may have inherited an early-onset variant of bipolar disorder that first presents with symptoms of ADHD (Faraone et al., 1997). Stimulants may lead to kindling or cause a *de novo* manic episode. The alternatives include atomoxetine; modafinil, an alpha-adrenergic agonist; bupropion; or a tricyclic antidepressant (TCA). Atomoxetine was found useful in treating ADHD in children with bipolar disorder who did not respond well to stimulants in an open case series (Hah & Chang, 2005). None of the children had a manic reaction, but one such reaction was reported for an adult with bipolar disorder (Steinberg & Chouinard, 1985). Modafinil has positive data for treating uncomplicated ADHD (Biederman et al., 2005; Greenhill et al., 2006), but its utility in the population with bipolar disorder and ADHD is unknown. Bupropion may be problematic for reasons described already, although less so than selective serotonin reuptake inhibitors (SSRIs). TCAs are not recommended in children secondary to cardiac concerns.

In general, the evidence is not overwhelming for prohibiting use of stimulants in this population. Furthermore, as the child has no unique manic symptoms (irritability is often associated with ADHD), there is little to point to an underlying bipolar disorder other than family history, which is not diagnostic. Therefore, it appears reasonable to begin a short-acting stimulant at low dose and with careful monitoring for any worsening of mood or new manic symptoms. A short-acting stimulant may be preferable initially, as longer acting stimulants have a greater risk of causing initial insomnia, which could be confused with an early symptom of mania. Problematic reactions would then spur discontinuation of the stimulant and a trial of atomoxetine, with guanfacine or modafinil third line. There are no data currently to support starting a mood stabilizer first to "protect" against a manic reaction and then adding a stimulant. In the only relevant study, 1/30 children with bipolar disorder and ADHD taking divalproex experienced a subsequent manic episode after mixed-salts amphetamine was added, which quickly resolved after discontinuation of the stimulant (Scheffer, Kowatch, Carmody, & Rush, 2005).

Antidepressants

Another class of medications that may be harmful to this population is the antidepressants, particularly SSRIs. There are now several reports of SSRIs triggering manic or mixed episodes (Cicero, El-Mallakh, Holman, & Robertson, 2003; Faedda, Baldessarini, Glovinsky, & Austin, 2004). Larger retrospective studies report that this phenomenon may occur in 25–50% of adolescents with bipolar disorder at some point in their treatment (Baumer et al., 2006). Furthermore, new-onset suicidal ideation may occur in up to 25%, which may have contributed to the Food and Drug Administration's (FDA) warnings now intrinsic to SSRIs (Baumer et al., 2006). It is not clear yet whether these agents, in causing such behavioral outcomes, also cause neurobiological changes that could be considered kindling. Indeed, some studies have found that stimulants and SSRIs do *not* lead to an earlier AAO of bipolar disorder (Saxena, Iorgova, Dienes, & Change, 2003; Tillman & Geller, 2006). However, fully manic episodes secondary to these agents likely do indicate episodes that are "for the worse."

If such agents are problematic in children with already declared or underlying bipolar disorder, then clinicians are faced with certain dilemmas. Should antidepressants be used to treat depression in children at high risk for bipolar disorder? An illustrative case may help illustrate this quandary.

Case 2

A 14-year-old female with a major depressive episode has significant dysphoric mood, low energy, anhedonia, hypersomnia, and suicidal ideation. She has been in individual psychotherapy for 1 year and has never taken psychotropic medications. Her mother has bipolar II disorder, responsive to lamotrigine and quetiapine, and her maternal grandfather had bipolar I disorder, treated with lithium. What medication should be prescribed?

For Antidepressants. There is no irrefutable evidence that this adolescent has underlying, undeclared bipolar disorder. An antidepressant could be started and the patient monitored carefully for any worsening or quick elevation of mood, increased agitation, or decreased sleep. If these symptoms appear, the antidepressant could be quickly stopped. Bupropion has been suggested as an antidepressant that may be less likely to cause a manic episode than SSRIs (Leverich et al., 2006). Fluoxetine, although having the most efficacy data in childhood depression, should be avoided due to its relatively long half-life. Starting a mood stabilizer or antipsychotic would require drawing labs and exposure to a higher possibility of more serious adverse effects. Finally, if the patient does not have an acute adverse reaction to the antidepressant, it might be useful to continue the antidepressant, as there are some data to suggest that long-term treatment with SSRIs may not hasten the development of bipolar disorder (Saxena et al., 2003) and in fact may guard against the development of mania in patients with psychotic unipolar depression (DelBello et al., 2003).

Against Antidepressants. There is little good evidence for the efficacy of SSRIs in children or adolescents with unipolar depression. This patient has high familial loading for bipolar disorder. She has clues for a bipolar depression: low energy, hypersomnia. The majority of adults with bipolar disorder report that their first mood episode consisted of depression, usually occurring during adolescence (Perlis et al., 2004). She is young, with a clear depressive episode—the risk of future mania approaches 30% (Geller et al., 1994). Labs should be drawn anyway to assess general medical condition and thyroid status. SSRIs may have generally fewer serious adverse effects (e.g., weight gain, extrapyramidal symptoms, metabolic concerns, serious rash, sedation) compared with mood stabilizers or antipsychotics, whereas the adverse effect of a manic or mixed episode may trump all others. However, what medication should be started? This area remains somewhat speculative but leans in the direction of lithium, lamotrigine, divalproex, or quetiapine (see the next section). Again, although very few data exist in this area, there are also few data that support the use of SSRIs in childhood. Therefore, there is no clear-cut "right" answer, but either option could be explored with the family and/or the child or adolescent in order to come up with a plan.

PSYCHOPHARMACOLOGICAL INTERVENTIONS

Pharmacological intervention in children at risk for bipolar disorder may achieve two things: amelioration of current symptoms and prevention of further progression to fully expressed bipolar disorder. However, identifying which child should receive such intervention is problematic. Due to the high heritability of bipolar disorder, offspring of parents with bipolar disorder are one group that have been thought to be at high risk for bipolar disorder, especially those who already have significant mood symptoms (depression or mood instability; Chang, Steiner, Dienes, Adleman, & Ketter, 2003). Such offspring may already present with mood disorders (depression, dysthymia, cyclothymia) that stop short of full bipolar disorder. Nevertheless, they may already be receiving medication treatment for these disorders, so the ethics involved in using psychotropic agents in this population are less problematic. More difficult to consider are children who show less symptomatology, such as these with only ADHD or anxiety or even mild depression. Until better diagnostic markers for bipolar disorder can be established (such as biological markers; Chang, Adleman, Wagner, Barnea-Goraly, & Garrett, 2006), it appears prudent to consider only the slightly more impaired offspring as being at high risk for bipolar disorder development. Even in these children it may be somewhat controversial to treat with such agents as mood stabilizers or antipsychotics.

Another issue to consider is how to define response in an individual or group of high-risk children. Should amelioration of manic symptoms be the goal? Decrease of depressive symptoms? Lowering aggression or improving overall functioning? As the ultimate goal may be prevention, it is difficult to know exactly which areas need to improve to achieve this goal. Furthermore, because there are multiple pathways to developing bipolar disorder, these children can present differently, leading to a heterogeneous group for study. This heterogeneity creates further difficulty in defining the optimal outcome, as each child may have different acute concerns. Despite these methodological concerns, there are some early data in this area.

Geller and colleagues performed the first study of pharmacological intervention in a high-risk population (Geller et al., 1998) (see Table 15.1). She studied 30 prepubertal children, all with MDD and family histories of mood disorder, with 40% having a parent with bipolar disorder, 40% having a more distant relative with bipolar disorder, and 20% having a history of only unipolar depression. Participants were randomized to lithium or placebo and evaluated over 6 weeks. No differences were found between the two groups in improvement in depressive symptoms. The final Children's Global Assessment Scale (CGAS) scores in both groups, though improved, were still below 60, indicating continuing clinical problems. However, there appeared to be a wide distribution of participants who responded well and those who responded poorly, suggesting that some participants may have had unique factors associated with response. Whether these factors were related to increased family history of bipolar disorder is unknown, as the authors did not report such a subanalysis of data grouped by family history. Furthermore, no longitudinal follow-up was done to investigate potential effects on bipolar outcome of these children, so the prophylactic qualities of lithium cannot be commented on. Thus, although lithium is likely effective in bipolar depression in adolescents (Patel et al., 2006), it is unclear whether it is as effective in children at risk for bipolar disorder who are depressed. It is possible that lithium may be more effective in depressed children who have either relatively high family histories of bipolar disorder or close relatives with lithium-responsive bipolar disorder (Duffy et al., 2002; Grof, 2002). The neuroprotective effects of lithium also make this a good candidate for early intervention (Manji, Moore, & Chen, 2000b; Moore, Bebchuk, Hasanet, et al., 2000; Moore, Bebchuk, Wilds, Chen, & Manji, 2000). However, further studies in these populations are necessary before definitive conclusions regarding lithium can be made.

In another early intervention study, we investigated the use of open divalproex in 24 bipolar offspring with mood and/or disruptive behavioral disorders (Chang, Dienes, et al., 2003). None of the participants, ages 7–17, had bipolar I or II disorder, but all had at least some mild affective symptoms as manifested by a minimum score of 12 on the Young Mania Rating Scale (YMRS) or Hamilton Rating Scale for Depression (HAM-D). Diagnoses included ADHD, MDD, cyclothymia, and dysthymia, and most participants had had previous trials of antidepressants and/or stimulants. Participants were tapered off of any current medications and then begun on divalproex monotherapy, eventually reaching a mean final dose of 821 mg/

TABLE 15.1. Studies of Intervention with Youth At Risk for Bipolar Disorder

First author (year)	n	Age range (years)	Diagnoses	Intervention	Study design	Findings
Geller (1998)	30	6–12	MDD (family history of mood disorder)	Lithium vs. placebo	Placebo-controlled, double-blind, 6-week study	No difference between groups in depressive symptom improvement.
Chang, Dienes, et al. (2003)	24	7–17	Bipolar offspring with mood and behavioral symptoms (ADHD, dysthymia, MDD, cyclothymia)	DVPX monotherapy	Open, 12-week study	78% responders by week 12 (reduction in manic or depressive symptoms by 50%); decreases in aggression
Findling (2000, 2007)	32	5–17	Bipolar offspring with cyclothymia, BD NOS	DVPX vs. placebo	Placebo-controlled, double-blind, maintenance study (up to 5 years)	No difference between groups in time to study discontinuation; subset of high familial BD loading with DVPX more effective than placebo
DelBello (2006)	20	12–18	Bipolar offspring with mood disorders (BD NOS, BD II, dysthymia, cyclothymia, MDD)	Quetiapine monotherapy	Single-blind, 12-week study	81% responders by week 12 (significant improvement of bipolar symptoms by clinician impression)

Note. BD, bipolar disorder; BD NOS, bipolar disorder, not otherwise specified; BD II, bipolar II disorder; ADHD, attention-deficit/hyperactivity disorder; MDD, major depressive disorder; DVPX, divalproex.

day (serum level = 79.0 ± 26.8 μg/ml). After 12 weeks, 78% of participants were considered responders by the Clinician's General Impression—Improvement (CGI-I) score, showing general improvement in mood and functioning, with the majority showing improvement by week 3. Furthermore, overall aggression was significantly decreased as well (Saxena, Howe, Simeonova, Steiner, & Chang, 2006). Of note was that responders had lower levels of plasma glutamate following divalproex treatment compared with nonresponders (Saxena et al., 2006). Thus this study demonstrated the potential of divalproex in treating acute symptoms of mania, depression, and aggression in children with putative prodromal bipolar disorder.

However, another similar but placebo-controlled study found no difference between divalproex and placebo in a maintenance study of bipolar offspring with subthreshold bipolar disorder. This study included 56 offspring of parents with bipolar disorder (mean age 10.7 years) who had either bipolar disorder NOS or cyclothymia. Participants were randomly assigned to receive either divalproex or placebo, with the divalproex group ultimately titrated up to 15 mg/kg of daily divalproex (mean serum level = 78 μg/mL at the end of the study). The primary outcome was time to discontinuation from the study due to any reason, and secondary outcome was time to discontinuation due to a mood event. The treatment groups did not differ in either primary (median time placebo = 83 days; median time divalproex = 78 days) or secondary outcome. Although changes in mood symptom ratings did not differ between groups, both groups did show improvements in mood symptoms and psychosocial functioning over time. Furthermore, divalproex was found superior to placebo in a small subset of participants who had at least three first- or second-degree relatives with emotional or behavioral problems (Findling et al., 2007). Thus, given these preliminary studies, and studies demonstrating in vitro neuroprotective effects (Manji, Moore, & Chen, 2000a), valproate may be most useful for early intervention in children with high familial loading for bipolar and other mood disorders.

Quetiapine has also been investigated for its utility in pediatric populations at high risk for bipolar disorder. DelBello and colleagues (2006) conducted a 12-week single-blind study of quetiapine for bipolar offspring with mood disorders (mean age = 14.7 years) that were considered subsyndromal to full bipolar disorder (no participants had histories of mania). Eleven (55%) had BD NOS, considered to be one criteria for mania—a symptom short of meeting criteria for mania, or meeting all criteria except duration. Three had bipolar II disorder, 3 (11%) had dysthymia, 2 cyclothymia, and 1 MDD. Thus almost all participants had a bipolar spectrum disorder, and as such these participants were farther along the progression line for bipolar disorder than those in the previously discussed studies involving valproate. Quetiapine was begun at 100 mg/day, then increased every day up to 400 mg/day, with flexible dosing thereafter to achieve 300–600 mg/day based on clinical need. Fifteen participants completed the study, and final mean dose was 460 mg/day. The indicator of showing response was a score of "1" or "2" (much or moderate improvement in bipolar symptoms) on the Clinical Global Impressions—Bipolar (CGI-BP) Scale. After 1 week there were 4 responders (25%), growing to 81% by week 12. YMRS scores decreased from 18.1 to 8.7, and mean Children's Depression Rating Scale—Revised (CDRS-R) score decreased from 38.2 to 27.7. The most common adverse effects were somnolence (55%), headache (25%), musculoskeletal pain (25%), and dyspepsia (25%).

Thus these bipolar offspring with subsyndromal bipolar disorder responded well acutely to quetiapine monotherapy. As for the previously discussed studies, it remains to be seen whether quetiapine is effective in preventing or delaying the onset of full bipolar disorder. Longitudinal studies lasting at least 3 years, with placebo-controlled arms, are necessary to better investigate the prophylactic potential of these agents. However, such a long study would naturally be difficult to conduct. Real-world variables, including psychosocial stressors, psychotherapeutic interventions, and substance abuse, could occur during that time. Participant attrition and the need for further medication could be problematic. One solution might be a survival design, in which a need for further intervention (psychosocial or pharmacological) would indicate dropping out of the study. Then survival curves could be compared between the two groups (placebo and active agent). Large numbers in each group would then be necessary to balance for various demographics, such as gender, age, and even phenomenological presentation.

PSYCHOTHERAPEUTIC/ PSYCHOSOCIAL INTERVENTIONS

In addition to pharmacological interventions, psychosocial interventions may have special utility for prevention of bipolar disorder. Psychotherapy may be more targeted than medications, without the potential for physical adverse effects. Furthermore, specific issues unique to the child and family can be addressed. These advantages make psychosocial interventions a less controversial and potentially more targeted form of early intervention in at-risk children.

For example, in a study addressing prevention of unipolar depression in children, group cognitive therapy was more effective than no specific intervention in reducing depressive symptoms in adolescent offspring of parents with depression (Clarke et al., 2001). Similarly, psychoeducation sessions for families with a depressed parent were found effective in reducing problematic behaviors of the children in the household (Beardslee &

Gladstone, 2001). These types of approaches to prevention of depression could be similarly applied to bipolar paradigms.

Goals of this type of intervention in children at risk for bipolar disorder would include decreasing the amount of stress the child is exposed to while improving the child's internal coping mechanisms. Psychoeducation is also extremely valuable in ensuring that the entire family is "on the same page." Topics discussed could include triggers for mood episodes; the importance of sleep, exercise, and schedule in mood regulation; the etiology and presentation of bipolar disorder; and medications and side effects. These strategies have begun to be used and studied in pediatric bipolar disorder (Fristad, Goldberg-Arnold, & Gavazzi, 2002; Miklowitz et al., 2004; Pavuluri et al., 2004). A logical extension is the implementation of these concepts in populations at risk for bipolar disorder. For example, family-focused therapy for adolescents (FFT-A) could be extended to deal with general issues of mood regulation in high-risk patients, such as patients with first-degree relatives with bipolar disorder (see Miklowitz, Mullen, & Chang, Chapter 9, this volume).

CONCLUSIONS

The future holds great promise for this area of preventative research in bipolar disorder. Brain imaging and genetic studies of pediatric bipolar disorder have already made inroads into understanding the development and etiology of this disorder and into finding biological markers that could be used for early detection. Pharmacological and psychotherapeutic interventions are beginning to be studied at the short-term level. Greater awareness of the early harbingers of bipolar disorder have been made. Thus, although we clearly do need additional information in order to create risk-quantification algorithms, we have already identified populations at high enough risk for bipolar disorder to warrant intervention. The ethical questions regarding intervention in an at-risk population remain unanswered; however, as more data emerge in this field and we have better diagnostic specificity and more long-term safety and efficacy data, those concerns should lessen. One ethical question, though, may be more difficult to answer, and that is what we are losing by preventing mania. For example, there has long been an association between creativity and mood disorders, and even some hint of heightened creativity in children with bipolar disorder (Simeonova, Chang, Strong, & Ketter, 2005). Yet this creativity appears to lessen with longer duration of illness (Simeonova et al., 2005), and repeated episodes are thought to impair functional creativity (Jamison, 1995). The majority of patients would seem to prefer never having had this tremendously disabling disorder, but perhaps a questionnaire addressing whether patients would have preferred early intervention and potential prevention of their bipolar disorder would be warranted. A similar such study found that 83% of parents favored acute medication intervention in their children, if the children were deemed at very high risk of developing bipolar disorder before the development of severe symptoms (Post, Leverich, Fergus, Miller, & Luckenbaugh, 2002). The majority of parents also favored psychotherapeutic intervention if their child was to have only moderate symptom severity.

However, no long-term longitudinal intervention studies are being conducted in populations at high risk for bipolar disorder. This type of study, with a control arm, a large sample, and multiyear duration, is expensive and unwieldy and thus may not receive much funding interest from the pharmaceutical industry, private foundations, or even the U.S. National Institute of Mental Health. Yet these types of studies may be the ones that eventually serve to significantly decrease the morbidity and mortality burden of bipolar disorder on society and individuals worldwide.

REFERENCES

Adler, C. M., DelBello, M. P., Mills, N. P., Schmithorst, V., Holland, S., & Strakowski, S. M. (2005). Comorbid ADHD is associated with altered patterns of neuronal activation in adolescents with bipolar disorder performing a simple attention task. *Bipolar Disorders, 7,* 577–588.

Baumer, F. M., Howe, M., Gallelli, K., Simeonova, D. I., Hallmayer, J., & Chang, K. D. (2006). A pilot study of antidepressant-induced mania in pediatric bipolar disorder: Characteristics, risk factors, and the serotonin transporter gene. *Biological Psychiatry, 60,* 1005–1012.

Beardslee, W. R., & Gladstone, T. R. (2001). Prevention of childhood depression: Recent findings and future prospects. *Biological Psychiatry, 49,* 1101–1110.

Biederman, J., Faraone, S., Mick, E., Wozniak, J., Chen, L., Ouellette, C., et al. (1996). Attention-deficit hyperactivity disorder and juvenile mania: An overlooked comorbidity? *Journal of the American Academy of Child and Adolescent Psychiatry, 35,* 997–1008.

Biederman, J., Swanson, J. M., Wigal, S. B., Kratochvil, C. J., Boellner, S. W., Earl, C. Q., et al. (2005). Efficacy and safety of modafinil film-coated tablets in children and adolescents with attention-deficit/hyperactivity disorder: Results of a randomized, double-blind, placebo-controlled, flexible-dose study. *Pediatrics, 116,* e777–e784.

Birmaher, B., Axelson, D., Strober, M., Gill, M. K., Valeri, S., Chiappetta, L., et al. (2006). Clinical course of children and adolescents with bipolar spectrum disorders. *Archives of General Psychiatry, 63,* 175–183.

Blumberg, H. P., Kaufman, J., Martin, A., Whiteman, R., Zhang, J. H., Gore, J. C., et al. (2003). Amygdala and hippocampal volumes in adolescents and adults with bipolar disorder. *Archives of General Psychiatry, 60,* 1201–1208.

Blumberg, H. P., Martin, A., Kaufman, J., Leung, H. C., Skudlarski, P., Lacadie, C., et al. (2003). Frontostriatal abnormalities in adolescents with bipolar disorder: Preliminary observations from functional MRI. *American Journal of Psychiatry, 160,* 1345–1347.

Cannon, T. D., Huttunen, M. O., Dahlstrom, M., Larmo, I., Rasanen, P., & Juriloo, A. (2002). Antipsychotic drug treatment in the prodromal phase of schizophrenia. *American Journal of Psychiatry, 159,* 1230–1232.

Carlson, G. A. (2005). Early onset bipolar disorder: Clinical and research considerations. *Journal of Clinical and Child Adolescent Psychology, 34,* 333–343.

Carlson, G. A., & Kelly, K. L. (2003). Stimulant rebound: How common is it and what does it mean? *Journal of Child and Adolescent Psychopharmacology, 13*, 137–142.

Carlson, G. A., Loney, J., Salisbury, H., Kramer, J. R., & Arthur, C. (2000). Stimulant treatment in young boys with symptoms suggesting childhood mania: A report from a longitudinal study. *Journal of Child and Adolescent Psychopharmacology, 10*, 175–184.

Carter, T. D., Mundo, E., Parikh, S. V., & Kennedy, J. L. (2003). Early age at onset as a risk factor for poor outcome of bipolar disorder. *Journal of Psychiatric Research, 37*, 297–303.

Caspi, A., Sugden, K., Moffitt, T. E., Taylor, A., Craig, I. W., Harrington, H., et al. (2003). Influence of life stress on depression: Moderation by a polymorphism in the 5-HTT gene. *Science, 301*, 386–389.

Chang, K. (2003). Stimulant use in pediatric bipolar disorder with attention-deficit/hyperactivity disorder: Pro. *Journal of Bipolar Disorders: Reviews and Commentaries, 2*, 16–17.

Chang, K., Adleman, N. E., Dienes, K., Simeonova, D. I., Menon, V., & Reiss, A. (2004). Anomalous prefrontal-subcortical activation in familial pediatric bipolar disorder: A functional magnetic resonance imaging investigation. *Archives of General Psychiatry, 61*, 781–792.

Chang, K., Adleman, N., Wagner, C., Barnea-Goraly, N., & Garrett, A. (2006). Will neuroimaging ever be used to diagnose pediatric bipolar disorder? *Developmental Psychopathology, 18*, 1133–1146.

Chang, K., Karchemskiy, A., Barnea-Goraly, N., Garrett, A., Simeonova, D. I., & Reiss, A. (2005). Reduced amygdalar gray matter volume in familial pediatric bipolar disorder. *Journal of the American Academy of Child and Adolescent Psychiatry, 44*, 565–573.

Chang, K., Steiner, H., Dienes, K., Adleman, N., & Ketter, T. (2003). Bipolar offspring: A window into bipolar disorder evolution. *Biological Psychiatry, 53*, 945–951.

Chang, K., Wagner, C., Gallelli, K., Howe, M., Karchemskiy, A., Garrett, A., et al. (2006). *Effects of divalproex on brain chemistry and function in adolescents at risk for bipolar disorder.* Paper presented at the 53rd Annual Meeting of the American Academy of Child and Adolescent Psychiatry, San Diego, CA.

Chang, K. D., Blasey, C. M., Ketter, T. A., & Steiner, H. (2003). Temperament characteristics of child and adolescent bipolar offspring. *Journal of Affective Disorders, 77*, 11–19.

Chang, K. D., Dienes, K., Blasey, C., Adleman, N., Ketter, T., & Steiner, H. (2003). Divalproex monotherapy in the treatment of bipolar offspring with mood and behavioral disorders and at least mild affective symptoms. *Journal of Clinical Psychiatry, 64*, 936–942.

Chang, K. D., & Steiner, H. (2003). Offspring studies in child and early adolescent bipolar disorder. In B. Geller & M. DelBello (Eds.), *Bipolar disorder in childhood and early adolescence* (pp. 107–129). New York: Guilford Press.

Chang, K. D., Steiner, H., & Ketter, T. A. (2000). Psychiatric phenomenology of child and adolescent bipolar offspring. *Journal of the American Academy of Child and Adolescent Psychiatry, 39*, 453–460.

Chen, B. K., Sassi, R., Axelson, D., Hatch, J. P., Sanches, M., Nicoletti, M., et al. (2004). Cross-sectional study of abnormal amygdala development in adolescents and young adults with bipolar disorder. *Biological Psychiatry, 56*, 399–405.

Cicero, D., El-Mallakh, R. S., Holman, J., & Robertson, J. (2003). Antidepressant exposure in bipolar children. *Psychiatry, 66*, 317–322.

Clarke, G. N., Hornbrook, M., Lynch, F., Polen, M., Gale, J., Beardslee, W., et al. (2001). A randomized trial of a group cognitive intervention for preventing depression in adolescent offspring of depressed parents. *Archives of General Psychiatry, 58*, 1127–1134.

DelBello, M. P., Carlson, G. A., Tohen, M., Bromet, E. J., Schwiers, M., & Strakowski, S. M. (2003). Rates and predictors of developing a manic or hypomanic episode 1 to 2 years following a first hospitalization for major depression with psychotic features. *Journal of Child and Adolescent Psychopharmacology, 13*(2), 173–185.

DelBello, M. P., & Geller, B. (2001). Review of studies of child and adolescent offspring of bipolar parents. *Bipolar Disorders, 3*, 325–334.

DelBello, M. P., Soutullo, C. A., Hendricks, W., Niemeier, R. T., McElroy, S. L., & Strakowski, S. M. (2001). Prior stimulant treatment in adolescents with bipolar disorder: Association with age at onset. *Bipolar Disorders, 3*, 53–57.

DelBello, M., Whitsel, R. M., Adler, C., Kowatch, R. A., Stanford, K., & Strakowski, S. M. (2006). *Quetiapine efficacy in adolescents with mood disorders and a family history of bipolar disorder.* Poster presented at the 53rd Annual Meeting of the American Academy of Child and Adolescent Psychiatry, San Diego, CA.

DelBello, M. P., Zimmerman, M. E., Mills, N. P., Getz, G. E., & Strakowski, S. M. (2004). Magnetic resonance imaging analysis of amygdala and other subcortical brain regions in adolescents with bipolar disorder. *Bipolar Disorders, 6*, 43–52.

Dickstein, D. P., Milham, M. P., Nugent, A. C., Drevets, W. C., Charney, D. S., Pine, D. S., et al. (2005). Frontotemporal alterations in pediatric bipolar disorder: Results of a voxel-based morphometry study. *Archives of General Psychiatry, 62*, 734–741.

Duffy, A., Alda, M., Kutcher, S., Cavazzoni, P., Robertson, C., Grof, E., et al. (2002). A prospective study of the offspring of bipolar parents responsive and nonresponsive to lithium treatment. *Journal of Clinical Psychiatry, 63*(12), 1171–1178.

Faedda, G. L., Baldessarini, R. J., Glovinsky, I. P., & Austin, N. B. (2004). Treatment-emergent mania in pediatric bipolar disorder: A retrospective case review. *Journal of Affective Disorders, 82*, 149–158.

Faraone, S. V., Biederman, J., Mennin, D., Wozniak, J., & Spencer, T. (1997). Attention-deficit hyperactivity disorder with bipolar disorder: A familial subtype? *Journal of the American Academy of Child and Adolescent Psychiatry, 36*, 1378–1390.

Findling, R. L., Frazier, T. W., Youngstrom, E. A., McNamara, N. K., Stansbrey, R. J., Gracious, B. L., et al. (2007). Double-blind, placebo-controlled trial of divalproex monotherapy in the treatment of symptomatic youth at high risk for developing bipolar disorder. *Journal of Clinical Psychiatry, 68*(5), 781–788.

Findling, R. L., Gracious, B. L., McNamara, N. K., & Calabrese, J. R. (2000). The rationale, design, and progress of two novel maintenance treatment studies in pediatric bipolarity. *Acta Neuropsychiatrica, 12*, 136–138.

Frazier, J. A., Breeze, J. L., Makris, N., Giuliano, A. S., Herbert, M. R., Seidman, L., et al. (2005). Cortical gray matter differences identified by structural magnetic resonance imaging in pediatric bipolar disorder. *Bipolar Disorders, 7*, 555–569.

Fristad, M. A., Goldberg-Arnold, J. S., & Gavazzi, S. M. (2002). Multifamily psychoeducation groups (MFPG) for families of children with bipolar disorder. *Bipolar Disorders, 4*, 254–262.

Galanter, C. A., Carlson, G. A., Jensen, P. S., Greenhill, L. L., Davies, M., Li, W., et al. (2003). Response to methylphenidate in children with attention deficit hyperactivity disorder and manic symptoms in the multimodal treatment study of children with attention deficit hyperactivity disorder titration trial. *Journal of Child and Adolescent Psychopharmacology, 13*, 123–136.

Geller, B., Badner, J. A., Tillman, R., Christian, S. L., Bolhofner, K., & Cook, E. H., Jr. (2004). Linkage disequilibrium of the brain-derived neurotrophic factor Val66Met polymorphism in children with a prepubertal and early adolescent bipolar disorder phenotype. *American Journal of Psychiatry, 161*, 1698–1700.

Geller, B., Cooper, T. B., Zimerman, B., Frazier, J., Williams, M., Heath, J., et al. (1998). Lithium for prepubertal depressed children with family history predictors of future bipolarity: A double-blind, placebo-controlled study. *Journal of Affective Disorders, 51*, 165–175.

Geller, B., Fox, L. W., & Clark, K. A. (1994). Rate and predictors of prepubertal bipolarity during follow-up of 6- to 12-year-old depressed children. *Journal of the American Academy of Child and Adolescent Psychiatry, 33*, 461–468.

Gotlib, I. H., Traill, S. K., Montoya, R. L., Joormann, J., & Chang, K. (2005). Attention and memory biases in the offspring of parents with bipolar disorder: Indications from a pilot study. *Journal of Child Psychology and Psychiatry, 46,* 84–93.

Greenhill, L. L., Biederman, J., Boellner, S. W., Rugino, T. A., Sangal, R. B., Earl, C. Q., et al. (2006). A randomized, double-blind, placebo-controlled study of modafinil film-coated tablets in children and adolescents with attention-deficit/hyperactivity disorder. *Journal of the American Academy of Child and Adolescent Psychiatry, 45,* 503–511.

Grof, P., Duffy, A., Cavazzoni, P., Grof, E., Garnham, J., MacDougall, M., et al. (2002). Is response to prophylactic lithium a familial trait? *Journal of Clinical Psychiatry, 63*(10), 942–947.

Hah, M., & Chang, K. (2005). Atomoxetine for the treatment of attention-deficit/hyperactivity disorder in children and adolescents with bipolar disorders. *Journal of Child and Adolescent Psychopharmacology, 15,* 996–1004.

Hechtman, L., & Greenfield, B. (2003). Long-term use of stimulants in children with attention deficit hyperactivity disorder: Safety, efficacy, and long-term outcome. *Paediatric Drugs, 5,* 787–794.

Henin, A., Biederman, J., Mick, E., Sachs, G. S., Hirshfeld-Becker, D. R., Siegel, R. S., et al. (2005). Psychopathology in the offspring of parents with bipolar disorder: A controlled study. *Biological Psychiatry, 58,* 554–561.

Howe, M., Karchemskiy, A., Yee, J., Beenhakker, J., Hallmayer, J., & Chang, K. (2006). *Prospective longitudinal study of offspring at risk for bipolar disorder: Three-year follow-up.* Poster presented at the 53rd Annual Meeting of the American Academy of Child and Adolescent Psychiatry, San Diego, CA.

Jamison, K. R. (1995). Manic-depressive illness and creativity. *Scientific American, 272,* 62–67.

Karchemskiy, A., Chang, M., Simeonova, D. I., Howe, M., Garrett, A., Reiss, A., et al. (2006). *Decreased amygdalar volume in familial subsyndromal bipolar disorder.* Poster presented at the 53rd Annual Meeting of the American Academy of Child and Adolescent Psychiatry, San Diego, CA.

Kessler, R. C., Chiu, W. T., Demler, O., Merikangas, K. R., & Walters, E. E. (2005). Prevalence, severity, and comorbidity of 12-month DSM-IV disorders in the National Comorbidity Survey Replication. *Archives of General Psychiatry, 62,* 617–627.

Kleinman, L., Lowin, A., Flood, E., Gandhi, G., Edgell, E., & Revicki, D. (2003). Costs of bipolar disorder. *Pharmacoeconomics, 21,* 601–622.

Kochman, F. J., Hantouche, E. G., Ferrari, P., Lancrenon, S., Bayart, D., & Akiskal, H. S. (2005). Cyclothymic temperament as a prospective predictor of bipolarity and suicidality in children and adolescents with major depressive disorder. *Journal of Affective Disorders, 85,* 181–189.

Kochler-Troy, C., Strober, M., & Malenbaum, R. (1986). Methylphenidate-induced mania in a prepubertal child. *Journal of Clinical Psychiatry, 47,* 566–567.

Leverich, G. S., Altshuler, L. L., Frye, M. A., Suppes, T., McElroy, S. L., Keck, P. E., Jr., et al. (2006). Risk of switch in mood polarity to hypomania or mania in patients with bipolar depression during acute and continuation trials of venlafaxine, sertraline, and bupropion as adjuncts to mood stabilizers. *American Journal of Psychiatry, 163,* 232–239.

Lewy, A. J., Nurnberger, J. I., Jr., Wehr, T. A., Pack, D., Becker, L. E., Powell, R. L., et al. (1985). Supersensitivity to light: Possible trait marker for manic-depressive illness. *American Journal of Psychiatry, 142,* 725–727.

Manji, H. K., Moore, G. J., & Chen, G. (2000a). Clinical and preclinical evidence for the neurotrophic effects of mood stabilizers: Implications for the pathophysiology and treatment of manic-depressive illness. *Biological Psychiatry, 48*(8), 740–754.

Manji, H. K., Moore, G. J., & Chen, G. (2000b). Lithium up-regulates the cytoprotective protein Bcl-2 in the CNS in vivo: A role for neurotrophic and neuroprotective effects in manic-depressive illness. *Journal of Clinical Psychiatry, 61*(Suppl. 9), 82–96.

McGorry, P. D., Yung, A. R., Phillips, L. J., Yuen, H. P., Francey, S., Cosgrave, E. M., et al. (2002).

Randomized controlled trial of interventions designed to reduce the risk of progression to first-episode psychosis in a clinical sample with subthreshold symptoms. *Archives of General Psychiatry, 59*, 921–928.

Meyer, S. E., Carlson, G. A., Wiggs, E. A., Martinez, P. E., Ronsaville, D. S., Klimes-Dougan, B., et al. (2004). A prospective study of the association among impaired executive functioning, childhood attentional problems, and the development of bipolar disorder. *Developmental Psychopathology, 16*, 461–476.

Miklowitz, D. J., George, E. L., Axelson, D. A., Kim, E. Y., Birmaher, B., Schneck, C., et al. (2004). Family-focused treatment for adolescents with bipolar disorder. *Journal of Affective Disorders, 82*(Suppl. 1), S113–S128.

Moore, G. J., Bebchuk, J. M., Hasanat, K., Chen, G., Seraji-Bozorgzad, N., Wilds, I. B., et al. (2000). Lithium increases N-acetyl-aspartate in the human brain: In vivo evidence in support of bcl-2's neurotrophic effects? *Biological Psychiatry, 48*(1), 1–8.

Moore, G. J., Bebchuk, J. M., Wilds, I. B., Chen, G., & Manji, H. K. (2000). Lithium-induced increase in human brain grey matter. *Lancet, 356*(9237), 1241–1242.

Nurnberger, J. I., Jr., Berrettini, W., Tamarkin, L., Hamovit, J., Norton, J., & Gershon, E. (1988). Supersensitivity to melatonin suppression by light in young people at high risk for affective disorder: A preliminary report. *Neuropsychopharmacology, 1*, 217–223.

Patel, N. C., DelBello, M. P., Bryan, H. S., Adler, C. M. Kowatch, R. A., Stanford, K., et al. (2006). Open-label lithium for the treatment of adolescents with bipolar depression. *Journal of the American Academy of Child and Adolescent Psychiatry, 45*(3), 289–297.

Pavuluri, M. N., Graczyk, P. A., Henry, D. B., Carbray, J. A., Heidenreich, J., & Miklowitz, D. J. (2004). Child- and family-focused cognitive-behavioral therapy for pediatric bipolar disorder: Development and preliminary results. *Journal of the American Academy of Child and Adolescent Psychiatry, 43*, 528–537.

Perlis, R. H., Miyahara, S., Marangell, L. B., Wisniewski, S. R., Ostacher, M., DelBello, M. P., et al. (2004). Long-term implications of early onset in bipolar disorder: Data from the first 1,000 participants in the systematic treatment enhancement program for bipolar disorder (STEP-BD). *Biological Psychiatry, 55*, 875–881.

Post, R. M. (1992). Transduction of psychosocial stress into the neurobiology of recurrent affective disorder. *American Journal of Psychiatry, 149*, 999–1010.

Post, R. M. Leverich, G. S., Fergus, E., Miller, R., & Luckenbaugh, D. (2002). Parental attitudes towards early intervention in children at high risk for affective disorders. *Journal of Affective Disorders, 70*(2), 117–124.

Post, R. M., Luckenbaugh, D. A., Leverich, G. S., Altshuler, L. L., Frye, M. A., Suppes, T., et al. (2006, October 6). *Increased rate of childhood onset bipolar illness in the U.S. compared with two European countries.* Paper presented at the International Conference on Bipolar Illness, Barcelona, Spain.

Raja, M., & Azzoni, A. (2004). Suicide attempts: Differences between unipolar and bipolar patients and among groups with different lethality risk. *Journal of Affective Disorders, 82*, 437–442.

Reichart, C. G., & Nolen, W. A. (2004). Earlier onset of bipolar disorder in children by antidepressants or stimulants? An hypothesis. *Journal of Affective Disorders, 78*, 81–84.

Rich, B. A., Vinton, D. T., Roberson-Nay, R., Hommer, R. E., Berghorst, L. H., McClure, E. B., et al. (2006). Limbic hyperactivation during processing of neutral facial expressions in children with bipolar disorder. *Proceeding of the National Academy of Sciences of the United States of America, 103*, 8900–8905.

Sachs, G. S., Baldassano, C. F., Truman, C. J., & Guille, C. (2000). Comorbidity of attention deficit hyperactivity disorder with early- and late-onset bipolar disorder. *American Journal of Psychiatry, 157*, 466–468.

Saxena, K., Howe, M., Simeonova, D., Steiner, H., & Chang, K. (2006). Divalproex sodium reduces overall aggression in youth at high risk for bipolar disorder. *Journal of Child and Adolescent Psychopharmacology, 16,* 252–259.

Saxena, K., Iorgova, D., Dienes, K., & Chang, K. (2003, May). *Medication exposure in bipolar offspring with ADHD or depression.* Poster presented at the 156th Annual Meeting of the American Psychiatric Association, San Francisco, CA.

Scheffer, R. E., Kowatch, R. A., Carmody, T., & Rush, A. J. (2005). Randomized, placebo-controlled trial of mixed amphetamine salts for symptoms of comorbid ADHD in pediatric bipolar disorder after mood stabilization with divalproex sodium. *American Journal of Psychiatry, 162,* 58–64.

Simeonova, D. I., Chang, K. D., Strong, C., & Ketter, T. A. (2005). Creativity in familial bipolar disorder. *Journal of Psychiatric Research, 39,* 623–631.

Soutullo, C. A., Chang, K. D., Diez-Suarez, A., Figueroa-Quintana, A., Escamilla-Canales, I., Rapado-Castro, M., et al. (2005). Bipolar disorder in children and adolescents: International perspective on epidemiology and phenomenology. *Bipolar Disorders, 7,* 497–506.

Soutullo, C. A., DelBello, M. P., Ochsner, J. E., McElroy, S. L., Taylor, S. A., Strakowski, S. M., et al. (2002). Severity of bipolarity in hospitalized manic adolescents with history of stimulant or antidepressant treatment. *Journal of Affective Disorders, 70,* 323–327.

Steinberg, S., & Chouinard, G. (1985). A case of mania associated with tomoxetine. *American Journal of Psychiatry, 142,* 1517–1518.

Tillman, R., & Geller, B. (2006). Controlled study of switching from attention-deficit/hyperactivity disorder to a prepubertal and early adolescent bipolar I disorder phenotype during 6-year prospective follow-up: Rate, risk, and predictors. *Developmental Psychopathology, 18,* 1037–1053.

Wilke, M., Kowatch, R. A., DelBello, M. P., Mills, N. P., & Holland, S. K. (2004). Voxel-based morphometry in adolescents with bipolar disorder: First results. *Psychiatry Research, 131,* 57–69.

CHAPTER 16

Treatment of Bipolar Depression

SHANNON RAE BARNETT, MARK A. RIDDLE, *and* JOHN T. WALKUP

The treatment of bipolar depression in children and adolescents can be extremely difficult. This chapter includes a discussion of five factors that complicate any conclusions about the best treatment of bipolar depression in children and adolescents: (1) the controversy about the diagnosis of bipolar disorder in youths; (2) the difficulty of generalizing data from the adult literature; (3) the mixed results about the efficacy of both antidepressants and mood stabilizers in the treatment of adult bipolar depression; (4) the risk of antidepressants inducing a switch to mania or inducing rapid cycling; and (5) the lack of data in the treatment of bipolar depression in youths. This chapter explores each of these factors. The chapter ends with some suggestions for treatment that should be taken in the context of the uncertainty that surrounds the treatment of bipolar depression in youths.

CONTROVERSY SURROUNDING THE DIAGNOSIS OF BIPOLAR DISORDER IN CHILDREN AND ADOLESCENTS

The diagnosis of bipolar depression in children and adolescents is complicated by two factors. First, researchers do not all agree on the best way to define bipolar disorder in this population. Researchers also generally define the target population in a way that increases specificity (they want to increase the percentage of enrolled participants who really have the disorder), but clinicians are still faced with the decision of what to do with patients who have a more ambiguous clinical picture. Second, in children and to a lesser extent adolescents with bipolar disorder, it is often difficult to differentiate between a manic episode and a mixed episode. It is therefore difficult to determine when it might be beneficial to begin treatment for the depressive symptoms.

As described in detail in other chapters in this volume, researchers do not all agree on the best way to diagnose bipolar depression in children and adolescents. Whereas adults often meet DSM diagnostic criteria—for example, a distinct period of elevated mood and/or irritability lasting at least 2 weeks, discrete cycles, and so forth—children frequently present with a different constellation of symptoms and course. Unlike adults, children and adolescents with bipolar disorder often present with a chronic, noncyclic course of symptoms that is characterized by severe irritability and symptoms of hyperarousal (Findling et al., 2001; Geller et al., 2001; Geller et al., 2002). Children and adolescents may experience frequent shifts in mood occurring many times per day; this has been referred to as ultra-rapid cycling (Geller et al., 2000a; Geller et al., 2000b). Some research studies require symptoms of euphoria and grandiosity to make the diagnosis in children and adolescents (Geller et al., 2000a), but others do not (Biederman et al., 2000). Others have defined a range of "bipolarity," including a narrow, an intermediate, and a broad phenotype (Leibenluft, Chamey, Towbin, Bhangoo, & Pine, 2003). Thus one expert might diagnose bipolar disorder, whereas another might describe the same child as having attention-deficit/ hyperactivity disorder (ADHD) plus oppositional defiant disorder (ODD) and/or mood disorder not otherwise specified (NOS). Because different studies define bipolar disorder in different ways, it is difficult for clinicians to generalize the outcomes of these studies to clinical practice.

Children and adolescents with bipolar disorder often present with a mixed state of depressive and manic symptoms. The difficulty for most clinicians is to differentiate between a manic episode and a mixed episode. The reason is that almost all children and adolescents with mania show marked irritability, psychomotor agitation, difficulties with sleep, and difficulties with concentration—four symptoms of the five that are necessary for the diagnosis of a depressive episode. One possible strategy for differentiating a mixed episode from a manic episode might be to use the adult criteria for a depressive episode: requiring either a significant depressed mood or anhedonia. However, further research is required to determine the appropriateness of this approach.

OBSTACLES FOR GENERALIZING THE LITERATURE FROM ADULT BIPOLAR DEPRESSION

Almost all of the data about the treatment of bipolar depression come from the adult literature. Unfortunately, it is not clear that pediatric bipolar depression will respond to the same treatment as does adult bipolar depression. For one thing, children and adolescents have a course of illness that is distinct from the classic episodic course of bipolar disorder that is typically represented in treatment studies of adult bipolar disorder. Second, the adult literature includes a number of subpopulations of bipolar disorder that may each have a distinct response to treatment. Finally, it appears that, at least with unipolar depression, children have a poorer response to antidepressants as compared with adults with unipolar depression. Even if antidepressants are useful in the treatment of adult bipolar depression, it is not known whether children and adolescents will have a similar positive response to antidepressants.

Course of Illness

Before a discussion about the treatment of bipolar depression can begin, it is first important to discuss what is meant by the term *bipolar depression*. Traditionally the treatment of bipolar depression has referred to the treatment of the depressive episodes that occur separate from manic episodes. These depressive episodes are a leading cause of long-term problems in the management of bipolar illness. In adults, bipolar I disorder (BP I), bipolar II disorder (BP II), and cyclothymia are all characterized by an episodic course consisting of both depressive episodes (or dysthymia in the case of cyclothymia) and episodes of mania (BP I) or hypomania (BP II). Patients with bipolar I and bipolar II disorders spend a greater proportion of time in a depressed state as compared with a manic state. For bipolar I, the ratio of depression to mania has been estimated at 3:1, and for bipolar II, this ratio has been estimated at 37:1 (Frye, Gitlin, & Altshuler, 2004; Post et al., 2003). Because many of these episodes occur apart from manic episodes, it is possible to study the treatment of depressive episodes in adults separately from the treatment of manic symptoms.

Unlike adults with bipolar disorder, children and adolescents rarely present with an episodic course that is characterized by distinct periods of depression that are separate from manic symptoms. It is therefore risky to extrapolate information from the adult literature to the treatment of children and adolescents with bipolar disorder. Children and adolescents are more likely to have a mixed and chronic course of illness characterized by frequent and severe mood swings that may include episodes of euphoria, although many clinicians also diagnose bipolar disorder in youths with a chronic course of irritability and anger outbursts (see Figure 16.1 for a comparison of the classic adult course of bipolar disorder with the course seen more commonly in children and adolescents). Whether or not this chronic and mixed course will respond similarly to treatments that are effective in the more classic episodic course is unknown at this time. Because there are no data on the treatment of depressive symptoms in children and adolescents with a chronic course of bipolar disorder, the following sections

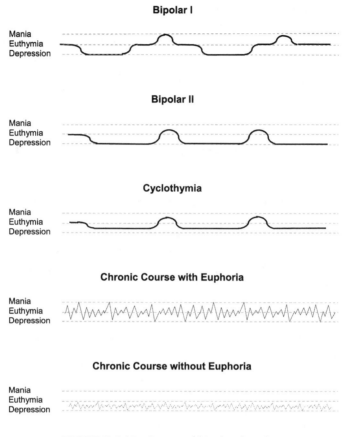

FIGURE 16.1. Course of bipolar disorder.

focus on the treatment of depression in adults with a more episodic course of illness. Implications for the treatment of children and adolescents are also discussed.

Characteristics of Bipolar Depression

Even in adults, there are differences in depressive episodes between unipolar depression, bipolar II depression, and bipolar I depression, leading some experts to believe that treatment studies that include one of these populations cannot be generalized to the other populations. In addition, because of the distinct treatment responses of these three populations, the results of treatment studies that include more than one of these populations must be interpreted with some caution. These populations differ in family history, in the female:male ratio, in treatment response, and in the frequency of atypical features of depression (Benazzi, 2001, 2003, 2004; Berk & Dodd,

2005). One of the biggest differences between bipolar depression and unipolar depression is the occurrence in bipolar depression of a mixed state that includes both depressive symptoms and symptoms of mania, including racing thoughts, irritability, distractibility, and increased speech (Benazzi, 2000). This mixed state most closely resembles that of youths with a chronic course of illness, but it is also the state with the least amount of adult treatment data.

TREATMENT OF BIPOLAR DEPRESSION IN ADULTS

The treatment of bipolar depression may include antidepressants, lamotrigine, the mood stabilizers, and the atypical antipsychotics (see Table 16.1 for a summary). In addition, there are some emerging data on the use of psychotherapy for the treatment of bipolar depression. The literature regarding the efficacy of each of these treatments is discussed in this section. In addition, alternative treatments, including electroconvulsant therapy (ECT) and rapid transcranial magnetic stimulation (rTMS), are briefly discussed.

Antidepressants

The antidepressants appear to be efficacious in the treatment of bipolar disorder in adults, even though the data are limited and no single antidepressant has been found to be effective in at least two adequately powered placebo-controlled studies (Kusumakar, 2002; Thase & Sachs, 2000). However, a meta-analysis of 12 randomized trials with a total of 1,088 patients found antidepressants to be more effective than placebo (Gijsman, Gessed, Rendell, Nolen, & Goodwin, 2004). One study has also demonstrated a similar short-term treatment response to antidepressants when inpatients with bipolar depression were compared with inpatients with unipolar depression (Möller, Bottlender, Grunze, Strauss, & Wittman, 2001).

In adults with bipolar I and II depression, there are data to support the efficacy of the tricyclic antidepressants (TCAs), monoamine oxidase inhibitors (MAOIs), fluoxetine, and bupropion (El-Mallakh & Karippot, 2002). In addition, paroxetine has been found to be effective when added to lithium when the lithium is less than 0.8 mEq/L but not when the lithium level is greater than 0.8 mEq/L (El-Mallakh & Karippot, 2002). There are almost no data on the efficacy of other antidepressants for bipolar depression, including nefazodone, mirtazapine, and reboxetine (Thase & Sachs, 2000).

Studies of bipolar II disorder have demonstrated a poor response to TCAs, MAOIs, and lithium. There are open data suggesting a positive response to fluoxetine and venlafaxine (Berk & Dodd, 2005; Hadjipavlou, Mok, & Yatham, 2004). There is also a pilot study suggesting a positive ef-

TABLE 16.1. Treatment of Bipolar Depression—Adults

Author/year	Inclusion diagnosis	Diagnostic tool	Type of study	Outcome measure	n	Treatment	Results
Nemeroff et al. (2001)	BP I	DSM-III-R Multiaxial evaluation	Randomized, double-blind, placebo controlled	HRSD/ CGI-S	117	Paroxetine vs. Imipramine. All patients were on lithium.	For Li level <.08meq/liter-paroxetine and imipramine were superior to placebo. At Li level > 0.8 meq/liter-paroxetine and imipramine were no better than placebo.
Young et al. (2000)	BP I/II	SCID	Randomized, single-blind	HRSD/ GAF/ YMRS	27	Paroxetine vs. second mood stabilizer (lithium or divalproex)	For completers, there was no difference between conditions, but there were significantly more completers in the paroxetine group.
Cohn, Collins, Ashbrook, & Wernicke (1989)	BPD (did not specify I or II)		Randomized, double-blind, placebo controlled	HRSD	89	Fluoxetine vs. imipramine Response rate: Fluoxetine 86% Imipramine 57% Placebo 38%	Response rate: Fluoxetine 86% Imipramine 57% Placebo 38%
McIntyre et al. (2002)	BP I/II	SCID	8-week, randomized, single-blind	HDRS	36	Topiramate vs. bupropion SR	Topiramate = bupropion SR
Davis, Bartolucci, & Petry (2005)	BP I	SCID	8-week, randomized, double-blind, placebo controlled	HRSD	25	Divalproex	Mean change from baseline: Divalproex –43.5 Placebo –27.00 Remission: Divalproex 46% Placebo 25% (Not statistically significant)

(continued)

311

TABLE 16.1. (*continued*)

Author/year	Inclusion diagnosis	Diagnostic tool	Type of study	Outcome measure	n	Treatment	Results
Evins et al. (2006)	BP I/II	SCID	6-week, randomized, double-blind, placebo controlled	HRSD, CGI-S	18	Inositol augmentation of lithium or valproate	Response rate: Inositol 44% vs. placebo 0
Frangou, Lewis, & McCrone (2006)	BP I/II	SCID	12-week, randomized, double-blind, placebo controlled	HRSD	75	Eicosapentaenoic acid (EPA) omega-3 fatty acid	EPA significantly better than placebo)
Goldberg, Burdick, & Endick (2004)	BPD (did not specify I or II)	SCID	Randomized, double-blind, placebo controlled (condition assigned by nonblind research assistant)	HDRS/ CGI	22	Pramipexole	Response: pramipexole 67% vs. placebo 20% Mean change in HDRS: pramipexole 48% vs. placebo 21%
Zarate et al. (2004)	BP II	SCID	6-week, randomized double-blind, placebo controlled	MADRS	21	Pramipexole	Response: pramipexole 60% vs. 9% Placebo ($p = .02$)
Calabrese et al. (2003)	BP I	SADS	52-week, randomized, double-blind, placebo controlled	HAM-D, MRS	463	Lamotrigine vs. Lithium	Median time to intervention for any mood sx with [95% confidence interval]: Placebo 93 [58–180] Lithium 170 [105–?] Lamotrigine 200 [146–399]
Calabrese et al. (1999)	BP I	SCID	Randomized, double-blind, placebo controlled	HRSD/ CGI-I	195	Lamotrigine	Response on CGI-I: 51% on 200mg/day, 41% on 50mg/day, 26% placebo. MADRS dropped 16–17 points on Lamotrigine vs. 10 points on placebo.

Study							
Tohen et al. (2003)	BP I	SCID	8-week, randomized, double-blind, placebo controlled	MADRS	833	Olanzapine vs. olanzapine-fluoxetine combination	Olanzapine-fluoxetine combination > olanzapine > placebo
Calabrese et al. (2005)	BP I/II	SCID	8-week, randomized, double-blind, placebo controlled	MADRS HDRS	542	Quentiapine (Quet)	Response: Quet 600mg/day 58.2% Quet 300mg/day 57.6% Placebo 36.1% Remission: Quet 52.9% Placebo 28.4%
Post et al. (2003;	BP I/II	SCID	Randomized, double-blind, placebo controlled	IDS	59	Eicosapentaenoic acid	Eicosapentaenoic acid = placebo
Chengappa et al. (2000)	BP I/II	SCID	Randomized, double-blind, placebo controlled	MADRS/ HRSD	24	Inositol	Response rate: Inositol 67% Placebo 33%
Stoll et al. (1999)	BP I/II	SCID	Randomized, double-blind, placebo controlled	Time to exit the study because of need to add medication for bipolar disorder	30	Omega-3 fatty acid ethyl esters	The omega-3 fatty acid group had a significantly lower dropout rate (3/14) when compared with placebo (10/16). Nine of the dropouts on placebo vs. none of the dropouts on omega-3 fatty acid dropped out for worsening depression.

Note. SCID, Structured Clinical Interview for DSM-IV; SADS, Schedule for Affective Disorders and Schizophrenia; HRSD, Hamilton Rating Scale for Depression; HDRS, Hamilton Depression Rating Scale; CGI-S, Clinical Global Impression Scale—Severity; CSI-I, Clinical Global Impression Scale—Improvement; YMRS, Young Mania Rating Scale; MADRS, Montgomery–Ashberg Depression Rating Scale; MRS, Mania Rating Scale.

fect of two dopamine agonists used to treat Parkinson's disease, prami-pexole and ropinizole (Berk & Dodd, 2005).

Antidepressants in Combination with Mood Stabilizers

Although most studies using antidepressants in bipolar disorder have al-lowed the concomitant use of mood stabilizers, a few studies have focused on the addition of antidepressants to mood stabilizers. Studying the addi-tive effect of antidepressants to mood stabilizers is important because some of the mood stabilizers appear to have antidepressant effects (discussed shortly) in patients with bipolar depression. In addition, some data suggest that patients with bipolar depression respond better to antidepressants when on either divalproex or lithium as compared with placebo (Bowden, 2005; Gyulai et al., 2003). There is one study that compared the addition of an antidepressant (paroxetine) with the addition of a mood stabilizer (lithium or divalproex) in patients who had significant depressive symp-toms with stable treatment on a first mood stabilizer. Both groups demon-strated similar improvements in depressive symptoms; however, there was a significantly higher dropout rate in the group with two mood stabilizers as opposed to the group in which paroxetine was added to a mood stabilizer (Young et al., 2000).

Long-Term Efficacy

Very few data exist on the long-term efficacy of using antidepressants in bi-polar disorder. It is possible that a small percentage of patients may benefit from long-term treatment with antidepressants. In patients with bipolar I disorder who have a positive response to antidepressants, there are data to suggest that these patients may have fewer relapses of depression when they are maintained on antidepressants. However, other data suggest that only a small proportion (19.2%) of patients who were successfully treated with antidepressants are still taking an antidepressant 1 year later. In this study most patients stopped their antidepressants because of either a return of de-pressive symptoms or the emergence of either hypomania or mania (Malhi, Mitchell, & Salim, 2003).

Adverse Drug Interactions

Most experts in bipolar depression recommend that antidepressants be used in combination with mood stabilizers during the treatment of bipolar depres-sion to reduce the likelihood that the patient will switch into a manic state. When using antidepressants in combination with mood stabilizers and anti-psychotics, there is a potential for adverse drug interactions. In particular, both paroxetine and fluoxetine inhibit cytochrome P450 3A4 that may lead to an increase in carbamazepine levels. When fluvoxamine and clozapine are coadministered, the dose of clozapine may need to be decreased because of an interaction mediated by the cytochrome P450 IA2 isoenzyme.

Lamotrigine

Lamotrigine is becoming increasingly popular in the treatment of adults with bipolar depression. However, the use of lamotrigine in children and adolescents is limited because a younger age is associated with an increased risk of developing a serious rash while on this medication. In adults, open data suggest that some patients with bipolar II disorder can be successfully treated long term with lamotrigine either alone or in combination with a mood stabilizer (Hadjipavlou et al., 2004; Manning et al., 2005). Lamotrigine has also been shown to be superior to placebo in two of three small studies of the treatment of bipolar depression in adults, but not in the treatment of mania. It has been found to be effective in both refractory rapid cycling and nonrapid-cycling bipolar depression (Frye et al., 2004; Keck & McElroy, 2003).

Mood Stabilizers

There is evidence that the mood stabilizers, particularly lithium, carbamazepine, and divalproex, all have moderate acute antidepressant properties in adults (Malhi et al., 2003). For example, a 1-year randomized, placebo-controlled study of patients with bipolar I disorder demonstrated that divalproex was superior to both lithium and placebo at preventing premature termination secondary to depression (Gyulai et al., 2003). There is also evidence that many patients with bipolar depression have a least a partial response to lithium (Frye et al., 2004). Retrospective studies have demonstrated that patients treated with lithium have fewer hospitalizations for suicide attempts when compared with patients treated with divalproex or carbamazepine. However, because of the retrospective nature of these data, there is no control for severity of illness (Bowden, 2005). In addition, lithium has proven prophylaxis of depression in bipolar I disorder in patients who were started on lithium at a time of normal functioning (Fieve, Kumbaraci, & Dunner, 1976). Carbamazepine has also been shown to be effective in the treatment of bipolar depression in three small studies in which it was used alone or in combination with lithium (Keck & McElroy, 2003). Gabapentin has no proven benefit for monotherapy, but some clinicians believe it may be useful as an adjunctive treatment (Malhi et al., 2003).

Antipsychotics

The only medication that currently has Food and Drug Administration (FDA) approval for the treatment of bipolar depression in adults is a combination of olanzapine and fluoxetine (Symbyax; Frye et al., 2004). Olanzapine alone appears to have some antidepressant effect on bipolar depression, but with the addition of fluoxetine, there is a greater antidepressant effect with no increase in the rate of switches to mania (Tohen et al., 2003).

Other data suggest that other atypical antipsychotics may have some antidepressant effects in bipolar depression. An open-label study has demonstrated favorable results for the use of quetiapine in bipolar depression (Malhi et al., 2003). There are no studies that test the efficacy of risperidone monotherapy, but when it is added to a mood stabilizer, some proven benefit occurs, although risperidone has also been linked to several reports of drug-induced mania (Kusumakar, 2002). Some data also demonstrate a benefit from clozapine (Kusumakar, 2002).

The data on the traditional antipsychotics are less favorable. Traditional antipsychotics have been associated with dysphoria after long-term use (Kusumakar, 2002). The use of depot neuroleptics has mixed results, with one study demonstrating an increase in depression with these medications, whereas a second showed a decrease in hospital days for mania, for depression, and for mixed episodes (Kusumakar, 2002).

Stimulants

Although many clinicians believe that stimulants may induce switching to mania, there is actually evidence that these medications may be effective in patients with bipolar depression. Some preliminary data suggest that stimulants may be effective at treating bipolar depression with a low rate of precipitation of switches to mania (El-Mallakh & Karippot, 2002).

Psychotherapy

Psychotherapy for bipolar depression has the potential to improve depressive symptoms with a theoretically low risk of causing a switch into mania or precipitating rapid cycling. However, very few studies have tested the efficacy of such treatments in this population. Cognitive-behavioral therapy (CBT) has the best data, and most of these studies target bipolar disorder in general as opposed to focusing on bipolar depression. However, there are four studies, two of which are randomized treatment-controlled trials (RTCs), that demonstrate improvements in depressive symptoms with CBT (Gonzalez-Pinto et al., 2004; Jones, 2004; Malhi et al., 2003).

Other Treatments

There are several other treatments that may in time prove useful in the treatment of bipolar depression in children and adolescents. Some of these treatments (such as ECT) have proven of benefit in adults with bipolar depression, whereas most of the other strategies discussed have only preliminary data about their efficacy in bipolar depression.

ECT has proven benefit in bipolar depression (Malhi et al., 2003; Thase & Sachs, 2000), but ECT is rarely used in adolescents and is almost never used in children. However, for severe refractory cases, ECT should be considered. A newer treatment, rTMS, may be an alternative to ECT, with fewer cognitive effects and no need for general anesthesia. Although the efficacy of rTMS has not been demonstrated in bipolar depression (Thase & Sachs, 2000), there is one case report of a 47-year-old man with bipolar depression who demonstrated response to rTMS, relapsed once treatment ended, and then responded to a second course of treatment with rTMS (George et al., 1998). There is also one case report in the literature of a patient taking venlafaxine who developed mania after three sessions of rTMS (Huang, Su, & Shan, 2004). The safety of this treatment in children and adolescents has not been tested. However, this treatment may be a beneficial alternative for children and adolescents if it is found to be effective at treating bipolar depression without leading to cognitive side effects.

Strategies for augmenting antidepressants have shown some promise in the treatment of unipolar depression, but these strategies have not been tested in the treatment of bipolar depression. These strategies include augmentation with thyroid hormone, with buspirone (a 5-HT_{1A} partial agonist), and with pindolol (a 5-HT_{1A} agonist; Thase & Sachs, 2000). One study has tested the efficacy of augmentation in the treatment of bipolar depression. The alpha-2 agonist idazoxan was compared with bupropion in a 6-week double-blind trial of 14 patients with bipolar depression, and there was a 50% reduction on the Hamilton Depression Rating Scale (HDR-S) in both groups (Goldberg, Burdick, & Endick, 2004).

Some open-label data suggest benefit from the use of the omega-3 fatty acids in the treatment of bipolar depression. However, a double-blind trial of the omega-3 fatty acid eicosapentaenoic acid (EPA) found no benefit over placebo for patients with either acute bipolar depression or with rapid cycling.

Phototherapy and sleep deprivation are not recommended treatment alternatives for the treatment of bipolar depression in children and adolescents. Phototherapy may alleviate depressive symptoms in patients with a seasonal pattern of bipolar disorder consisting of depression in the fall and mania in the spring. However, this treatment may lead to sleep disruption and switches to mania. Sleep deprivation may also have some short-lived benefit, but it can also precipitate switches to mania (Thase & Sachs, 2000).

RISK OF ANTIDEPRESSANTS INDUCING A SWITCH TO MANIA OR RAPID CYCLING

Risk of Switching to Mania

One of the major concerns about the use of antidepressants in patients with bipolar disorder is the risk of precipitating a switch in the mood state to mania or hypomania (see Table 16.2). The actual risk associated with the use of antidepressants is difficult to ascertain but appears to be low for the selective serotonin reuptake inhibitors (SSRIs) and bupropion. Patients with bipolar disorder may spontaneously switch from depression to mania, with some patients doing so at a high rate, whereas others may never switch. Unless studies control for the rate of switching that occurred prior to the initiation of antidepressants, it impossible to make a definitive statement as to whether or not antidepressants increase the likelihood of switching to mania. In addition, the use of a mood stabilizer may alter the results of studies. Some studies with adults have demonstrated that mood stabilizers such as lithium, carbamazepine, and divalproex offer some protection from switching to mania when antidepressants are added (Bottlender, Rudolf, Strauss, & Möller, 2001), although they may not completely eliminate this risk (Keck & McElroy, 2003). If mood stabilizers offer some protection against switching to mania, studies that allow concurrent treatment with a mood stabilizer may not be able to detect an increased switch rate by antidepressants.

Of the antidepressants, the SSRIs and bupropion are associated with the lowest rates of antidepressant-induced mania. Several studies suggest that, in general, antidepressants increase the risk of switching to mania by 2–3 times the spontaneous rate (El-Mallakh & Karippot, 2002; Ghaemi, Hsu, Soldani, & Goodwin, 2003; Kusumakar, 2002). However, other studies have not demonstrated an increased rate of switching in patients receiving antidepressants with or without a mood stabilizer (Bauer et al., 2005; Boerlin, Gitlin, Zoellner, & Hammen, 1998; Frankle et al., 2002). The TCAs and MAOIs are thought to present a clear risk of switching, whereas less evidence exists that the SSRIs induce switching (Parker & Parker, 2003; Gijsman et al., 2004). In a meta-analysis of all available clinical trial data, the rate of manic switches for SSRIs was 3.8%, which was equal to placebo (4.7%). Both the SSRI and placebo rates were significantly lower than the rate for TCAs (10%; Gijsman et al., 2004). Bupropion is another antidepressant that has been shown to have a low risk for switching a patient into mania (El-Mallakh & Karippot, 2002; Erfurth, Michael, Stadtland, & Arolt, 2002). The data about venlafaxine are mixed, with some studies finding a higher rate of mania (Bowden, 2005), whereas other studies have found no manic switches in patients treated with venlafaxine (Frye et al., 2004).

Risk of Developing Rapid Cycling

A final risk associated with antidepressants is the development of a pattern of rapid cycling. The induction of rapid cycling is difficult to evaluate because of the need for long-term studies with patients matched for similar number of previous episodes. The current evidence that antidepressants may induce

TABLE 16.2. Rates of Antidepressant-Induced Switches to Mania

Author/year	Treatment	Placebo controlled	Rate of switching	Factors that predict switching
Leverich et al. (2006)	Bupropion Sertraline Venlafaxine	No	Acute phase of treatment: Hypomania 11.4%/ Mania 7.9% Continuation phase of treatment: Hypomania 21.8%/ Mania 14.9%	Venlafaxine had the highest rate of subthreshold brief hypomanic episodes. Bupropion had the lowest switch rate.
Keck & McElroy (2005)	Olanzapine Olanzapine/ fluoxetine combination	Yes	Olanzapine 5.7% Olanzapine/ fluoxetine 6.4% Placebo 6.7%	
Joffe et al. (2002)	SSRI Bupropion	No	SSRI 15.8% Bupropion 7.8% (nonsignificant)	Antidepressant-induced mania and cycle acceleration occurred more frequently in BP I vs. BP II.
Erfurth, Michael, Stadtland, & Arolt (2002)	Bupropion	No	No switches to mania/ hypomania during 6-week trial	
Goldberg & Whiteside (2002)	Any antidepressant	No	39.6% of antidepressant trials associated with a switch to mania	Increased risk associated with increased number of previous antidepressant trials and with substance abuse or dependence. Mood stabilizers were not uniformly protective.
Henry, Sorbara, Lacoste, Gindre, & Leboyer (2001)	Any antidepressant	No	Hypomania 11% Mania 16%	No association with sex, age BP I vs. BP II, or anticonvulsants, or number of previous manic episodes. Lithium associated with a decreased rate vs. no lithium (15% vs. 44%).

(continued)

TABLE 16.2. (*continued*)

Author/year	Treatment	Placebo controlled	Rate of switching	Factors that predict switching
Boerlin, Gitlin, Zoellner, & Hammen (1998)	Any antidepressant	No	10% had disruptive switch, 28% had any switch	Higher number of previous manic episodes associated with switching. TCAs/ MAOIs associated with switching. Mood stabilizer + antidepressant had the same switch rate as mood stabilizer alone.
Sachs, Lafer, Stoll, & Banov (1994)	Desipramine, bupropion	No	Long-term switch-rate: Desipriamine 50% vs. bupropion 11%	
Peet (1994)	SSRI vs. TCA	Meta-analysis, compared to placebo	TCA—11.2% SSRI—3.7% Placebo—4.2%	

rapid cycling is dominated by case series that include small numbers of patients without a control group and by retrospective chart reviews.

Rapid cycling was first introduced as a qualifier in DSM for patients with four or more affective episodes in any one year. More recently patients with a chronic course of continuous cycling have also been classified as rapid cycling, as have patients who have severe affective dysregulation (Papolos, 2003). Some writers define patients who cycle within weeks to days as ultra-rapid cyclers and those who have distinct, abrupt mood shifts that are shorter than 24 hours in duration as ultra-ultra rapid, or ultradian (Papolos, 2003). Because of the variety of definitions of rapid cycling, it is difficult to interpret the results of studies that attempt to evaluate the development of rapid cycling. It is unclear whether antidepressants increase the risk of all types of rapid cycling or only induce one or two subtypes. The definitions also make it difficult to interpret results that do not show an increase in rapid cycling, because these studies may use more restrictive definitions of rapid cycling.

The evidence as to whether or not antidepressants can induce rapid cycling is mixed. There is some evidence that antidepressants may lead to an increase in rapid cycling, with estimates that they may increase the risk of developing rapid cycling fivefold (El-Mallakh & Karippot, 2002; Ghaemi et al., 2004; Wehr & Goodwin, 1979). In addition, there are reports of rapid cycling reverting back to a pattern of nonrapid cycling after the antidepressant has been discontinued (El-Mallakh & Karippot, 2002). However, other studies do not show any relationship between TCAs and mood shifts in patients with rapid cycling (Coryell et al., 2003). In addition, other authors state that when participants are matched based on the number of previous episodes, there is no evidence that antidepressants increase the risk of developing rapid cycling, particularly for patients with long symptom-free periods between episodes (Papolos, 2003).

Although some evidence exists that antidepressants may induce a chronic dysphoric state, there are no controlled data that support this link. There are case reports of patients with bipolar I disorder who have an initial benefit from TCA antidepressants but who, over time, develop a chronic dysphoric state that gradually improves once the antidepressant has been discontinued (El-Mallakh & Karippot, 2002). Other authors have concluded that antidepressants have a small risk of inducing mood instability (Malhi et al., 2003). Clinicians should be aware of this potential effect of antidepressants and consider discontinuing the antidepressant when patients develop a chronic dysphoric state or demonstrate a significant increase in mood lability.

DATA FOR TREATING BIPOLAR DEPRESSION IN CHILDREN AND ADOLESCENTS

Treatment of Unipolar Depression in Children and Adolescents

In adults, there are several classes of antidepressants with proven efficacy for unipolar depression: heterocyclic compounds, including TCAs; MAOIs; SSRIs; bupropion; mirtazapine; nefazodone; trazodone; and venlafaxine. Unfortunately, the efficacy in children and adolescents with unipolar depression is not as clear. Studies in children and adolescents have found no superiority of the TCAs over placebo. The data on the efficacy of the SSRIs are mixed, with the strongest data being available for fluoxetine, which has an FDA indication for unipolar depression in children and adolescents. There are also data from two placebo-controlled studies of sertraline that, when combined, demonstrate a small but significant difference between active and placebo groups (Wagner et al., 2003). There are no published large placebo-controlled studies on any other medication for the treatment of unipolar depression in children and adolescents (Ambrosini, 2000).

Treatment of Bipolar Depression in Children and Adolescents

Data on the use of antidepressants in children with bipolar depression is extremely limited (see Table 16.3). There are no data about the efficacy of using antidepressants in youths with bipolar disorder and only indirect evidence about the possibility that antidepressants may induce mania in children and adolescents with bipolar disorder. In youths who are treated with SSRIs for obsessive–compulsive disorder (OCD) and major depressive disorder (MDD), there is some evidence to suggest that the SSRIs may cause psychiatric adverse events, including changes in mood and sleep disturbance (see Table 16.4). The median time to onset of the symptoms was estimated to be 91 days. When the SSRI was stopped, the symptoms resolved in approximately half of the patients by day 28 and in three-quarters of the patients by day 49 (Wilens et al., 2003). However, there is also evidence that antidepressants can be used safely in children and adolescents with bipolar disorder. Drug-induced behavioral disinhibition is more likely to be observed in patients with disruptive behavioral disorders as opposed to those with bipolar disorder (Carlson & Mick, 2003; Craney & Geller, 2003). In addition, the use of neither antidepressants nor stimulants changes the rate of recovery from or relapse back to mania during a 2-year follow-up.

Psychotherapy may prove to be an effective adjunct to the psychopharmacological treatment of children and adolescents with bipolar depression. One pilot study has tested a combination of family-focused treatment and CBT in children and adolescents with bipolar disorder. This study did not have a control group, but a significant improvement in depressive symptoms, as well as other symptoms, occurred during the course of treatment (Pavuluri et al., 2004). Further study is needed to determine the role that psychotherapy should play in the treatment of children and adolescents with bipolar depression.

As mentioned earlier, some adult literature suggests that stimulants may be an effective treatment for bipolar depression. Because of the high

TABLE 16.3. Treatment of Bipolar Depression—Children and Adolescents

Author/ year	Inclusion diagnosis	Diagnostic tool	Type of study	Outcome measure	N (age)	Treatment	Results
Patel et al. (2006)	BP-I, Depression	WASH-U-KSADS	Open treatment	CDRS	27 (12–18 year-olds)	Lithium	> = 50% decrease in CDRS 48% CDRS < = 28 and CGI-BP Improvement of 1 or 2—30%
Chang, Saxena, & Howe (2006)	BP-I, II, NOS, Depression	CDRS/ YMRS	Open treatment	CDRS-R and CGI-I	20 (12–17 year-olds)	Lamotrigine	CGI-I 1 or 2—84% > = 50% improvement of CDRS-R—63%

TABLE 16.4. Disinhibition in Children and Adolescents with Antidepressants

Author/year	Diagnoses included	Type of study	Medication	Definition of disinhibition	Rate
Safer & Zito (2006)	All	Meta-analysis of all published double-blind studies that separate adverse events by age	All	Activation	Activation 2–3 fold more prevalent in children vs. adolescents. Activation rare in adults. SSRI related insomnia is not always accompanied by activation
Treatment of Adolescents With Depression Study (TADS) Team (2004)	MDD	Randomized, placebo controlled	Fluoxetine	Mania Hypomania Elevated mood Irritability Anger Agitation Hyperactivity All behavioral changes	Fluoxetine + CBT vs. fluoxetine vs. CBT vs. placebo 0% vs. 0.92% vs. 0% vs. 0.89% 0.93% vs. 1.83% vs. 0% vs. 0.89% 0% vs. 0.92% vs. 0% vs. 0% 0.93% vs. 0.92% vs. 0% vs. 0% 0% vs. 0.92% vs. 0% vs. 0% 0% vs. 0% vs. 0% vs. 0.89% 0% vs. 0.92% vs. 0% vs. 0% 16% (12 pts) vs. 23% (20 pts) vs. 1% (1 pt) vs. 11% (9 pts)
Geller et al. (2004)	OCD	Randomized, placebo controlled	Paroxetine	Hyperkinesia Hostility Agitation	All paroxetine vs. placebo; children paroxetine vs. placebo; adolescents paroxetine vs. placebo All: 12.2% vs 5.7%; Child: 17.2% vs. 7.0%; Adolescent: 5.0% vs. 4.2% All: 9.2% vs. 1.0%; Child: 12.1% vs. 1.8%; Adolescent: 7.5% vs. 0% All : 5.1% vs. 1.9%; Child: 5.2% vs. 0%; Adolescent: 5.0% vs. 4.2%
Wagner, Berard, et al. (2004)	Social Anxiety	Randomized, placebo controlled	Paroxetine	Hyperkinesia Hostility	Paroxetine vs. placebo children 8.7% vs. 0 adolescents 1.7% vs. 0 total 3.7% vs. 0 children 6.5% vs. 0 adolescents 1.7% vs. 1.8% total 3.1% vs. 1.3%

(continued)

323

TABLE 16.4. (*continued*)

Author/year	Diagnoses included	Type of study	Medication	Definition of disinhibition	Rate
Wagner, Robb, et al. (2004)	MDD	Randomized, placebo controlled	Citalopram	Mania Agitated depression Agitation	No patients 2 of 85 patients on placebo 2 of 89 patients on citalopram
Wilens et al. (2003)	MDD/ OCD	Chart review	SSRIs	Irritable Manic Aggression	15% 6% 1% No association found with age or diagnosis
Carlson & Mick (2003)	Any	Retrospective	Any	Drug-induced behavioral disinhibition (DIBD) (defined as an increase in time-outs)	20 of 267 patients met criteria. Increase risk associated with a diagnosis of ADHD or PDD and with SSRI use. Decreased risk associated with older age and stimulant use. 15% improved with no medication change; 40% improved when the drug was stopped; 45% had an adverse response to many medications. DIBD was definitely linked to medication in 4.4% of patients.
Wagner et al. (2003)	MDD	Randomized, placebo controlled	Sertraline	Agitation	Children: 8.1% serrtraline vs. 2.3% placebo Adolescents: sertraline similar to placebo
Walkup et al. (2002)	Separation anxiety; social phobia; GAD	Open Extension	Fluvoxamine and fluoxetine	Need to stop medication	7 of 48 placebo nonresponders put on fluvoxamine; 0 of 48 fluvoxamine responders continued on fluvoxamine; 0 of 14 fluvoxamine nonresponders changed to fluoxetine
Liebowitz et al. (2002)	OCD	Randomized, placebo controlled	Fluoxetine	Irritability Anger Outbursts Excitability	Fluoxetine vs. placebo 23.8% vs. 13.6 % 19.0% vs. 13.6% 28.6% vs. 18.2 5

324

Study	Diagnosis	Design	Drug	Adverse effect	Results
Emslie et al. (2002)	MDD	Randomized, placebo controlled	Fluoxetine	Mania	Fluoxetine vs. placebo 1 pt (o.9%) vs. 0%
Seedat et al. (2002)	PTSD	Open	Citalopram	Activation	None reported
Walkup et al. (2001)	Social phobia, separation anxiety, GAD	Randomized, placebo controlled	Fluvoxamine	Increased motor activity	Fluvoxamine vs. placebo 27% vs. 12%
Riddle et al. (2001)	OCD	Randomized, placebo controlled	Fluvoxamine	Agitation Hyperkinesia	Fluvoxamine vs. placebo 12.3% vs. 3.2% 12.3% vs. 3.2%
Keller et al. (2001)	MDD	Randomized, placebo controlled	Paroxetine/imipravine	Emotional lability Hostility	Paroxetine vs. imipramine vs. placebo 6.5% vs. 3.2% vs. 1.1% 7.5% vs. 3.2% vs. 0%
Geller et al. (2001)	OCD	Rancomized, placebo controlled	Fluoxetine	Hyperkinesia	Fluoxetine vs. placebo 12.7% vs. 3.1%
Cook et al. (2001)	OCD	Open extension	Sertraline	Hyperkinesia	All patients vs. 6–12-year-olds vs. 13–18-year-olds 11.7% vs. 16.7% vs. 6.2%
Biederman et al. (1999)	BPD + ADHD	Chart review	TCA	Mania	TCAs increased the incidence of mania, but when they did not induce mania, they were associated with improved ADHD symptoms (even when compared to a stimulant).
March et al. (1998)	OCD	Randomized, placebo controlled	Sertraline	Agitation	Sertraline vs. placebo 13% vs. 2%
Emslie et al. (1998)	MDD	Follow-up	Fluoxetine	Adverse events not described	

rates of comorbid ADHD in children and adolescents with bipolar disorder, many children with pediatric bipolar disorder are treated with stimulants. It will be important to determine whether or not the stimulants can also be used to treat bipolar depression in children and adolescents.

SUMMARY AND RECOMMENDATIONS

There is a continuing debate about the best way to treat bipolar depression in adults. In children and adolescents, this confusion is enhanced because of the chronic course of mood lability, often without discrete periods of mania or depression, that may or may not respond to treatments that are clearly helpful to adults. In addition, the efficacy of the antidepressants in unipolar depression appears to be less robust in children and adolescents when compared with adults. There is also uncertainty about the risk of inducing mania or rapid cycling when using antidepressants to treat bipolar depression in children and adolescents. Finally, it is very difficult to study the long-term outcomes in children and adolescents in such a way as to learn about both positive and negative results of treatment.

When clinicians are confident about the diagnosis of bipolar disorder, it is recommended that the treatment of bipolar depression begin with a trial of a mood stabilizer. If the symptoms continue after treatment with a mood stabilizer, the clinician may consider the addition of an antidepressant, particularly an SSRI or bupropion. Stimulants may also be tried, particularly when there is a comorbid diagnosis of ADHD. Whenever antidepressants are added to the treatment regimen of bipolar depression, clinicians should first educate parents and caregivers about the symptoms of mania. The clinician should also follow symptoms closely over time to monitor for a worsening of symptoms, either secondary to a switch to mania or secondary to the development of a rapid-cycling course. Whenever an antidepressant is used in a youth with bipolar disorder, it is suggested that the clinician pay close attention to a worsening of symptoms both immediately after starting the antidepressant and for at least the first 3 months after initiating treatment with an antidepressant. Clinicians should also monitor patterns of aggression, suicidal ideation, psychosis, and disinhibition. If these symptoms increase, stopping the antidepressant will usually result in an improvement of the symptoms (Craney & Geller, 2003; Papolos, 2003). In patients with significant depressive symptoms who cannot tolerate an antidepressant, clinicians may consider the addition of an atypical antipsychotic.

Children and adolescents with bipolar depression may also benefit from adjunctive CBT. Although there are limited data to support the efficacy of this treatment in children and adolescents with bipolar depression, there is a potential for benefit with this treatment, with a low risk of adverse events.

For children and adolescents with refractory bipolar depression, clinicians may consider the use of lamotrigine or ECT. Other treatments for bipolar depression do not have enough data to support their use in children and adolescents at this time.

REFERENCES

Ambrosini, P. J. (2000). A review of pharmacotherapy of major depression in children and adolescents. *Psychiatric Services*, *51*, 627–633.

Bauer, M., Rasgon, N., Grof, P., Altshuler, L., Gyulai, L., Lapp, M., et al. (2005). Mood changes related to antidepressants: A longitudinal study of patients with bipolar disorder in a naturalistic setting. *Psychiatry Research*, *133*, 73–80.

Benazzi, F. (2000). Depressive mixed states: Unipolar and bipolar II. *European Archives of Psychiatry and Clinical Neuroscience*, *250*, 249–253.

Benazzi, F. (2001). Factor analysis of the Montgomery Asberg Depression Rating Scale in 251 bipolar II and 306 unipolar depressed outpatients. *Progress in Neuro-Psychopharmacology and Biological Psychiatry*, *25*, 1369–1376.

Benazzi, F. (2003). How could antidepressants worsen unipolar depression? *Psychotherapy and Psychosomatics*, *72*, 107–108.

Benazzi, F. (2004). Intra-episode hypomanic symptoms during major depression and their correlates. *Psychiatry and Clinical Neurosciences*, *58*, 289–294.

Berk, M., & Dodd, S. (2005). Bipolar II disorder: A review. *Bipolar Disorders*, *7*, 11–21.

Biederman, J., Mick, E., Faraone, S. V., Spencer, T., Wilens, T. E., & Wozniak, J. (2000). Pediatric mania: A developmental subtype of bipolar disorder? *Biological Psychiatry*, *48*, 458–466.

Boerlin, H. L., Gitlin, M J., Zoellner, L. A., & Hammen, C. L. (1998). Bipolar depression and antidepressant-induced mania: A naturalistic study. *Journal of Clinical Psychiatry*, *59*, 374–379.

Bottlender, R., Rudolf, D., Strauss, A., & Möller, H. (2001). Mood-stabilisers reduce the risk of developing antidepressant-induced maniform states in acute treatment of bipolar I depressed patients. *Journal of Affective Disorders*, *63*, 79–83.

Bowden, C. L. (2005). Treatment options for bipolar depression. *Journal of Clinical Psychiatry*, *66*, 3–6.

Carlson, G. A., & Mick, E. (2003). Drug-induced disinhibition in psychiatrically hospitalized children. *Journal of Child and Adolescent Psychopharmacology*, *13*, 153–163.

Coryell, W., Solomon, D., Turvey, C., Keller, M., Leon, A. C., Endicott, J., et al. (2003). The long-term course of rapid-cycling bipolar disorder. *Archives of General Psychiatry*, *60*, 914–920.

Craney, J., & Geller, B. (2003). Clinical implications of antidepressant and stimulant use on switching from depression to mania in children. *Journal of Child and Adolescent Psychopharmacology*, *13*, 201–204.

El-Mallakh, R. S., & Karippot, A. (2002). Reply: Antidepressants for bipolar depression. *Psychiatric Services*, *53*, 1331.

Erfurth, A., Michael, N., Stadtland, C., & Arolt, V. (2002). Bupropion as add-on strategy in difficult-to-treat bipolar depressive patients. *Neuropsychobiology*, *45*, 33–36.

Fieve, R. R., Kumbaraci, T., & Dunner, D. L. (1976). Lithium prophylaxis of depression in bipolar I, bipolar II, and unipolar patients. *American Journal of Psychiatry*, *133*, 925–929.

Findling, R. L., Gracious, B. L., McNamara, N. K., Youngstrom, E. A., Demeter, C. A., Branicky,

L. A., et al. (2001). Rapid, continuous cycling and psychiatric co-morbidity in pediatric bipolar I disorder. *Bipolar Disorders, 3*, 202–10.

Frankle, W. G., Perlis, R. H., Deckersbach, T., Grandin, L. D., Gray, S. M., Sachs, G. S., et al. (2002). Bipolar depression: Relationship between episode length and antidepressant treatment. *Psychological Medicine, 32*, 1417–1423.

Frye, M. A., Gitlin, M. J., & Altshuler, L. L. (2004). Unmet needs in bipolar depression. *Depression and Anxiety, 19*, 199–208.

Geller, B., Craney, J. L., Bolhofner, K., DelBello, M. P., Williams, M., & Zimerman, B. (2001). One-year recovery and relapse rates of children with a prepubertal and early adolescent bipolar disorder phenotype. *American Journal of Psychiatry, 158*, 303–335.

Geller, B., Craney, J. L., Bolhofner, K., Nickelsburg, M. J., Williams, M., & Zimerman, B. (2002). Two-year prospective follow-up of children with a prepubertal and early adolescent bipolar disorder phenotype. *American Journal of Psychiatry, 159*, 927–933.

Geller, B., Zimerman, B., Williams, M., Bolhofner, K., Craney, J. L., DelBello, M. P., et al. (2000a). Diagnostic characteristics of 93 cases of a prepubertal and early adolescent bipolar disorder phenotype by gender, puberty and comorbid attention deficit hyperactivity disorder. *Journal of Child and Adolescent Psychopharmacology, 10*, 157–164.

Geller, B., Zimerman, B., Williams, M., Bolhofner, K., Craney, J. L., DelBello, M. P., et al. (2000b). Six-month stability and outcome of a prepubertal and early adolescent bipolar disorder phenotype. *Journal of Child and Adolescent Psychopharmacology, 10*, 165–173.

George, M. S., Speer, A. M., Molloy, M., Nahas, Z., Teneback, C. C., Risch, S. C., et al. (1998). Low frequency daily left prefrontal rTMS improves mood in bipolar depression: A placebo-controlled case report. *Human Psychopharmacology: Clinical and Experimental, 13*, 271–275.

Ghaemi, S. N., Hsu, D. J., Soldani, F., & Goodwin, F. K. (2003). Antidepressants in bipolar disorder: The case for caution. *Bipolar Disorders, 5*, 421–433.

Ghaemi, S. N., Rosenquist, K. J., Ko, J. Y., Baldassano, C. F., Kontos, N. J., & Baldessarini, R. J. (2004). Antidepressant treatment in bipolar versus unipolar depression. *American Journal of Psychiatry, 161*, 163–165.

Gijsman, H. J., Geddes, J. R., Rendell, J. M., Nolen, W. A., & Goodwin, G. M. (2004). Antidepressants for bipolar depression: A systematic review of randomized, controlled trials. *American Journal of Psychiatry, 161*, 1537–1547.

Goldberg, J. F., Burdick, K. E., & Endick, C. J. (2004). Preliminary randomized, double-blind, placebo-controlled trial of pramipexole to mood stabilizers for treatment-resistant bipolar depression. *American Journal of Psychiatry, 161*, 564–566.

Gonzalez-Pinto, A., Gonzalez, C., Enjuto de Corres, S., Fernandez, B., Lopez, P., Palomo, J., et al. (2004). Psychoeducation-and cognitive-behavioral therapy in bipolar disorder: An update. *Acta Psychiatrica Scandinavica, 109*, 83–90.

Gyulai, L., Bowden, C. L., McElroy, S. L., Calabrese, J. R., Petty, F., Swann, A. C., et al. (2003). Maintenance efficacy of divalproex in the prevention of bipolar depression. *Neuropsychopharmacology, 28*, 1374–1382.

Hadjipavlou, G., Mok, H., & Yatham, L. N. (2004). Pharmacotherapy of bipolar II disorder: A critical review of current evidence. *Bipolar Disorders, 6*, 14–25.

Huang, C., Su, T., & Shan, I. (2004). A case report of repetitive transcranial magnetic stimulation-induced mania. *Bipolar Disorders, 6*, 444–445.

Jones, S. (2004). Psychotherapy of bipolar disorder: A review. *Journal of Affective Disorders, 80*(2–3), 101–114.

Keck, P. E. J., Jr., & McElroy, S. L. (2003). New approaches in managing bipolar depression. *Journal of Clinical Psychiatry, 64*, 13–18.

Kusumakar, V. (2002). Antidepressants and antipsychotics in the long-term treatment of bipolar disorder. *Journal of Clinical Psychiatry, 63*, 23–28.

Leibenluft, E., Charney, D. S., Towbin, K., Bhangoo, R. K., & Pine, D. S. (2003). Defining clinical phenotypes of juvenile mania. *American Journal of Psychiatry, 160,* 430–437.

Malhi, G. S., Mitchell, P. B., & Salim, S. (2003). Bipolar depression: Management options. *CNS Drugs, 17,* 9–25.

Manning, J. S., Haykal, R. F., Connor, P. D., Cunningham, P. D., Jackson, W. L., & Long, S. (2005). Sustained remission with lamotrigine augmentation or monotherapy in female resistant depressives with mixed cyclothymic–dysthymic temperament. *Journal of Affective Disorders, 84,* 259–266.

Möller, J., Bottlender, R., Grunze, H., Strauss, A., & Wittman, J. (2001). Are antidepressants less effective in the acute treatment of bipolar I compared to unipolar depression? *Journal of Affective Disorders, 61,* 141–146.

Papolos, D. F. (2003). Switching, cycling, and antidepressant-induced effects on cycle frequency and course of illness in adult bipolar disorder: A brief review and commentary. *Journal of Child and Adolescent Psychopharmacology, 13,* 165–171.

Parker, G., & Parker, K. (2003). Which antidepressants flick the switch? *Australian and New Zealand Journal of Psychiatry, 37,* 464–468.

Pavuluri, M. N., Graczyk, P. A., Henry, D. B., Carbray, J. A., Heidenreich, J., & Miklowitz, D. J. (2004). Child- and family-focused cognitive-behavioral therapy for pediatric bipolar disorder: Development and preliminary results. *Journal of the American Academy of Child and Adolescent Psychiatry, 43,* 528–537.

Post, R. M., Leverich, G. S., Altshuler, L. L., Frye, M. A., Suppes, T. M., Keck, P. E., Jr., et al. (2003). An overview of recent findings of the Stanley Foundation Bipolar Network: Part I. *Bipolar Disorders, 5,* 310–319.

Thase, M. E., & Sachs, G. S. (2000). Bipolar depression: Pharmacotherapy and related therapeutic strategies. *Biological Psychiatry, 48,* 558–572.

Tohen, M., Vieta, E., Calabrese, J., Ketter, T. A., Sachs, G., Bowden, C., et al. (2003). Efficacy of olanzapine and olanzapine-fluoxetine combination in the treatment of bipolar I depression. *Archives of General Psychiatry, 60,* 1079–1088.

Wagner, K. D., Amborsini, P., Rynn, M., Wohlberg, C., Yang, R., Greenbaum, M. S., et al. (2003). Efficacy of sertraline in the treatment of children and adolescents with major depressive disorder: Two randomized controlled trials. *Journal of the America Medical Association, 290,* 1033–1041.

Wehr, T. A., & Goodwin, F. K. (1979). Rapid cycling in manic-depressives induced by tricyclic antidepressants. *Archives of General Psychiatry, 36,* 555–559.

Wilens, T. E., Biederman, J., Kwon, A., Chase, R., Greenberg, L., Mick, E., et al. (2003). A systematic chart review of the nature of psychiatric adverse events in children and adolescents treated with selective serotonin reuptake inhibitors. *Journal of Child and Adolescent Psychopharmacology, 13,* 143–152.

Young, L. T., Joffe, R. T., Robb, J. C., MacQueen, G. M., Marriott, M., & Patelis-Siotis, I. (2000). Double-blind comparison of addition of a second mood stabilizer for treatment of patients with bipolar depression. *American Journal of Psychiatry, 157,* 124–126.

PART III

OTHER ISSUES

CHAPTER 17

Polycystic Ovary Syndrome

PARAMJIT T. JOSHI *and* ADELAIDE S. ROBB

Polycystic ovary syndrome (PCOS) is a common, complex, and serious endocrine disorder that affects women in their reproductive years. The disorder was first recognized in 1935 by two gynecologists, Stein and Leventhal (1935). They described a group of women who had a constellation of infertility and several menstrual irregularities and were obese. They were also found to have enlarged ovaries with multiple cysts at laparotomy (Zawadski & Dunaif, 1992). Although it has come to be known as PCOS, the ovarian morphology is a nonspecific finding. Approximately 20% of normal women can have classic polycystic ovarian morphology on ultrasound examination (Dunaif, 1997). Subsequently, others have reported PCOS to be a disorder characterized by ovulatory dysfunction and hyperandrogenism that is thought to have a higher prevalence in women with epilepsy and, perhaps, bipolar disorder.

Unlike the earlier reports by Stein and Leventhal (1935), others have noted that women with PCOS can be lean, and the symptoms of androgen excess may be absent. PCOS is the leading cause of hormonally related infertility and hirsutism and has been associated with multiple reproductive and metabolic disorders. Approximately 80% of women with oligomenorrhea, the clinical consequence of chronic anovulation, have PCOS (Dunaif, 1997). PCOS is also a major risk factor for type 2 diabetes mellitus (DM) in women (Legro et al., 1999).

An association between the development of PCOS and the use of antiepileptic drugs was first suggested by Isojärvi et al. (1993). This suggestion was based on clinical observations that women with epilepsy who received an antiepileptic drug experienced an increased rate of menstrual abnormalities. Although there are no reports of PCOS in teenage girls, use of mood stabilizers such as valproate is increasing for the treatment of bipolar disorders in children and adolescents. Three letters to the editor of the *Journal of the American Academy of Child and Adolescent Psychiatry* (Garland & Behr, 1996; Eberle, 1998; Johnston, 1999) draw attention to this potential association between use of valproate and development of PCOS in teenage girls. They stimulate awareness for both clinicians and researchers and ask for prospective studies to be conducted to shed light on this possible association between the use of mood stabilizers (specifically valproate), other antiepileptic medications, and PCOS.

PCOS is associated with several reproductive, metabolic, and general health disorders, including increased risk of miscarriage, insulin resistance, hyperlipidemia, and cardiovascular disease. Endometrial, ovarian, and breast cancer have all been reported to be more common in women with PCOS (Hardiman, Pillay, & Atiomo, 2003; Balen, 2001; Coulam, Annegers, & Kranz, 1983; Schildkraut et al., 1996). Elevated levels of circulating estrogen and the lack of cycling shedding of the endometrium are considered to be the likely etiology of the increased risk for endometrial carcinoma in women with PCOS (Rasgon, 2004; Hardiman et al., 2003; Siiteri, 1987). In a large case control study examining the relationship between endogenous steroid hormones and endometrial cancer, Potischman and colleagues (1996) found increased risk of endometrial cancer in women with decreased sex-hormone-binding globulin (SHBG) and increased androgen levels.

Although obesity is not always present in women with PCOS, it is a common finding, with reports of up to 50% of women with PCOS being obese, described primarily as the android-type obesity, with an increase in the waist–hip ratio (Lobo & Carmina, 2000). It has been postulated that obesity within itself may promote the development of PCOS through peripheral aromatization of androgen to estrogen within adipose tissue (Franks, 1995; Siiteri, 1987). Subsequently this obesity contributes to the high rates of type 2 diabetes and hyperlipidemia and increases the risk of cardiovascular disease in women with PCOS (Rasgon, 2004).

DEFINITION

PCOS is characterized by both hormonal and metabolic abnormalities. Disparate definitions of this syndrome have been proposed. A contemporary working definition is hyperandrogenism and chronic anovulation (i.e., menstrual abnormalities and reproductive morbidity) in the absence of identifiable pituitary or adrenal pathology. Interestingly, polycystic ovaries are not necessary for the diagnosis to be made (Dunaif & Thomas, 2001; Lobo & Carmina, 2000).

Many of these women have endocrine abnormalities such as elevated testosterone and/or luteinizing hormone (LH) levels (Franks, 1995). However, some women with polycystic ovaries can be entirely endocrinologically normal. Moreover, approximately 10% of women with all the features of the endocrine syndrome have normal-appearing ovaries by ultrasound examination (Ehrmann et al., 1995). Accordingly, the recommended diagnostic criteria for PCOS at the 1990 National Institutes of Health (NIH) conference on polycystic ovary syndrome (Zawadski & Dunaif, 1992) were hyperandrogenism and chronic anovulation in the absence of specific diseases of the ovaries, adrenals, or pituitary. It is important to differentiate this endocrine syndrome from the ovarian morphological change of polycystic ovaries. Outside the United States, it is still typical to diagnose women by the appearance of their ovaries on ultrasound examination. These differing diagnostic criteria for PCOS account for many of the discrepant findings in the literature. It appears, however, that polycystic ovaries function abnormally, even in the absence of the peripheral endocrine syndrome, both in the steroidogenic activity of the theca interna and in the follicular responses to exogenous follicle-stimulating hormone (FSH; Franks, 1995).

Therefore, the definition of PCOS differs in the United States and in Europe in the following ways:

- In the United States, PCOS is defined as a metabolic syndrome, and anatomical changes need not be present to establish diagnosis.
- In Europe, on the other hand, PCOS is defined as polycystic ovaries in the presence of one or more clinical signs of endocrine dysfunction, such as menstrual irregularities, hirsutism, or infertility.

The diagnostic criteria for PCOS on which participants agreed at the 1990 NIH–PCOS consensus conference (Zawadski & Dunaif, 1992; Duncan, 2001; Ernst & Goldberg, 2002), are as follows:

- The presence of ovulatory dysfunction (polymenorrhea, oligomenorrhea, or amenorrhea).
- Clinical evidence of hyperandrogenism and/or hyperandrogenemia.
- Exclusion of other endocrinopathies affecting adrenal or thyroid function, such as hyperprolactinemia, hypothyroidism, adrenal hyperplasia, or Cushing's syndrome.
- Exclusion of anatomical findings of polycystic ovaries, multifollicular ovaries, or hyperandrogenism in isolation.

However, as suggested by Chappell, Markowitz, and Jackson (1999), the diagnosis of PCOS is generally made through a combination of clinical, biochemical, and ultrasonographic findings.

DIFFERENCES BETWEEN PCOS AND POLYCYSTIC OVARIES

Whereas PCOS is a complex endocrine disorder characterized by metabolic and endocrine abnormalities that affects women in their reproductive years, polycystic ovaries are a common but not intrinsically pathological occurrence in 22–30% of the general female population (Luef, Abraham, Haslinger, et al., 2002; Genton et al., 2001). The accepted definition of polycystic ovaries by ultrasonographic and anatomical criteria is the presence of at least 10 subcapsular follicular cysts, measuring 2–8 mm in diameter, arranged around or within thickened ovarian stroma (Adams et al., 1985; Adams, Polson, & Franks, 1986; Duncan, 2001). As many as 25% of women with radiological findings of polycystic ovaries have no endocrine or menstrual irregularities, suggesting that an isolated finding of polycystic ovaries may be a normal variation and may not necessarily imply altered fertility (Genton et al., 2001). It is therefore important to distinguish between these two conditions when interpreting clinical studies (Ernst & Goldberg, 2002). A case control study of 258 women with and without other hormonal or metabolic symptoms of PCOS, showed that there was no significant effect on fertility (Hassan & Killick, 2003). Therefore, the finding of polycystic ovaries in otherwise healthy women may not necessarily predict reproductive dysfunction (Rasgon, 2004).

Other disorders that need to be considered in the differential for PCOS include: nonclassic adrenal 21-hydroxylase deficiency (prevalence 1–5%), hyperprolactinemia and Cushing's syndrome (occasional occurrence), surreptitious androgen use (rare), extreme insulin resistance syndromes, for example, type A (rare), and ovarian and adrenal androgen-secreting neoplasms (very rare).

PREVALENCE

Only recently have there been studies of the prevalence of the classic endocrine syndrome of hyperandrogenism and chronic anovulation. The prevalence of PCOS in the general population of reproductive-age women has been estimated to be between 4 and 12%, without any differences in prevalence between Caucasian and African American women (Dunaif & Thomas, 2001; Lobo & Carmina, 2000; Knochenhauer et al., 1998). However, most reports show a higher prevalence (10.5–26%) of PCOS in women with epilepsy than in the general population (Bauer et al., 2000; Bilo et al., 2001). Franks (1995) reported that 37% of women with amenorrhea and 90% with oliomenorrhea had PCOS. Bauer et al. (2000) studied 93 women with epilepsy and found that the incidence of PCOS was 10.5% in an untreated group, 11.1% in a valproate-treated group, and 10% in a carbamazepine-treated group. There are no prevalence studies in females under the age of 18 years.

Valproate is an approved treatment for epilepsy syndrome. Bipolar treatment guidelines from Canada and the United States recommend valproate as a first-line strategy in the acute treatment of bipolar disorder (O'Donovan et al., 2002). Most persons with bipolar disorder require maintenance treatment, which necessitates the need for careful appraisal of long-term tolerability and safety issues. There have been reports of valproic acid inducing PCOS in females with epilepsy (Franks, 1995). These observations have initiated preliminary investigation in bipolar disorder (Dunaif & Thomas, 2001; Knochenhauer et al., 1998; Yen, 1991). Recently, O'Donovan et al. (2002) reported that valproate-treated females with bipolar disorder exhibited a high prevalence of menstrual irregularities and exhibited ultrasonographically confirmed polycystic ovaries (41%). A study of ambulatory females with DSM-IV-defined bipolar disorder between the ages of 18 and 45 (10 receiving valproate monotherapy) failed to identify any biochemical or ultrasonographic evidence of PCOS in females receiving valproate or lithium (Rasgon et al., 2000). It was noted by both groups that bipolar females exhibited a higher prevalence of menstrual disturbances than the general population. Others have described the potential associations between PCOS and valproate (Herzog, 1996; Post et al., 2001).

Although it awaits to be established whether females with bipolar disorder manifest a higher prevalence of primary reproductive endocrine disorders, they appear to be more overweight or obese than the general population (Suppes, Leverich, & Keck, 2001). Valproate and several other psychotropic agents impart substantial weight gain (Ferriman & Gallwey, 1961; Roste et al., 2001). Excess weight gain may independently predispose and portend risk for subsequent reproductive endocrine and metabolic disorders. Various theories have been offered to explain this higher prevalence of PCOS and other reproductive disorders in these patient populations, including the effects of the disease itself and of antiepileptic drugs, especially valproate, which may directly cause PCOS or indirectly lead to the disorder by causing weight gain that triggers insulin resistance, increased testosterone levels, and other reproductive abnormalities.

CLINICAL FEATURES

Hyperandrogenism and anovulation are the key features of PCOS, as defined by the National Institutes of Health (NIH) consensus diagnostic criteria. The common clinical manifestations of these abnormalities, therefore, are as follows:

Menstrual Irregularities

These may manifest themselves at puberty either with delayed menarche followed by the onset of irregular periods or as the breakdown of a previously regular menstrual cycle within a few years. Chronic anovulation in PCOS is associated with disordered gonadotropin secretion and presents as oligomenorrhea (8–10 menstrual cycles/year) or amenorrhea (the absence of menstrual cycles) before menopausal onset (Lobo & Carmina, 2000). Women with PCOS often are infertile, and for the few PCOS patients who become pregnant, there are increased risks of miscarriage, gestational diabetes, and pregnancy-induced hypertension (Duncan, 2001; Lobo & Carmina, 2000; Ernst, 2002).

These menstrual irregularities are also associated with weight gain, and it is reported that approximately half of the women with PCOS are obese and that 20% of them will have either impaired glucose tolerance or type 2 diabetes by the time they reach 40 years of age (Duncan, 2001). Other risks associated with PCOS are endometrial hyperplasia or malignancy, hypertension, coronary heart disease, and unhealthy lipid profiles, that is, elevated levels of triglycerides and low-density lipoproteins (LDLs).

Hyperandrogenism

Hyperandrogenism may appear clinically as hirsutism, acne, male pattern balding, and/or male distribution of body hair or alopecia (Lobo & Carmina, 2000). The virilizing features of this illness are due to the elevated androgens (testosterone and androstenedione) and their precursors dehydroepiandrosterone (DHEA) and dehydroepiandrosterone-sulfate (DHEAS; Herzog, 1996). The excess androgens are associated with subtle hyperestrogenism (Lobo & Carmina, 2000; Dahlgren et al., 1992).

It is thought that the disorder may be caused by increased steroidogenic activity that is an intrinsic defect in the ovary (Dunaif & Thomas, 2001). *In vitro* studies show that women with PCOS secrete increased amounts of androstenedione (an androgen) and increased amounts of 17-hydroxyprogesterone (a steroid that is an intermediate in the androgen and glucocorticoid biosynthetic pathway) from thecal cells (the androgen-producing cells of the ovary). This increased secretion by thecal cells may be a result of dysregulation of the rate-limiting enzyme in androgen biosynthesis, cytochrome P-450c17α.

Reproductive Endocrine Abnormalities

Reproductive endocrine abnormalities are often present, but none are pathonomonic or found in all women with the disorder. The common endocrine abnormalities include: elevation of LH in urine and serum and low normal plasma FSH, leading to an increased LH/FSH ratio (Duncan, 2001). This go-nadotropin hormonal imbalance leads to an increase in LH-stimulated ovar-ian steroidogenesis and a decrease in follicle maturation (Franks, Mason, & Willis, 2000; Rasgon, 2004). This incomplete follicle maturation in turn is thought to lead to the formation of a larger number of small, immature folli-cles and, subsequently, the formation of follicular cysts (Rasgon, 2004).

Furthermore, decreases in SHBG as a result of hyperinsulinemia and hyperandrogenism, are commonly seen in this syndrome. The decreased SHBG concentration increases the bioavailable fraction of androgens and estrogens, which may increase free testosterone levels. In general, however, estrogen and FSH levels remain in the normal range (Isojärvi et al., 1995; Bauer et al., 2000; Herzog, 1996).

Metabolic Abnormalities

Metabolic abnormalities such as hyperinsulinemia and insulin resistance occur at greater frequency and intensity in women with PCOS. Approxi-mately 40% of women with PCOS have been shown to have impaired glu-cose tolerance tests (Ehrmann et al., 1999; Legro et al., 1999). The rates of impaired glucose tolerance vary from 31 to 35%, versus 7.8% when com-pared with the general U.S. female population (Ehrmann et al., 1999; Legro et al., 1999). Consequently, up to 20% of obese women may exhibit type 2 diabetes by age 40 years (Dunaif, 1995). Insulin resistance is independent of the effect of obesity and may occur regardless of whether the women are lean or obese compared with normal women (Franks, 1995). Further, Lobo and Carmina (2000) have shown that insulin resistance has been found to be more pronounced in women with chronic anovulation than in those who have ovulatory cycles.

In women with PCOS, insulin resistance is characterized by decreased sensitivity to insulin in peripheral tissues but not hepatic resistance, unlike insulin resistance in type 2 diabetes. Hopkinson and colleagues (1998) re-ported that there was support for suggesting that decreased peripheral insu-lin sensitivity and, consequently, hyperinsulinemia were pivotal to the pathogenesis of PCOS. Hopkinson hypothesized that insulin acts in the liver to inhibit the production of insulin-like growth factor 1 (IGF-1) binding protein and SHBG, with the latter leading to an increase in free testoster-one. Therefore, according to Hopkinson, insulin resistance not only in-creases the secretion of ovarian androgen but also promotes an increase in the proportion of free (biologically active) hormone.

Lipid and Lipoprotein Abnormalities

These abnormalities include elevated LDLs and triglycerides, decreased lev-els of high-density lipoproteins (HDL), and apolipoproteins A-1 (Legro,

Kunselman, & Dunaif, 2001; Lobo & Carmina, 2000). Additionally, impaired fibrinolytic activity has also been reported, as assessed by measurements of elevated levels of circulating plasminogen activator inhibitor levels (a potent inhibitor of fibrinolysis), which has been shown to be a risk factor for the occurrence of hypertension and myocardial infarction (Dahlgren et al., 1992; Hopkinson et al., 1998). However, decreased levels of HDL is considered to be the most characteristic lipid abnormality in women with PCOS (Hopkinson et al., 1998).

Reproductive Abnormalities

These abnormalities can often develop shortly after menarche in many women and can last most of their reproductive lives. In others it may appear as a breakdown of a previously regular menstrual cycle, which is often associated with weight gain (Duncan, 2001). However, the most pressing concern is the occurrence of varying degrees of infertility, with PCOS identified in 75% of women with anovulatory infertility (Legro et al., 2001). Women have also been reported to be at much greater risk of having multiple pregnancies through ovulation induction or after in vitro fertilization (Legro et al., 2001).

ETIOLOGY

The etiology of PCOS is not fully understood, though several authors have suggested that PCOS is caused by interactions between a variety of genetic, neuroendocrine, metabolic, and environmental factors (Rasgon, 2004; Dunaif & Thomas, 2001).

Genetic Factors

Familial aggregation of PCOS has been clearly established, suggesting genetic susceptibility (Franks, 1995; Legro & Strauss et al., 1998). Various modes of transmission have been discussed, including an autosomal dominant inheritance pattern based on familial aggregation of hyperandrogenism in first-degree relatives of patients with PCOS (Legro, Strauss, et al., 1998; Ernst & Goldberg, 2002). In addition, brothers of women with PCOS often show evidence of insulin resistance and elevated dehydroepiandrosterone levels, findings that might suggest their reproductive and metabolic phenotypes resemble those of their sisters with PCOS (Dunaif & Thomas, 2001). There is also evidence that there may be a genetic defect in ovarian and adrenal androgen biosynthesis that may synergize with a metabolic abnormality (Rasgon, 2004; Lobo & Carmina, 2000). Studies on women with PCOS suggest that the disorder may be caused by increased steroidogenic activity that is intrinsic, presumably a genetic defect in the ovary (Dunaif & Thomas, 2001). *In vitro* studies have shown that women with PCOS secrete increased amounts of androstenedione (an adrogen) and 17-hydroxyprogesterone (a steroid that is an intermediate in the androgen and glucocorticoid biosynthetic pathway) from thecal cells (the androgen producing cells of the ovary). This increased secretion by thecal cells may be a result of dysregulation of the rate-limiting enzyme in androgen biosynthesis, cytochrome P-450c17a (Franks, 1995).

In order to determine whether there was a biochemical reproductive endocrine phenotype, Legro, Spielman, et al. (1998) studied the sisters of women with PCOS and found that there was familial aggregation of hyperandrogenemia in PCOS kindreds, with 46% of 115 sisters thus affected. Only one-half of these sisters fulfilled diagnostic criteria for PCOS with chronic anovulation and hyperandrogenemia. The remaining affected sisters had hyperandrogenemia with regular menses. The affected sisters also had a significant elevation of DHEAS levels, suggesting that there was an adrenal component to the hyperandrogenemia. The distribution of testosterone levels in the sisters appeared to be bimodal. Although the sample size was relatively small, this suggested that testosterone levels in PCOS families reflected a monogenic trait controlled by two alleles at an autosomal locus.

A genetic defect may be responsible for the insulin resistance found in women with PCOS (Ernst & Goldberg, 2002). Defects in insulin receptors have been reported in up to half of women with PCOS who also may have a decrease in tyrosine phosphorylation and an increase in serine phosphorylation. These factors can all contribute to impaired insulin activity (Dunaif, 1995).

Neurological Factors

The incidence of menstrual irregularities and PCOS both appear to be more common among women with epilepsy than among women without epilepsy (Bilo et al., 1988). PCOS has been reported to occur in 20% of women with temporal lobe epilepsy and 25% of women with complex partial seizures (Herzog et al., 1986). Another study described PCOS in 15% of women with primary generalized epilepsy (Bilo et al., 2001). In general, it has been reported that PCOS occurs in 10.5–26% of women with epilepsy (Bauer et al., 2000; Bilo et al., 2001). Some authors have suggested that epilepsy may play an intrinsic role in the development of PCOS (Herzog et al., 1986; Ernst & Goldberg, 2002) and postulate that epileptic discharges from the amygdala to the hippocampus may affect the secretion of gonadotropin-releasing hormone (GnRH). Increased GnRH pulse frequency in turn promotes LH secretion over FSH secretion and leads to an elevated LH/FSH ratio (Knobil, 1980).

Furthermore, studies have demonstrated higher LH pulse frequencies with left-sided than with right-sided temporal foci (Drislane et al., 1994), and PCOS may be more common with left temporolimbic epileptiform discharges than with right temporolimbic epileptiform discharges. In turn, anovulatory cycles can trigger limbic seizure discharges (Herzog, 1993). Levels of progesterone, a hormone that can raise the seizure threshold, are low in anovulatory women, including those with PCOS (Herzog et al., 1986). Therefore, it is postulated that temporolimbic structures in anovulatory women are primarily exposed to estrogen, which has a known proseizure effect. In addition, limbic seizure discharges may also reduce levels of serum dopamine, leading to increased LH and prolactin secretion by the pituitary (Herzog et al., 1986; Ernst & Goldberg, 2002). Alternatively, a dysfunction in neurotransmission or genetic vulnerability common to both epilepsy and reproductive endocrine disorders may account for the link between PCOS and epilepsy (Herzog et al., 1986; Ernst & Goldberg, 2002).

Endocrine Factors

The possible endocrine factors that may contribute to the development of PCOS include an increased LH/FSH ratio and increased insulin and androgen concentrations. Increased levels of 17-hydroxyprogesterone levels in thecal cells have also been implicated in playing a role in the development of PCOS. Abbott, Dumesic, and Franks (2002) propose a developmental theory in understanding some of these endocrine etiological factors. Accordingly, they postulated that during gestation, placental human chorionic gonadotrophin (hCG), fetal pituitary LH, and genes regulating folliculogenesis and steroidogenesis, individually or together, result in fetal ovarian hyperandrogenemia that leads to prenatal, and possibly prepubertal, exposure to excess androgen. Postpubertally, this early exposure to excess androgen diminishes steroid hormone negative feedback on pituitary LH, resulting in abnormal LH secretion and predisposing women to accumulation of abdominal adiposity that exaggerates insulin resistance. The resulting hyperinsulinemia interacts with LH hypersecretion to augment ovarian steroidogenesis and to induce premature arrest of the follicle development and anovulation.

Metabolic Factors

The insulin resistance that has been described in patients with PCOS decreases the release of SHBG in the liver, which in turn increases free androgen levels that have been implicated in PCOS (Duncan, 2001). When present, obesity worsens insulin resistance (Dunaif & Thomas, 2001) further making the patients more vulnerable to develop PCOS by the mechanism described herein, as obesity independently is associated with decreased levels of SHBG and elevated estrogen levels (Ernst & Goldberg, 2002). Research has shown that experimentally raising insulin levels can directly stimulate ovarian androgen production in women with PCOS (Dunaif & Thomas, 2001). Insulin can also stimulate steroidogenesis by enhancing the sensitivity to adrenocorticotropic hormone and thereby increasing pituitary LH release. These reproductive effects of insulin appear to be limited to women with PCOS. It is important to note that insulin-lowering therapies can restore menstrual cycles in some chronically anovulatory women with PCOS (Dunaif & Thomas, 2001).

Environmental Factors

A number of investigators have recognized that PCOS-like symptoms may be manifested in response to environmental cues, such as prenatal exposure to androgens and weight gain (Adams et al., 1985; Adams et al., 1986). Further, anabolic steroids and antiepileptic drugs (AEDs) have also been implicated in the development of PCOS. Investigators have reported an increased frequency of reproductive disorders in patients with epilepsy (Franks, 1995; Wang, Davies, & Norman, 2001). Thus it is also possible that this population of patients is more likely to be treated with valproate, and, as a consequence, investigators observed a higher incidence of PCOS-like symptoms. However, the finding that valproate increases steroid biosynthesis in theca cells isolated from both normal-cycling and PCOS patients suggests that valproate treatment could independently induce PCOS-like symptoms in the absence of a genetic predisposition for PCOS (Herzog & Schachter, 2001; Ernst & Goldberg, 2002).

CORRELATION BETWEEN BIPOLAR DISORDER AND PCOS

Reproductive disorders have also been reported to have an increased prevalence in women with bipolar disorder. Similar to epilepsy, controversy exists as to whether these abnormalities are caused by the bipolar disorder or by treatment (Rasgon et al., 2000; O'Donovan et al., 2002). The high rate of reported menstrual disturbances may indicate a preexisting compromise in reproductive endocrine function in women with bipolar disorder. This preexisting potential compromise, in turn, may be a marker for dysregulation of the hypothalamic–pituitary–gonadal (HPG) axis. Matsunaga and Sarai (1993) evaluated the HPG axis in 12 women with bipolar disorder. They reported elevated basal LH in 8 women and decreased basal FSH in 6 women. Polycystic ovaries were observed by ultrasonography in 8 of 12 cases, suggesting that a relationship might exist between bipolar disorder and the PCOS-associated hormonal abnormalities in these cases. In a study by Rasgon et al. (2005), 80 women ages 18–45 years being treated for bipolar disorder and not taking steroid contraceptives were recruited to complete questionnaires about their menstrual cycles and to provide blood samples for measurement for a range of reproductive endocrine and metabolic hormone levels. All women received antimanic medications for bipolar disorder. The investigators reported that 50% of women reported current menstrual abnormalities that preceded the diagnosis of bipolar disorder. Fifteen percent reported developing menstrual abnormalities since treatment for bipolar disorder, of which 80% reported changes in menstrual flow (heavy or prolonged bleeding) and 33% reported changes in cycle frequency. These results were consistent with an earlier report by Rasgon and colleagues (2000) indicating that menstrual abnormalities are common in women with bipolar disorder and that the HPG axis may be compromised in some women with bipolar disorder. In the latter study the participants received antimanic medications, and 35% also were taking oral contraceptives. Although it is possible that long menstrual cycles resulted from the pharmacological treatment of bipolar disorder, the observations that menstrual abnormalities precede the onset of bipolar symptoms and that simultaneous oral contraceptive use is associated with long menstrual cycles suggest that women with bipolar disorder may have an underlying predisposition to long or abnormal menstrual cycles (Matsunaga & Sarai, 1993; Rasgon et al., 2000). A recent study examined 300 women ages 18–45 years with bipolar disorder who were evaluated for PCOS. A comparison was made between the incidence of hyperandrogenism and oligomenorrhea that developed while taking valproate versus other anticonvulsants (lamotrigine, topiramate, gabapentin, carbamaxepine, and oxcarbazepine) and also lithium. Of the 230 women who completed the evaluation, results showed that hyperandrogenism with oligomenorrhea developed in 9 (10.5%) of 86 women on valproate and 2 (1.4%) of 144 women on a nonvalproate anticonvulsant or lithium (relative risk 7.5%; $p = .002$). Oligomenorrhea always began within 12 months of valproate use (Joffe et al., 2006).

Others have suggested screening for bipolar disorder in women with PCOS. In a pilot study of 78 women identified with PCOS, Klipstein and Goldberg (2006) reported that 28% had either been previously diagnosed with bipolar disorder or had met Mood Disorder Questionnaire (MDQ) threshold criteria for bipolar disorder. These authors concluded that there is likely a higher rate of women with PCOS who screen positive for bipolar disorder than is expected in the general population. Further, they postulated that there could be a link between PCOS and bipolar disorder secondary to a possible shared HPG axis abnormality.

CORRELATION BETWEEN ANTIEPILEPTIC
DRUGS AND PCOS

In Patients with Epilepsy

It has been suggested that use of anticonvulsants in general and sodium valproate in particular leads to an increased incidence of polycystic ovaries and PCOS (Isojärvi et al., 1993; Isojärvi et al., 1995; Isojärvi et al., 1996; Isojärvi et al., 1998). In their initial study of 238 women with epilepsy, Isojärvi and colleagues (1993) reported some symptoms of PCOS in 96 women, such as irregular menstrual cycles and hyperandrogenism, although the criteria used were not as defined by the NIH. Twenty-nine (12%) were treated with valproate alone, 120 (50%) with carbamazepine alone, and 12 (5%) with a combination of valproate and carbamazepine; 62 (26%) were treated with other AEDs; and 15 (6%) received no medication. Menstrual irregularities were reported by 45% of women receiving valproate, by 19% of those receiving carbamazepine, by 25% of those receiving a combination of both, by 13% receiving other medications, and by none who were untreated. Results of vaginal ultrasonography completed on the 96 women with histories of menstrual irregularities and epilepsy revealed polycystic ovaries in 43% of those treated with valproate, in 22% of those treated with carbamazepine, and in 50% of the combination group.

In a subsequent study, Isojärvi et al. (1995) studied 8 women with epilepsy before and after 1 and 5 years of carbamazepine treatment. All of the women had regular menstrual cycles before the study. Of these 8 women, 2 reported menstrual irregularities, and 3, including these 2 women, had elevated SHBG levels after 5 years of carbamazepine therapy.

In a 1996 study, Isojärvi et al. compared 22 women with epilepsy receiving valproate monotherapy, 43 women receiving carbamazepine monotherapy, and a normal control group without epilepsy. Polycystic ovaries, hyperandrogenism, or both were found in 64% of the valproate group, 21% of the carbamazepine group, and 19% of the control participants. Further, polycystic ovaries and hyperandrogenism occurred more often in obese women on valproate (about 40%) than in lean women on valproate (about 20%). These women also had slightly higher fasting insulin levels (valproate-treated group, 16.9 ± 10.5; carbamazepine group, 15.4 ± 10.5; control group, 9.6 ± 5.1). The investigators also reported that half of the valproate-treated group had progressive weight gain (mean = 21 kg) and lower insulin-like growth factor binding protein levels (Duncan, 2001). This weight gain is thought to perhaps lead to the development of the metabolic syndrome, including hyperinsulinemia, which has been shown to stimulate polycystic ovaries and androgen synthesis. The diagnostic criteria used in the preceding two studies did not meet NIH criteria, and no distinction was made by the authors between polycystic ovaries and PCOS. No information was available about ovarian structure and function prior to treatment with AEDs.

To examine whether discontinuing valproate would reverse its apparent effects on weight, menstrual irregularities, frequency of polycystic ovaries, testosterone levels, HDL-C, and triglycerides, Isojärvi et al. (1998) studied 16 women with epilepsy who had polycystic ovaries or hyperandrogenism and were obese and who were switched to lamotrigine. Over the next year, 12 women who remained in the study lost weight, decreased their waist and hip circumference, and showed a decrease in their body mass index (BMI). In addition, insulin and testosterone levels decreased, and the lipid profiles improved. Ultrasonography revealed that the number of follicles per ovary decreased and the number of women who had menstrual abnormalities decreased. The small sample size, lack of control group, selection of only obese women, and nonrandomization were among the limitations of this study.

In a larger cohort of women with epilepsy being treated with either valproate or carbamazepine, Isojärvi et al. (2001) further assessed the frequency of metabolic and reproductive endocrine disorders. The authors studied 72 women and noted that neither the duration of epilepsy, treatment with valproate, nor dose was associated with polycystic ovaries or hyperandrogenism. Similar to their previous study (Isojärvi et al., 1996), polycystic ovaries and hyperandrogenism were seen in 79% of obese women and 65% of lean women treated with valproate. This information was not reported for the carbamazapine group or control group. The frequency of polycystic ovaries and hyperandrogenism in the carbamazepine-treated group was 20% and, among the normal controls, 19%. Menstrual disorders were seen in 79% of the obese valproate-treated women and in 48% of the lean valproate-treated women, in comparison with 13% of the obese control participants and 17% of the lean control participants who had menstrual irregularities. This information was not reported for the carbamazepine-treated women, though this group had a slightly lower frequency of menstrual disorders than controls. The authors also did not report separate hormone values for lean or obese carbamazepine-treated or control-group participants.

Compared with controls in the same study, women on valproate had higher testosterone levels and lower ratios of HDL-C to total cholesterol. As expected, obese valproate-treated women had higher BMI, higher insulin, and higher lipid profiles and lower HDL-C to total cholesterol ratios than the lean valproate-treated women. However, the contribution of valproate versus obesity to metabolic and hormonal abnormalities in this sample was unclear as only 14 (38%) of 37 women taking valproate were obese. Furthermore, LH levels in valproate-treated women were not significantly different from those of the control group. Although at first glance these data appear to support the hypothesis that the metabolic abnormalities induced by valproate may contribute to the development of the symptoms of PCOS, it is difficult to make generalizations because of the study design and unreported data sets. The effects of obesity versus those of AEDs on the development of polycystic ovaries and hyperandrogenism need to be studied independently.

Several other investigators have conducted studies to replicate the findings reported by Isojärvi and colleagues. Pylvanen et al. (2002) demonstrated that the rates of obesity were the same in patients with epilepsy taking valproate as in normal control participants. However, both lean and obese patients receiving valproate had higher insulin levels than controls, but there was no difference in leptin levels between any of the groups. In reviewing this study, Rasgon (2004) concluded that these data support a causative role for valproate rather than obesity in the development of hyperinsulinemia and suggest that valproate may be directly linked to insulin-stimulated hyperandrogenism in women with epilepsy. However, it is important to note that no untreated patients with epilepsy were included in the study, and the effect of epilepsy on hyperinsulinemia could not be independently assessed (Rasgon, 2004).

It can be argued that early exposure to valproate may increase the risk of PCOS secondary to earlier changes in cellular mechanisms that are thought to be the potential mechanisms for valproate dependent changes that can have an effect on follicular development in the young ovaries of developing girls. Because increased androgen production is a stable phenotype of PCOS theca cells, it is possible that the earlier these biochemical and perhaps structural changes occur, the more irreversible they may be, leading to a greater susceptibility and risk for the development of PCOS secondary to valproate treatment.

In another study examining the effects of AEDs in women with and without epilepsy, Betts, Yarrow, Dutton, Greenhill, and Rolfe (2003) studied 105 women, 54 of whom had been treated only with valproate and 51 of whom had either been treated with lamotrigine or carbamazepine for at least 1 year. They were compared with 50 women without epilepsy. Measurements of FSH, LH, testosterone, and prolactin were obtained from days 2 to 6 of their menstrual cycle, along with magnetic resonance image (MRI) scans of their pelvises. Women with epilepsy in general were significantly more likely to exhibit polycystic ovaries on their scans. Women taking valproate but not an oral contraceptive were also significantly more likely to have clinical biochemical evidence of PCOS with raised LH and/or testosterone than women who did not have epilepsy. This was not the case with women on either lamotrigine or carbamazepine. The investigators concluded that women with epilepsy—particularly if they are not taking oral contraceptives—are more likely than those without epilepsy to have polycystic ovaries by the European definition. Second, they concluded that women with epilepsy who are not taking oral contraceptives are significantly more likely to have PCOS if they have ever taken valproate (but not lamotrigine or carbamazepine; p = .003). Based on this finding, they suggested that perhaps oral contraceptives protect against polycystic ovaries in women who take valproate as an anticonvulsant. They reason that this increased risk with valproate is due to valproate being the only anticonvulsant to be associated with an increase in insulin resistance, which is one of the many factors to be associated with polycystic ovaries. Betts et al. (2003) recommended that valproate should be avoided in women of childbearing age.

Murialdo et al. (1997) studied 101 women with epilepsy between the ages of 16 and 50 years who were treated with a number of different AEDs that included phenobarbitol, phenytoin, and primidone, in addition to valproate and carbamazepine. They reported the occurrence of polycystic ovaries in 12% of the phenobarbitol group; 21% of the carbamazepine group; 0% of the valproate group; 40% of those receiving polytherapy that included valproate; and 13% of the group receiving polytherapy that did not include valproate. None of the women with polycystic ovaries exhibited any PCOS. A subsequent study by the same investigators (Murialdo et al., 1998) of 65 women with epilepsy being treated with valproate, carbamazepine, or phenobarbitol reported that the rates of polycystic ovaries, ovary volume, and hirsutism did not differ significantly among the three treatment groups.

In a study of 50 women with various forms of epilepsy, Bilo et al. (2001) found no significant association between reproductive endocrine disorders such as PCOS, hypothalamic amenorrhea, and luteal phase deficiency based on epilepsy type or AED treatment with or without valproate. They concluded that PCOS preceded the use of any AEDs and was increased in women with epilepsy independent of any drug treatment effects.

In an international multicenter study, 222 women with epilepsy of reproductive age were examined for the presence of menstrual irregularities and endocrine changes related to treatment with AEDs. Their results showed that although testosterone levels were within normal range for both groups (valproate or lamotrigine monotherapy), they were somewhat higher in the valproate group. On the other hand, total cholesterol and LDL levels were lower in the valproate group, and there was no difference in the insulin levels (Taylor, 2001).

Similarly, Bauer et al. (2000), in a prospective study, found no association between PCOS and valproate or carbamazapine treatment in a study of 93 women with epilepsy, refuting the earlier results of Isojärvi and colleagues (1993; Isojärvi et al., 1995; Isojärvi et al., 1996; Isojärvi et al., 1998). In this study the diagnosis of PCOS was made using the NIH criteria and hence distinguished between polycystic ovaries and PCOS. Comparisons were made between four groups of women: untreated, valproate treated, carbamazepine treated, and polytherapy treated.

In a longer term study following 43 women with epilepsy for 3 years who were being treated with valproate ($n = 22$), lamotrigine, or carbamazepine ($n = 21$), Luef, Abraham, Trink, et al. (2002) also found no association between valproate treatment and the frequency of menstrual disorders, polycystic ovaries, or both. However, they did report increased androgen levels in women on valproate. A larger study of 105 women with epilepsy, completed by the same authors (Luef, Abraham, Trinka, et al., 2002), also reaffirmed the findings reported in the earlier study. Patients in this study treated with valproate ($n = 52$) had a slightly lower incidence of menstrual disturbance (11%) and polycystic ovaries (12%) than those treated with carbamazepine ($n = 53$; 16% and 14%, respectively). These differences were not found to be significant. The rate of incidence of polycystic ovaries in the patients was 27%, compared with the rate of 20–30% in the general population, indicating no increase in the incidence of polycystic ovaries with valproate treatment.

Examining the relationship between ovulatory function and treatment with AEDs, Morrell et al. (2002) conducted a study on 94 women with epilepsy and 23 controls. The AEDs used were carbamazepine, valproate, phenytoin, phenobarbitol, lamotrigine, or gabapentine as monotherapy for 6 months or more. There were no statistically significant differences in the frequency of polycystic ovaries between any of the AED treatment groups. However, women with epilepsy were more likely to be obese than the controls, and obesity was higher in patients receiving valproate or lamotrigine. The authors acknowledged, however, that they were unable to control for previous use of AEDs prior to 6 months or for medication change and that the numbers of participants in any of the AED groups were variable, because the AED was selected based on the type of seizure.

A year later Morrell and colleagues (2003) published the results of an open-label, cross-sectional multicenter study of 198 women under the age of 35 years with a history of epilepsy who had been menstruating for at least 4 years and had been treated with lamotrigine or valproate for at least 8 months but no more than 60 months and who were not taking oral contraceptives (lamotrigine, $n = 106$; valproate, $n = 92$). Their results showed that compared with lamotrigine monotherapy, valproate monotherapy was associated with weight gain and higher androgen levels, hyperandrogenism, and longer menstrual cycles that were less likely to be regular, suggesting that these endocrine changes observed in some women using valproate for epilepsy may be secondary to drug therapy.

There is a paucity of studies examining the long-term reproductive endocrine health of young women with epilepsy during puberty. Little is known about the long-term effects of the use of AEDs during childhood and adolescence on reproductive endocrine health. Mikkonen et al. (2004)

studied 69 patients and 51 control participants over a period of time. At entry to the study, the age range was 8–18.5 years, and at follow-up, 12.5–25.8 years. Initially 35 patients were taking valproate, 17, carbamazepine, and 17, oxcarbazepine, as monotherapy. At follow-up only 42 of the 69 patients were on medications. All the participants were examined clinically, medical and menstrual histories were obtained, ovarian ultrasonography was examined, and serum reproductive hormone concentrations were analyzed. The results revealed no significant differences in laboratory or clinical findings between patients off medication and the controls. Postpubertal patients still on medication had higher serum testosterone and androstenedione levels than patients off medication, All the patients still on valproate had elevated serum androstenedione levels. PCOS was more common in 38% of the patients on medication (63% on valproate, 25% on other AEDs) than in patients off medication (6%) or in controls (11%; p = .0005). The investigators concluded that epilepsy during pubertal maturation does not affect reproductive endocrine health in participants who discontinue the medication before adulthood. However, an increased prevalence of endocrine disorders is detected if the patients remain on AEDs, especially valproate, until adulthood.

In an attempt to resolve the controversy and difficulty in separating menstrual and metabolic disturbances in women with epilepsy from effects of the AEDs, Ferin et al. (2003) studied the endocrine and metabolic response to long-term therapy with valproate on the normally cycling rhesus monkey. They compared two groups of 7 monkeys in each group, one free of medication and the other receiving valproate for a duration of 12.7–15.7 months. The results showed no difference in testosterone or LH levels between the two groups; both groups also had similar glucose and insulin responses to a glucose tolerance test. Examination of all 14 ovaries showed no histological evidence of PCOS. The investigators concluded that their results "did not support the hypothesis that treatment with valproate per se is responsible for the induction of PCOS" (Ferin et al., 2003, p. 2915).

In contrast, Nelson-DeGrave et al. (2004) published a study reporting that valproate potentiates androgen biosynthesis in human ovarian theca cells. The theca cells were isolated from follicles of normal-cycling women. The cells were treated for 72 hours with sodium valproate. Whereas low doses (i.e., 30–300 ug) had no effect on basal and forskolin-stimulated progesterone production, higher doses (1000–3000 ug) inhibited progesterone production. The most pronounced effect of valproate on androgen biosynthesis was observed in the dose range of 300–3000 ug, which represents therapeutic levels in the treatment of epilepsy and bipolar disorder. The investigators reported that valproate increased both basal and forskolin-stimulated P459c17 and P450scc protein levels, whereas the amount of steroidogenic acute regulatory protein was unaffected. Consistent with the ability of valproate to act as a histone deacetylase (HDAC) inhibitor in other cell systems, valproate (500 µg) treatment was observed to increase histone H3 acetylation and P450 17 alpha-hyroxylase mRNA accumulation. The HDAC inhibitor butyric acid (500 µM) similarly increased histone H3 acetylation and DHE biosynthesis, whereas valproate derivative valpromide (500 µM), which lacks HDAC inhibitory activity, has no effect on histone acetylation of DHEA biosythesis. The authors of this study concluded that these findings suggest that valproate-induced ovarian androgen biosynthesis results from changes in chromatin modifications (histone acetylation) that augment transcription of steroidogenic genes. This is the first study of its kind to provide biochemical evidence to support the role of valproate in the genesis of PCOS-like symptoms and to establish a direct link between valproate and increased ovarian androgen biosynthesis.

On the other hand, animal experiments have confirmed that in patients with unilateral amygdaloid seizures, the amygdala ipsilaterally activates neurons in the medial preoptic area, ventrolateral part of the ventromedial area, and premammillary nuclei of the hypothalamus, areas that are specifically involved in reproductive neuroendocrine function (Silveira et al., 2000). Furthermore, induction of seizures in the amygdala leads to a decrease in ipsilateral GnRH neuron fiber number (Friedman et al., 2002). These findings further support the hypothesis that unilateral limbic seizures may modulate reproductive endocrine function in a laterally asymmetric manner.

In Patients with Bipolar Disorder

Several investigators have also examined the occurrence of PCOS in patients with bipolar disorder (See Table 17.1). As is the case with patients with epilepsy, with whom there is controversy about whether PCOS occurs independent of the treatment with AEDs, so is the case in patients with bipolar disorders, with whom AEDs are often used as mood stabilizers to treat bipolar disorder. Rasgon et al. (2000) conducted a pilot study to determine whether PCOS is associated with valproate use in the treatment of bipolar disorder. The study evaluated the clinical and hormonal characteristics of PCOS in 22 women with DSM-IV diagnoses of bipolar disorder between the ages of 18 and 45 years. None of the patients met the NIH criteria of PCOS at the beginning of the study. Ten patients were receiving lithium monotherapy, another 10, valproate monotherapy, and 2, lithium-valproate combination therapy. Patients had a mean exposure of 5 years to lithium, 3 years to valproate, and 1 year to combination therapy.

All patients on lithium monotherapy or combination therapy and 60% of patients on valproate monotherapy reported menstrual disturbances preceding the start of medication, again suggesting that, as in the case of patients with epilepsy, some women with bipolar disorder may have compromised HPG axis independent of therapeutic agents used. There were no significant differences in BMI or hirsutism, and hormone levels were within normative values in the three treatment groups. Ovarian ultrasound revealed more follicles in one patient receiving lithium monotherapy and none in the patients on valproate monotherapy. The authors concluded that there was no significant association between PCOS and valproate or lithium therapy in women with bipolar disorder (Rasgon et al., 2000).

Another study in women with bipolar disorder, conducted by O'Donovan et al. (2002), studied 32 women who were either receiving valproate therapy (n = 17) or no drug therapy (n = 15) for bipolar mood disorder. The control group consisted of 22 women who had never been diagnosed with or treated for a psychiatric illness. At the start of treatment women receiving valproate had a significantly greater rate of menstrual abnormalities (47%) than women receiving no drug therapy (13%) and the control women (0%). Because the information about menstrual irregularities relied on a mailed questionnaire, there may have been some recall bias, and hence the authors suggested that the interpretation of data must be done with caution. Seven of the 8 women receiving valproate currently had menstrual problems, 2 had high BMI, and 5 had hirsutism. Two of the latter reported that the hirsutism began after valproate treatment was initiated. None of the women in the study had abnormal FSH or dehydro-epiandrosterone levels, although all the women had hyperandrogenism, 4 women had elevated LH/FSH ratio, and 5 women had polycystic ovaries, as determined by ultrasound. The authors concluded that these 7 women had clinical PCOS and estimated that PCOS was present in 41% of all valproate-treated women in the study. However, the authors did not assess the clinical characteristics of PCOS in all women in the study, making it difficult to justify their claim of a higher prevalence of PCOS in women receiving valproate than in women receiving no drug treatment or normal women. In looking at obesity in the three groups (BMI > 25), the rates were 43% in the valproate group, 57% in the nonmedication group, and 46% in the control group. There was no statistical difference between the three groups. The authors concluded that "this finding argues against a causal link between valproate, obesity and the presence of PCOS features" (O'Donovan et al., 2002, p. 328).

McIntyre et al. (2003) conducted a cross-sectional study of 38 women with bipolar disorder who had been receiving valproate or lithium monotherapy for at least 2 years. Metabolic, hormonal, and reproductive effects of treatment were assessed. They measured FSH, LH, and SHBG, which are often abnormal in women with PCOS. Among the valproate-treated patients, menstrual irregularities were reported by 50% of the patients compared with 15% of the lithium-treated patients, and they were more prevalent in obese patients than in lean patients. The lipid profiles were within reference ranges for both groups. Free testosterone and androstenedione levels were significantly higher in the valproate-treated patients, and LH was elevated in both groups. The data suggested that valproate may have an adverse impact and result in some aspects of the metabolic syndrome in some women with bipolar disorder. However, among the limitations of this study were the relatively small sample size, the cross-sectional design, and the lack of a control group.

Insulin resistance and hyperinsulinemia are hallmarks of the metabolic disorder and have been associated with the development of polycystic ovaries and hyperandrogenism (Glueck et al., 2003). In yet another study, Rasgon et al. (2002) presented data that assessed the association of insulin resistance and bipolar disorder in 39 women who were receiving lithium, valproate, other anticonvulsants, or antipsychotics. Seventeen women had BMIs over 27, and increased insulin resistance occurred in 19 of them. The distribution of insulin resistance was not associated with the type of mood stabilizer used. However, the authors did not report on the type of medication being taken by the women who showed insulin resistance. The authors concluded that their data suggest that insulin resistance is common among women with bipolar disorder, regardless of treatment.

Thirty women with bipolar disorder who were receiving valproate monotherapy, lithium monotherapy, or valproate-lithium combination therapy were compared with 15 women with idiopathic generalized epilepsy (IGE) receiving valproate monotherapy by Akdeniz et al. (2003). The mean duration of treatment in the valproate monotherapy group was less than 3 years in bipolar women and less than 5 years in women with IGE. No menstrual abnormalities were reported in the lithium group, which had had no previous exposure to valproate. In contrast, menstrual disturbances were reported in 20% of bipolar patients on valproate therapy and in 46.7% of patients with IGE on valproate therapy. Hirsutism was reported in 1 patient with bipolar disorder treated with lithium and in 4 patients with IGE receiving valproate. Total testosterone levels were significantly higher in patients with IGE receiving valproate compared with patients with bipolar disorder receiving lithium, and the LH/FSH ratio was significantly elevated in patients with IGE receiving valproate. There were no significant differences in the BMI, waist/hip ratio, and fasting lipid levels among the three study groups. However, fasting glucose was significantly elevated in patients with bipolar disorder and IGE receiving valproate. Other characteristics of PCOS, including hirsutism and an elevated LH/FSH ratio, were more prevalent in women with IGE receiving valproate than in women with bipolar disorder receiving valproate. Again, the results of this study suggest that valproate is more likely to be associated with certain symptoms of PCOS than is lithium. Furthermore, menstrual disorders in women with IGE receiving valproate had a higher incidence compared with women with bipolar disorder also receiving valproate. This suggests that perhaps neurological disorders may differentially contribute to the development of PCOS symptoms, independent of treatment.

TABLE 17.1. Studies of Women with Bipolar Disorder

Study	Population	Type	Number of participants	Drugs	Results
Rasgon et al. (2000)	BP	OL	22	10: Li (5 years) 10: VPA (3 years) 2: Li + VPA (1 year)	- BMI & hirsutism: no significant difference in three groups - Hormone levels WNL's in three groups - Increased ovarian follicles in 1 patient on Li & none on VPA monotherapy
O'Donovan et al. (2002)	BP	CG	32 active; 22 control	17/32: VPA 15/32: no drug	- No difference in obesity between three groups - No causal link between VPA, obesity, & presence of PCOS features
Rasgon et al. (2002)	BP	OL	39	Li, VPA, other AC & AP	- 17 had BMI > 27 - 19 had increased insulin resistance - No difference between drugs
McIntyre et al. (2003)	BP	CS	38	VPA or Li	Menstrual irregularities: - 50% with VPA - 15% with Li
Akdeniz et al. (2003)	BP: 30 IGE: 15	OL	45	VPA, Li, or combination	- VPA more likely to be associated with PCOS Sxs (Symptoms) than Li - IGE patients had higher incidence than BP patients (46.7% vs. 20%)

Note. AC, anti-convulsants; AP, antipsychotics; BP, bipolar; CG, control group; CS, cross-sectional; IGE, idiopathic generalized epilepsy; Li, lithium; OL, open label; VPA, valproic acid; WNL's, within normal limits.

SUMMARY

The studies reviewed in this chapter present several separate viewpoints regarding the association of AEDs (valproate in particular), epilepsy, bipolar disorder, and PCOS. These are summarized in the following list.

- AEDs such as valproate directly cause polycystic ovaries and/or hyperandrogenism.
- Although the evidence regarding AED-induced weight gain and its effects on reproductive function is mixed, several studies concluded that the weight gain from AEDs (in particular valproate) leads to insulin resistance, hyperandrogenism, and other reproductive abnormalities of PCOS.
- Based on the observation that there is overrepresentation of PCOS in women with temporal lobe epilepsy and bipolar disorders, an alternative hypothesis is that the underlying disorder (epilepsy or mood disorder) independently leads to the development of PCOS.
- Women with epilepsy and bipolar disorder may react differently to valproate treatment in terms of weight gain and thus be more or less predisposed to developing the metabolic syndrome, hyperinsulinemia, polycystic ovaries, or hyperandrogenism.
- Alternatively, women with epilepsy may have an underlying reproductive abnormality caused by factors independent of valproate treatment that is aggravated by weight gain. However, because the prevalence of polycystic ovaries and hyperandrogenism was not consistently reported for lean or obese women treated with other AEDs or for normal women, these studies did not demonstrate whether obese control participants or obese women with epilepsy taking other AEDs also had a higher or lower prevalence of polycystic ovaries or hyperandrogenism.

CONCLUSIONS

As increasing numbers of patients with bipolar disorder are in long-term treatment with valproate, there is an important need for further research that clarifies the relationship between long-term administration of valproate and other AEDs used as mood stabilizers and the potential development of reproductive endocrinological abnormalities. There is need for increased awareness among clinicians and patients of the unknown potential for these worrisome side effects. Some authors have suggested that if clinicians are concerned about the literature on PCOS and valproate, they can use valproate with caution, especially in young women with family histories suggestive of PCOS. Further, in women with epilepsy who are overweight or have menstrual irregularities, an endocrine assessment should be completed before starting treatment with valproate.

Some studies have strongly supported an association between valproate or AEDs and PCOS, but none of the studies have established a direct link between these medications and the development of the pituitary endocrinopathies underlying PCOS. Taken together, the studies summarized in this chapter fail to resolve the controversy regarding AED use and the development of the symptoms of PCOS. Some of the limitations of most of these studies include relatively small sample size, cross-sectional design, the lack of use of controls in many, the retrospective nature of the studies, and different definitions of what is considered to be PCOS. In addition, most of these studies did not include newly diagnosed patients who were untreated and thus were unable to distinguish between the disorder itself and AED use as the causal factor in the development of menstrual abnormalities, hyperandrogenism, and polycystic ovaries. Therefore, for the future, large, longitudinal, prospective studies are needed to resolve the issue surrounding AED use and PCOS. These studies should be conducted on newly diagnosed drug-naive patients with epilepsy or bipolar disorder to help characterize the causal connection between epilepsy, bipolar disorder, AEDs, and development of PCOS symptoms. Further, given the number of children and adolescents who are now being prescribed AEDs both for the treatment of epilepsy and bipolar disorder, this age group should also be included in future studies.

Until we understand more about the associations between epilepsy and bipolar disorders, AED therapies, and PCOS, clinicians prescribing AEDs should at least be aware of the possibility of valproate-induced PCOS and monitor patients accordingly. Women with preexisting menstrual abnormalities may represent a group at risk for development of reproductive dysfunction while being treated for bipolar disorder. Histories of menstrual irregularities, prior exposure to medications, and metabolic and hormonal status should be enquired about. Females with bipolar disorder receiving valproate who have any of these menstrual irregularities and obesity should have a reproductive endocrine workup and lipid profile. If blood testing is abnormal, they should be considered for gynecologic/endocrinological consultation. These findings suggest that clinicians may wish to discuss potential for menstrual cycle changes and metabolic issues in the informed-consent process when prescribing valproate. The treatment of obesity should be a major focus of preventive health care for patients with PCOS, epilepsy, and bipolar disorder. To date, there is no reason to contraindicate the use of valproate for the treatment of either epilepsy or bipolar disorder in women. Although the choice of the use of an AED for the treatment of epilepsy or bipolar disorder in women in their reproductive years should be based on the most effective agent for controlling the symptoms of the underlying disorder, patients should be informed about the reproductive endocrine and metabolic risks and consequences.

REFERENCES

Abbott, D. H., Dumesic, D. A., & Franks, S. (2002). Developmental origin of polycystic ovary syndrome: A hypothesis. *Journal of Endocrinology, 174*, 1–5.

Adams, J., Franks, S., Polson, D. W., et al. (1985). Multifollicular ovaries: Clinical and endocrine features and response to pulsatile gonadotropin releasing hormone. *Lancet, 2*(8469–8470), 1375–1379.

Adams, J., Polson, D. W., & Franks, S. (1986). Prevalence of polycystic ovaries in women with anovulation and idiopathic hirsutism. *British Medical Journal (Clinical Research Edition), 293*(6543), 355–359.

Akdeniz, F., Taneli, F., Noyan, A., et al. (2003). Valproate-associated reproductive and metabolic abnormalities: Are epileptic women at greater risk than bipolar women? *Progress in Neuropsychopharmacology and Biological Psychiatry, 27*(1), 115–121.

Balen, A. (2001). Polycystic ovary syndrome and cancer. *Human Reproduction Update, 7*(6), 522–525.

Bauer, J., Jarre, A., Klingmuller, D., et al. (2000). Polycystic ovary syndrome in patients with focal epilepsy: A study in 93 women. *Epilepsy Research, 41*(2), 163–167.

Betts, T., Yarrow, H., Dutton, N., Greenhill, L., & Rolfe, T. (2003). A study of anti-convulsant medication on ovarian function in a group of women with epilepsy who have only ever taken one anticonvulsant compared with a group of women without epilepsy. *Seizure, 12*, 323–329.

Bilo, L., Meo, R., Nappi, C., et al. (1988). Reproductive endocrine disorders in women with primary generalized epilepsy. *Epilepsia, 29*(5), 612–619.

Bilo, L., Meo, R., Valentino, R., et al. (2001). Characterization of reproductive endocrine disorders in women with epilepsy. *Journal of Clinical Endocrinology and Metabolism, 86*(7), 2950–2956.

Chappell, K. A., Markowitz, J. S., & Jackson, C. W. (1999). Is valproate pharmacotherapy associated with polycystic ovaries? *Annals of Pharmacotherapy, 33*, 1211–1216.

Coulam, C. B., Annegers, J. F., & Kranz, J. S. (1983). Chronic anovulation syndrome and associated neoplasia. *Obstetrics and Gynecology, 61*(4), 403–407.

Dahlgren, E., Janson, P. O., Johansson, S., et al. (1992). Polycystic ovary syndrome and risk for myocardial infarction: Evaluated from a risk factor model based on a prospective population study of women. *Acta Obstetricia et Gynecologica Scandinavica, 71*(8), 599–604.

Drislane, F. W., Coleman, A. E., Schomer, D. L., et al. (1994). Altered pulsatile secretion of luteinizing hormone in women with epilepsy. *Neurology, 44*(2), 306–310.

Dunaif, A. (1995). Hyperandrogenic anovulation (PCOS): A unique disorder of insulin action associated with an increased risk of non-insulin-dependent diabetes mellitus. *American Journal of Medicine, 98*(1A), 33S–39S.

Dunaif, A. (1997). Insulin resistance and the polycystic ovary syndrome: Mechanism and implications for pathogenesis. *Endocrine Reviews, 18*(6), 774–800.

Dunaif, A., & Thomas, A. (2001). Current concepts in the polycystic ovary syndrome. *Annual Review of Medicine, 52*, 401–419.

Duncan, S. (2001). Polycystic ovarian syndrome in women with epilepsy: A review. *Epilepsia, 42*(Suppl. 3), 60–65.

Eberle, A. (1998). Valproate and polycystic ovaries. *Journal of the American Academy of Child and Adolescent Psychiatry, 37*(10), 1009.

Ehrmann, D. A., Barnes, R. B., Rosenfield, R. L., et al. (1999). Prevalence of impaired glucose tolerance and diabetes in women with polycystic ovary syndrome. *Diabetes Care, 22*(1), 141–146.

Ernst, C. L., & Goldberg, J. F. (2002). The reproductive safety profile of mood stabilizers, atypical antipsychotics, and broad-spectrum psychotropics. *Journal of Clinical Psychiatry, 63*(Suppl. 4), 42–55.

Ferin, M., Morrell, M., Xiao, E., et al. (2003). Endocrine and metabolic responses to long term monotherapy with antiepileptic drug valproate in the normally cycling rhesus monkey. *Journal of Clinical Endocrinology and Metabolism, 88*, 2908–2915.

Ferriman, D., & Gallwey, J. D. (1961). Clinical assessment of body hair growth in women. *Journal of Clinical Endocrinology, 21*, 1440–1447.

Franks, S. (1995). Polycystic ovary syndrome. *New England Journal of Medicine, 333*(13), 853–861.

Franks, S., Mason, H., & Willis, D. (2000). Follicular dynamics in the polycystic ovary syndrome. *Molecular and Cellular Endocrinology, 163*(1–2), 49–52.

Friedman, M. N., Geula, C., Holmes, G. L., et al. (2002). GnRH-immunoreactive fiber changes with unilateral amygdala-kindled seizures. *Epilepsy Research, 52*(2), 73–77.

Garland, E. J., & Behr, R. (1996). Hormonal effects of valproic acid? *Journal of the American Academy of Child and Adolescent Psychiatry, 35*(11), 1424–1425.

Genton, P., Bauer, J., Duncan, S., et al. (2001). On the association between valproate and polycystic ovary syndrome. *Epilepsia, 42*, 295–304.

Glueck, C. J., Papanna, R., Wang, P., et al. (2003). Incidence and treatment of metabolic syndrome in newly referred women with confirmed polycystic ovarian syndrome. *Metabolism, 52*(7), 908–915.

Hardiman, P., Pillay, O. S., & Atiomo, W. (2003). Polycystic ovary syndrome and endometrial carcinoma. *Lancet, 361*(9371), 1810–1812.

Hassan, M. A., & Killick, S. R. (2003). Ultrasound diagnosis of polycystic ovaries in women who have no symptoms of polycystic ovary syndrome is not associated with subfecundity or subfertility. *Fertility and Sterility, 80*(4), 966–975.

Herzog, A. G. (1993). A relationship between particular reproductive endocrine disorders and the laterality of epileptiform discharges in women with epilepsy. *Neurology, 43*(10), 1907–1910.

Herzog, A. G. (1996). Polycystic ovarian syndrome in women with epilepsy: Epileptic or iatrogenic? *Annals of Neurology, 39*(5), 559–560.

Herzog, A. G., & Schachter, S. C. (2001). Valproate and the polycyctic ovarian syndrome: Final thoughts. *Epilepsia, 42*, 311–315.

Herzog, A. G., Seibel, M. M., Schomer, D. L., et al. (1986). Reproductive endocrine disorders in women with partial seizures of temporal lobe origin. *Archives of Neurology, 43*(4), 341–346.

Hopkinson, Z. E., Sattar, N., Fleming, R., et al. (1998). Polycystic ovarian syndrome: The metabolic syndrome comes to gynaecology. *British Medical Journal, 317*(7154), 329–332.

Isojärvi, J. I., Laatikainen, T. J., Knip, M., et al. (1996). Obesity and endocrine disorders in women taking valproate for epilepsy. *Annals of Neurology, 39*(5), 579–584.

Isojärvi, J. I., Laatikainen, T. J., Pakarinen, A. J., et al. (1993). Polycystic ovaries and hyperandrogenism in women taking valproate for epilepsy. *New England Journal of Medicine, 329*(19), 1383–1388.

Isojärvi, J. I., Laatikainen, T. J., Pakarinen, A. J., et al. (1995). Menstrual disorders in women with epilepsy receiving carbamazepine. *Epilepsia, 36*(7), 676–681.

Isojärvi, J. I., Rattya, J., Myllyla, V. V., et al. (1998). Valproate, lamotrigine, and insulin-mediated risks in women with epilepsy. *Annal of Neurology, 43*(4), 446–451.

Isojärvi, J. I., Tauboll, E., Pakarinen, A. J., et al. (2001). Altered ovarian function and cardiovascular risk factors in valproate-treated women. *American Journal of Medicine*, *111*(4), 290–296.

Joffe, H., Cohen, L. S., Suppes, T., et al. (2006). Valproate is associated with new-onset oligomenorrhea with hyerandrogenism in women with bipolar disorder. *Biological Psychiatry*, *59*, 1078–1086.

Johnston, H. F. (1999). More on valproate and polysystic ovaries. *Journal of the American Academy of Child and Adolescent Psychiatry*, *38*(4), 355.

Klipstein, K. G., & Goldberg, J. F. (2006). Screening for bipolar disorder in women with polycystic ovary syndrome: A pilot study. *Journal of Affective Disorders*, *91*, 205–209.

Knobil, E. (1980). The neuroendocrine control of the menstrual cycle. *Recent Progress in Hormone Research*, *36*, 53–88.

Knochenhauer, E. S., Key, T. J., Kahsar-Miller, M., et al. (1998). Prevalence of the polycystic ovary syndrome in unselected black and white women of the southeastern United States: A prospective study. *Journal of Clinical Endocrinology and Metabolism*, *83*(9), 3078–3082.

Legro, R. S., Kunselman, A. R., Dodson, W. C., et al. (1999). Prevalence and predictors of risk for type 2 diabetes mellitus and impaired glucose tolerance in polycystic ovary syndrome: A prospective, controlled study in 254 affected women. *Journal of Clinical Endocrinology and Metabolism*, *84*(1), 165–169.

Legro, R. S., Kunselman, A. R., & Dunaif, A. (2001). Prevalence and predictors of dyslipidemia in women with polycystic ovary syndrome. *American Journal of Medicine*, *111*(8), 607–613.

Legro, R. S., Spielman, R., Urbanek, M., et al. (1998). Phenotype and genotype in polycystic ovary syndrome. *Recent Progress in Hormone Research*, *53*, 217–256.

Legro, R. S., Strauss, J. F., III, Fox, J., et al. (1998). Evidence for a genetic basis for hyperandrogenemia in polycystic ovary syndrome. *Proceedings of the National Academy of Sciences of the USA*, *95*(25), 14956–14960.

Lobo, R. A., & Carmina, E. (2000). The importance of diagnosing the polycystic ovary syndrome. *Annals of Internal Medicine*, *132*(12), 989–993.

Luef, G., Abraham, I., Haslinger, M., et al. (2002). Polycystic ovaries, obesity and insulin resistance in women with epilepsy: A comparative study of carbamazepine and valproic acid in 105 women. *Journal of Neurology*, *249*(7), 835–841.

Luef, G., Abraham, I., Trinka, E., et al. (2002). Hyperandrogenism, postprandial hyperinsulinism and the risk of PCOS in a cross sectional study of women with epilepsy treated with valproate. *Epilepsy Research*, *48*(1–2), 91–102.

Matsunaga, H., & Sarai, M. (1993). Elevated serum LH and androgens in affective disorder related to the menstrual cycle: With reference to polycystic ovary syndrome. *Japanese Journal of Psychiatry and Neurology*, *47*(4), 825–842.

McIntyre, R. S., Mancini, D. A., McCann, S., et al. (2003). Valproate, bipolar disorder and polycystic ovarian syndrome. *Bipolar Disorders*, *5*(1), 28–35.

Mikkonen, K., Vainionpaa, L. K., Pakarinen, A. J., et al. (2004). Long term reproductive endocrine health in young women with epilepsy during puberty. *Neurology*, *62*, 445–450.

Morrell, M. J., Giudice, L., Flynn, K. L., et al. (2002). Predictors of ovulatory failure in women with epilepsy. *Annals of Neurology*, *52*, 704–711.

Morrell, M., Isojärvi, J., Taylor, A. E., et al. (2003). Higher androgens and weight gain with valproate compared with lamotrigine for epilepsy. *Epilepsy Research*, *54*, 189–199.

Murialdo, G., Galimberti, C. A., Gianelli, M. V., et al. (1998). Effects of valproate, phenobarbital, and carbamazepine on sex steroid setup in women with epilepsy. *Clinical Neuropharmacology*, *21*(1), 52–58.

Murialdo, G., Galimberti, C. A., Magri, F., et al. (1997). Menstrual cycle and ovary alterations in women with epilepsy on antiepileptic therapy. *Journal of Endocrinological Investigation*, *20*(9), 519–526.

Nelson-DeGrave, V. L., Wickenheisser, J. K., Cockrell, J. E., et al. (2004). Valproate potentiates androgen biosynthesis in human ovarian theca cells. *Endocrinology, 145,* 799–808.

O'Donovan, C., Kusumakar, V., Graves, G. R., et al. (2002). Menstrual abnormalities and polycystic ovary syndrome in women taking valproate for bipolar mood disorder. *Journal of Clinical Psychiatry, 63*(4), 322–330.

Post, R. M., Nolen, W. A., Kupka, R. W., et al. (2001). The Stanley Foundation Bipolar Network: 1. Rationale and methods. *British Journal of Psychiatry, 178*(Suppl. 41), 169–176.

Potischman, N., Hoover, R. N., Brinton, L. A., et al. (1996). Case-control study of endogenous steroid hormones and endometrial cancer. *Journal of the National Cancer Institute, 88*(16), 1127–1135.

Pylvanen, V., Knip, M., Pakarinen, A., et al. (2002). Serum insulin and leptin levels in valproate-associated obesity. *Epilepsia, 43*(5), 514–517.

Rasgon, N. (2004). The relationship between polycystic ovarian syndrome and antiepileptic drugs. *Journal of Clinical Psychopharmacology, 24*(33), 322–334.

Rasgon, N. L., Altshuler, L. L., Elman, S., et al. (2002, May). *Increased insulin resistance in women with bipolar disorder.* Poster presented at the annual meeting of the American Psychiatric Association, Philadelphia, PA.

Rasgon, N. L., Altshuler, L. L., Fairbanks, L., et al. (2005). Reproductive function and risk for PCOS on women treated for bipolar disorder. *Bipolar Disorders, 7,* 246–259.

Rasgon, N. L., Altshuler, L. L., Gudeman, D., et al. (2000). Medication status and polycystic ovary syndrome in women with bipolar disorder: A preliminary report. *Journal of Clinical Psychiatry, 61*(3), 173–178.

Roste, L. S., Tauboll, E., Berner, A., et al. (2001). Valproate but not lamotrigine induces ovarian morphological changes in Wistar rats. *Experimental and Toxicologic Pathology, 52,* 545–552.

Schildkraut, J. M., Schwingl, P. J., Bastos, E., et al. (1996). Epithelial ovarian cancer risk among women with polycystic ovary syndrome. *Obstetrics and Gynecology, 88,* 554–559.

Siiteri, P. K. (1987). Adipose tissue as a source of hormones. *American Journal of Clinical Nutrition, 45*(Suppl. 1), 277–282.

Silveira, D. C., Klein, P., Ransil, B. J., et al. (2000). Lateral asymmetry in activation of hypothalamic neurons with unilateral amygdaloid seizures. *Epilepsia, 41*(1), 34–41.

Stein, I. F., & Leventhal, M. L. (1935). Amenorrhea associated with bilateral polycystic ovaries. *American Journal of Obstetrics and Gynecology, 29,* 181–191.

Suppes, T., Leverich, G. S., & Keck, P. E. (2001). The Stanley Foundation Bipolar Treatment Outcome Network: 2. Demographics and illness characteristics of the first 261 patients. *Journal of Affective Disorders, 67,* 45–59.

Taylor, A. (2001, May). *Cross-sectional study comparing weight-pain and androgen levels in women with epilepsy taking lamotrigine (LTG) or valproate (VPA) monotherapy.* Poster presented at the Annual Meeting of the American Psychiatric Association, New Orleans, LA.

Wang, J. X., Davies, M. J., & Norman, R. J. (2001). Polycystic ovarian syndrome and the risk of spontaneous abortion following assisted reproductive technology treatment. *Human Reproduction, 16*(12), 2606–2609.

Yen, S. S. C. (1991). Chronic anovulation caused by peripheral endocrine disorders. In S. S. C. Yen & R. B. Jade (Eds.), *Reproductive endocrinology: Physiology, pathophysiology and clinical management* (3rd ed., pp. 576–630). Philadelphia: Saunders.

Zawadski, J. K., & Dunaif, A. (1992). Diagnostic criteria for polycystic ovary syndrome: Towards a rational approach. In A. Dunaif, J. R. Givens, & F. P. Haseltine (Eds.), *Polycystic ovary syndrome* (pp. 377–384). Oxford, UK: Blackwell Scientific.

CHAPTER 18

Weight Gain and Metabolic Abnormalities in Pediatric Bipolar Disorder

CHRISTOPH U. CORRELL

Bipolar disorder is a severe, often recurrent psychiatric illness that affects all aspects of behavior and functioning (Calabrese et al., 2003; Goldberg & Harrow, 2004; Post et al., 2003). Unfortunately, the correct diagnosis and adequate mood-stabilizer treatment of bipolar disorder are typically delayed by 8–10 years (Goldberg & Ernst, 2002; Lish, Dime-Meenan, Whybrow, Price, & Hirschfeld, 1994). Whereas adult-onset bipolar disorder has been well studied, less attention has focused on childhood-onset bipolar disorder (Leibenluft, Charney, & Pine, 2003). Importantly, between 59% (Lish et al., 1994) and 65% (Perlis et al., 2004) of individuals with bipolar disorder report having their first onset of symptoms before age 18 years. Moreover, the early-onset bipolar variant appears to be more severe and treatment-refractory than its adult-onset counterpart (Biederman et al., 2004; Carlson & Meyer, 2000; Findling & Calabrese, 2000; Findling et al., 2001; Geller et al., 2002; Wozniak, 2005).

Psychotropic medications have been the mainstay of bipolar disorder treatment. Over the past decade, the use of psychotropic medications and, especially, of second-generation antipsychotics (SGAs) in children and adolescents has increased (Cooper et al., 2006; Cooper, Hickson, Fuchs, Arbogast, & Ray, 2004; Olfson, Blanco, Liu, Moreno, & Laje, 2006; Zito et al., 2003). In a recent study, antipsychotic prescription frequency increased from 8.6 per 1,000 U.S. children in 1995–1996 to 39.4 per 1,000 U.S. children in 2001–2002 (rate ratio 4.89, 95% CI, 2.50–9.55). Almost one-third (32.4%) of the prescriptions were associated with visits to non-mental health providers, and 53% of prescriptions were for behavioral indications or affective disorders. Across all age groups, increases in prescriptions were more pronounced for less studied indications (Cooper et al., 2006). These data are reconfirmed by another recent study of outpatient visits to physicians in office-based practice, finding a more than six-fold increase of antipsychotic prescribing for persons age 20 years and younger between 1993 and 2002 (Olfson et al., 2006). Such increased use despite lack of evidence from large, controlled studies for efficacy and safety in pediatric populations is, at least, partly due to reduced rates of acute (Kane, 2001) and chronic (Correll, Leucht, & Kane, 2004) neuromotor effects, coupled with emerging evidence of improved and broader efficacy (Findling, 2005; Findling, Steiner, & Weller, 2005). However, despite these possible advantages, SGAs are at greater risk to cause weight gain and related abnormalities in lipid and glucose metabolism compared with first-generation antipsychotics (FGAs) in adult (Allison et al., 1999; Newcomer, 2005) and pediatric (Correll & Carlson, 2006; Fedorowicz & Fombonne, 2005) populations. This has caused concern because of the known associations between weight gain and obesity with diabetes, dyslipidemia, and hypertension, all of which are leading risk factors for future cardiovascular morbidity and mortality (American Diabetes Association et al., 2004).

The aims of this chapter are to (1) increase the awareness and knowledge of anthropometric and metabolic adverse events associated with treatments used to manage bipolar disorder in children and adolescents and (2) provide clinicians with tools to monitor and manage weight gain and metabolic complications in this vulnerable patient group.

METHODOLOGICAL ISSUES REGARDING THE MEASUREMENT OF BODY COMPOSITION AND METABOLISM DURING DEVELOPMENT

As recently discussed in the context of antipsychotic drug prescribing for children and adolescents (Correll, 2005; Correll & Carlson, 2006), the measurement of medication-induced changes in body composition, blood pressure, and metabolic indices in youths is complicated by the fact that children and adolescents are in a phase of physical development that involves physiological changes that are different across age groups and gender. Therefore, clinicians need to be aware of tools (Table 18.1) and "pathological" thresholds (Table 18.2) that differ from those used in adults.

Although pediatricians routinely evaluate the height, weight, and body mass index (BMI) of their patients according to sex- and age-adjusted growth curves, the use of BMI percentiles and z scores has not been

TABLE 18.1. Resources for Obtaining Sex- and Age-Adjusted Body Mass Index, Waist Circumference, and Blood Pressure for Children and Adolescents

Sex- and age-adjusted parameters	Resource for calculation
Body mass index percentile	Growth charts: *www.cdc.gov/growthcharts/*
Body mass index percentile and z scores	Web-based calculator: *www.kidsnutrition.org/ bodycomp/bmiz2.html*
Waist circumference percentile	Tables: Fernandez et al. (2004)
Blood pressure percentiles	Tables: "Fourth Report on the Diagnosis, Evaluation, and Treatment of High Blood Pressure in Children and Adolescents" (2004)

Note. From Correll and Carlson (2006). Copyright 2006 by the American Academy of Child and Adolescent Psychiatry. Reprinted by permission.

adopted widely in psychiatric practice involving youngsters. Whereas in adults the BMI is calculated either as weight in kg/height in meters^2 or weight in pounds × 703/height in inches^2, in children and adolescents BMI values vary too much during development to be useful for the monitoring of body composition changes over longer periods of time. Therefore, the use of sex- and age-adjusted BMI percentiles and z scores is crucial. These can be obtained from tables and charts from the Centers for Disease Control (*www.cdc.gov/growthcharts/*). Alternatively, a Web-based calculator (*www.kidsnutrition.org/bodycomp/bmiz2.html*) can be used.

By definition, < 5th BMI percentile is considered "underweight"; ≥ 5th–< 85th BMI percentile is considered "normal weight"; ≥ 85th–< 95th BMI percentile is considered "at risk"; and ≥ 95th BMI percentile is "overweight" (Krebs & Jacobson, 2003). As with BMI, blood pressure and waist circumference values need to be adjusted for age and sex, and tables with norm values are available for both these parameters ("Fourth report on the diagnosis, evaluation, and treatment," 2004; Fernandez, Redden, Pietrobelli, & Allison, 2004). These measures are also relevant for the definition of the metabolic syndrome in youngsters, a high-risk state for future cardiovascular morbidity and mortality (see the next section).

RELEVANCE OF AGE-INAPPROPRIATE WEIGHT GAIN IN CHILDREN AND ADOLESCENTS

Age-inappropriate weight gain seems to have particularly deleterious effects when it occurs early on in life (Cook, Weitzman, Auinger, Nguyen, & Dietz, 2003; Dietz & Robinson, 2005; Sinha et al., 2002; Weiss et al., 2004). Multiple prospective studies have reported that obesity, metabolic abnormalities, and weight gain during childhood strongly predict obesity, metabolic syndrome, hypertension, cardiovascular morbidity, sleep apnea, osteoarthritis, and malignancy risk in adulthood (Bao, Srinivasan, Wattig-

TABLE 18.2. Widely Used Pathological Thresholds in Adults versus Children and Adolescents

Variable	Adults	Children and adolescents
Body composition[a]		
Underweight (BMI)	< 18.5 kg/m^2	< 5th percentile
Normal weight (BMI)	18.5–24.9 kg/m^2	5th–< 85th percentile
Elevated (BMI)	"Overweight": 25–29.9 kg/m^2	"At-risk": 85th–< 95th percentile
Very elevated (BMI)	"Obese": ≥ 30 kg/m^2	"Overweight": ≥ 95th percentile
Abdominal obesity[b]		
Waist circumference: Male	≥ 102 cm (= > 40 inches)	≥ 90th percentile
Waist circumference: Female	> 88 cm (= > 35 inches)	≥ 90th percentile
Glucose metabolism (fasting)[c]		
Glucose intolerance/prediabetes		≥ 100–125.9 mg/dL
Fasting	≥ 100–125.9 mg/dL	≥ 140–199.9 mg/dL
2-hour postglucose load	≥ 140–199.9 mg/dL	
Diabetes mellitus		≥ 126 mg/dL
Fasting on two occasions	≥ 126 mg/dL	≥ 200 mg/dL
2-hour postglucose load	≥ 200 mg/dL	
Hyperinsulinemia[d]	? ≥ 20 μmol/L	? ≥ 20 μmol/L
Lipid metabolism (fasting)[e]		
Hypertriglyceridemia	≥ 150 mg/dL	≥ 110 mg/dL
Hypertension[e]		
Blood pressure	≥ 130/85 mm/Hg	≥ 90th percentile

[a]Krebs and Jacobson (2003).
[b]Fernandez et al. (2004).
[c]American Diabetes Association (2006).
[d]Insulin assays are not standardized in the United States and can vary between laboratories (Williams et al., 2002).
[e]Cook et al. (2003).

ney, & Berenson, 1994; Ebbeling, Pawlak, & Ludwig, 2002; Freedman et al., 2005; Guo, Roche, Chumlea, Gardner, & Siervogel, 1994; Guo, Wu, Chumlea, & Roche, 2002; Must, Jacques, Dallal, Bajema, & Dietz, 1992; Must & Strauss, 1999; Sinaiko, Donahue, Jacobs, & Prineas, 1999; Srinivasan, Myers, & Berenson, 2002; Vanhala, Vanhala, Keinanen-Kiukaanniemi, Kumpusalo, & Takala, 1999). An additional reason for concern about age-inappropriate weight gain and obesity during childhood and adolescence are findings from the general population indicating that the effect of obesity on diabetes and cardiovascular morbidity is strongest in adults younger than 40 years of age (Fontaine, Redden, Wang, Westfall, & Allison, 2003). This suggests that onset of obesity and metabolic abnormalities secondary to SGA and other mood-stabilizer treatment in childhood could lead to an accelerated development of such metabolic outcomes compared with individuals who start on antipsychotics later in life.

Weight gain and obesity are also associated with the metabolic syndrome, a constellation of physical and laboratory features that is more common in obese patients and that predisposes individuals with the syndrome to atherosclerotic cardiovascular disease (Bray, 2004; Grundy, 2004). The features of the metabolic syndrome are: abdominal obesity, dyslipidemia (principally elevated serum triglycerides and low HDL cholesterol), glucose intolerance, and hypertension. A common cause of all features of the metabolic syndrome appears to be insulin resistance, which can result from weight gain.

Several criteria have been used to define the syndrome in adults, but the most widely accepted is from the National Cholesterol Education Program's definition ("Executive Summary," 2001) that requires the presence of at least three of five criteria (see Table 18.3). Because, as discussed previously, normal values for the parameters that are part of the metabolic syndrome change with age, height, and gender, modified criteria have been proposed for use in children and adolescents (Table 18.3; Cook et al., 2003; de Ferranti et al., 2004; Weiss et al., 2004).

The metabolic syndrome has been reported to occur in about 5–10% of adolescents in the United States and in more than 30% of those who are overweight (Cook et al., 2003; de Ferranti et al., 2004; Duncan, Li, & Zhou, 2004). Importantly, the occurrence of the metabolic syndrome in

TABLE 18.3. Criteria for the Metabolic Syndrome in Adults and in Children and Adolescents

Metabolic syndrome criteria in adults ("Executive Summary," 2001)	Metabolic syndrome criteria in children and adolescents (Cook et al., 2003; Weiss et al., 2004)
Abdominal obesity, i.e., waist circumference ≥ 102 cm (= > 40 inches) in males and ≥ 88 cm (= > 35 inches) in females	Waist circumference ≥ 90th percentile, or BMI ≥ 95th percentile (i.e., "overweight")
Fasting serum triglyceride levels ≥ 150 mg/dL	Fasting serum triglyceride levels ≥ 110 mg/dL
Fasting high-density lipoprotein (HDL) cholesterol < 40 mg/dL in males and < 50 mg/dL in females	Fasting high-density lipoprotein (HDL) cholesterol < 40 mg/dL in males and females
Blood pressure ≥ 130/85 mm/Hg	Blood pressure ≥ 90th percentile for sex and age
Fasting glucose ≥ 110 mg/dL*	Fasting glucose ≥ 110 mg/dL*

Note. At least three criteria must be met. From Correll and Carlson (2006). Copyright 2006 by the American Academy of Child and Adolescent Psychiatry. Reprinted by permission.
*Adapted criterion: Fasting glucose ≥ 100 mg/dL (Grundy et al., 2005).

young individuals predicts early atherosclerosis and vascular disease as adults (Berenson et al., 1998; Li et al., 2003; Raitakari et al., 2003).

In addition to potential physical consequences, excessive weight gain can also have several deleterious psychosocial effects in patients, including stigmatization and further social withdrawal, poorer quality of life, and noncompliance with medication (Allison & Casey, 2001; Robinson, Chang, Haydel, & Killen, 2001; Strassnig, Brar, & Ganguli, 2003; Weiden, Daniel, Simpson, & Romano, 2003). Although some of these data exist in adults and nonpsychiatric child and adolescent populations, information on the psychosocial burden of weight gain in youths with bipolar disorder and other pediatric psychiatric populations is absent.

Although an association between weight gain and clinical response to antipsychotic medications has been described in adults (Ascher-Svanum, Stensland, Zhao, & Kinon, 2005; Czobor et al., 2002) and children (Masi, Cosenza, Mucci, & Brovedani, 2003; Sporn et al., 2005), this association can be explained by the inappropriate use of the last-observation-carried-forward method for efficacy, as well as weight gain assessments. Patients with less or inadequate response are more likely to drop out early during the trial and have less time to gain weight compared with patients who are considered responders and who stay in the trial longer and have more exposure to the drug and more time to gain weight. Taking exposure to the medication into account, studies have not reconfirmed an independent relationship of clinical relevance between weight gain and efficacy (Hennen, Perlis, Sachs, Tohen, & Baldessarini, 2004; Zipursky et al., 2005).

BIPOLAR DISORDER, OBESITY, AND METABOLIC ABNORMALITIES

To date, very little is known about prevalence rates of obesity and metabolic abnormalities in children and adolescents with bipolar disorder. In adults, however, rates of obesity and abnormalities of glucose and lipid parameters appear to be higher in patients with bipolar disorder compared with the general public (Keck & McElroy, 2003; McIntyre, Konarski, Misener, & Kennedy, 2005; Simon et al., 2006). A systematic review of 45 studies concluded that patients with bipolar disorder are at greater risk than the general population for being overweight and obese. The data suggested that comorbid binge-eating disorder; the number of depressive episodes; treatment with medications associated with weight gain, alone or in combination; excessive carbohydrate consumption; and low rates of exercise may be risk factors for weight gain and obesity in patients with bipolar disorder (Keck & McElroy, 2003). In a more recent systematic search of Medline and the Cochrane Collaboration, mortality from cardiovascular causes and pulmonary embolism (standardized mortality ratio approximately 2.0) and morbidity from obesity and type 2 diabetes mellitus may be increased in bipolar disorder compared with the general population (Morriss & Mohammed, 2005). Another recent Medline review of all English-language articles from 1966 to 2004 (using the key words *bipolar disorder, major depressive disorder, diabetes mellitus, glucose metabolism, mortality, overweight, obesity,* and *body mass index*) also concluded that subpopulations of patients with bipolar disorder are at high risk for diabetes mellitus, a risk that may be up to three times greater than in the general population (McIntyre et al., 2005). Although much less is known about the prevalence of dyslipidemia, the assumption is that due to the strong associations between overweight, obesity, and diabetes with lipid abnormalities, the latter are also highly likely to be more prevalent in patients with bipolar disorder.

However, despite these associations, the reasons and mechanisms for the higher rates of obesity and metabolic abnormalities in patients with bipolar disorder, which match similar results in other severe mental disorders (Brown, Inskip, & Barraclough, 2000; Osby, Correia, Brandt, Ekbom, & Sparen, 2000), is still unclear. Most likely, reasons are complex and include reduced exercise and poor diet, frequent depressive episodes, comorbidity with substance misuse, and poor quality of general medical care, in addition to treatment with medications that can increase appetite and weight. To date, however, there is no clear evidence that patients with bipolar disorder are more sensitive than other patients to weight gain and medical problems associated with long-term use of psychotropic medication (Morriss & Mohammed, 2005), suggesting that the type of medication and duration of treatment are major contributing factors.

CHANGES IN BODY COMPOSITION ASSOCIATED WITH CONVENTIONAL MOOD STABILIZERS AND SECOND-GENERATION ANTIPSYCHOTICS

Despite high utilization rates of SGAs and other mood-stabilizing medications in youths, data on weight gain due to these agents in children and adolescents, particularly from prospective studies, are still limited. This is problematic, as preliminary data suggest that pediatric populations may be at higher risk for SGA-induced weight gain than adults (Ratzoni et al., 2002; Safer, 2004; Sikich, Hamer, Bashford, Sheitman, & Lieberman, 2004).

In this section the published evidence for the weight-gain potential of conventional mood stabilizers and SGAs is summarized. The differences in trial duration and in patients' ages and baseline body compositions, as well as lack of reporting of changes in a metric (i.e., BMI z scores or percentiles) that would allow pooling of the data despite these fundamental disparities, make a direct comparison of the individual trial results impossible. However, except for three trials in which weight loss was observed (topiramate: $n = 2$; aripiprazole: $n = 1$) and three trials in which the weight gain was not significant compared with baseline (lamotrigine: $n = 1$; quetiapine: $n = 1$) or growth-adjusted weight gain (lithium and lithium plus risperidone: $n = 1$), significant and/or substantial weight gain was observed in the majority of 21 trials of mood-stabilizing agents in pediatric populations with bipolar disorder (Correll, 2007).

Conventional Mood Stabilizers

Eleven published trials of conventional mood stabilizers provide data on weight change in youths with bipolar disorder (Table 18.4).

Divalproex

Three studies reported on weight changes with divalproex in youths with bipolar disorder. In these studies, divalproex treatment was associated with 3.6 ± 6.0 kg over 4 weeks in 25 adolescents (mean age = 15.0 years; DelBello et al., 2006), 2.5 ± 2.1 kg over 6 weeks in 15 adolescents (mean age = 14.3), and 5.6 ± 4.3 kg (or approximately one standard deviation) over 24 weeks in 34 children and adolescents (mean age = 12.3 years; Pavuluri, Henry, Carbray, Naylor, & Janicak, 2005).

Lamotrigine

Only one recent open-label study in 20 youths with bipolar disorder and depression reported on weight gain with lamotrigine. In this study of 20 children and adolescents (mean age = 15.8 years), 8 weeks of treatment with lamotrigine was associated with nonsignificant increase in weight of 0.42 ± 1.9 kg (Chang, Saxena, & Howe, 2006).

Lithium

Despite the fact that lithium is among the oldest of mood-stabilizing agents, only three trials in youths with bipolar disorder have reported on weight changes in this population. In the largest mood-stabilizer trial to date of 100 adolescents (mean age = 15.2 years), 55.5% of the lithium-treated youngsters gained between 0.45 and 5.5 kg (mean weight gain was not reported). In a recent 6-week trial of 27 adolescents with bipolar disorder and depression (mean age = 15.6 years), lithium was associated with 1.7 ± 3.2 kg weight increase that was statistically significant. By contrast, the mean weight gain of 3.3 kg in 17 lithium-treated children and adolescents (mean age = 12.5 years) over a 1-year period was not significant after adjustment for age-appropriate weight gain secondary to growth (Pavuluri et al., 2006; Pavuluri, personal communication, July 12, 2006).

TABLE 18.4. Studies Reporting on Mood-Stabilizer-Induced Weight Gain in Pediatric Patients with Bipolar Disorder

Mood stabilizer (N = 12, n = 459)	First authors (year)	Design	N[a]	Age in years (range)	Duration in weeks[b] (mean)	Drop-out (%)	Dose (mg/day)	Weight gain (kg)	Comparator	p
					Mood stabilizer monotherapy (N = 10, n = 331)					
Divalproex (N = 74)	DelBello, Schweirs (2002)	DBRC	15	14.3 (12–18)	6 (5.7[c])	6.7	NR (102 µg/mL)	2.5 ± 2.1	DVPX + QTP: 4.2 ± 3.2 kg	NS
	Pavuluri (2005)	OL	34	12.3 (5–18)	24 (20.2)	NR	950 ± 355 (109 µg/mL)	5.6 ± 4.3 (~1 SD or 50th–70th BMI %ile)	Baseline	NR
	DelBello (2006)	DBRC	25	15.0 (12–18)	4 (3.3[c])	24.0	NR (101 µg/mL)	3.6 ± 6.0	QTP: 4.4 ± 5.0 kg	.2
Lamotrigine (N = 20)	Chang (2006)[d]	OL	20	15.8 (12–17)	8 NR	5.0	132 ± 31	0.42 ± 1.9 (0.26%[c])	Baseline	.32
Lithium (N = 144)	Patel et al. (2006)[d]	OL	27	15.6 (12–18)	6 5.1	25.9	1356 ± 335 (0.9 ± 0.3 mEq/L)	1.7 ± 3.2	Baseline	< .01
	Kafantaris (2003)	OL	100	15.2 (12–18)	4 (3.8[c])	7.0	1355 ± 389 (0.93 ± 0.21 mEq/L)	0.45–5.5 (range)	Baseline	NR
	Pavuluri (2006)	OL	17	12.5 (4–17)	48 (46.6[c])	NR	825 ± 350 (0.92 mEq/L)	3.3[e]	CDC growth curve Li + Ris: 3.7 kg	NS .34
Oxcarbazepine (N = 55)	Wagner (2006)	DBRPC	55	10.2[c] (7–18)	7 (NR)	29.1	1,515	0.83	PBO: –0.13	.025

(cont.)

TABLE 18.4. (*continued*)

Mood stabilizer (N = 12, n = 459)	First authors (year)	Design	N^a	Age in years (range)	Duration in weeks^b (mean)	Drop-out (%)	Dose (mg/day)	Weight gain (kg)	Comparator	p
Topiramate (N = 38)	DelBello (2005)	DBRPC	29	13.9 (6–17)	4 (NR)	17.2	278 ± 121	−1.8 ± 2.0 (−2.7%)	PBO: 0.9 ±1.4 (1.4%)	< .001 < .001
	DelBello, Kowatch (2002)	CR	9	14.0 (5–20)	28 (28)	N/A	104 ± 77	−5.0 ± 7.0	Baseline	.05
Mood-stabilizer combination therapy (N = 2, n = 128)										
Divalproex + lithium (N = 128)	Findling (2006)	OL	38	10.5 (5–17)	8 (NR)	7.9	Li: 872 ± 22.2 (0.83 ± 0.28 mEq/L) VPA: 833 ± 21 (75.5 ± 18.9 μg/mL)	1.2	Baseline	< .0001
	Findling (2003)	OL	90	10.9 (5–17)	20 (11.3)	NR	Li: 923 ± 280 (0.9 ± 0.3 mEq/L) VPA: 862 ± 25.9 (79.8 ± 25.9 μg/mL)	3.1 (0.3 ± 0.4/ week in 1st 8 weeks, 0.2 ± 0.5/week in next 8 weeks)	Baseline	< .0001

Note. Adapted from Correll (2007). Copyright 2007 by the American Academy of Child and Adolescent Psychiatry. Adapted by permission. CR, chart review; DBRC, double-blind randomized controlled; DBRPC, double-blind randomized placebo controlled; N/A, not applicable; NR, not reported; NS, not significant; OL, open label; OLR, open label randomized; DVPX, divalproex; QTP, quetiapine; Li, lithium; Ris, risperidone; CDC, Center for Disease Control; PEO, placebo.

^{a}Patient *n* may be larger in a given study, but only patients on index medication with data on weight gain are included.

^{b}In ascending order of trial duration.

^{c}Calculated.

^{d}In patients with bipolar depression.

^{e}Individual data for lithium monotherapy group provided by the author (Pavuluri, personal communication, July 12, 2006).

Oxcarbazepine

In a recent placebo-controlled study, 7 weeks of oxcarbazepine treatment was associated with significant weight gain of 0.83 kg in 55 children and adolescents (mean age = 10.2 years) compared with 55 placebo-treated youngsters who lost 0.13 kg (Wagner et al., 2006).

Topiramate

In the two trials with topiramate, children and adolescents lost significant weight. In a 4-week randomized, placebo-controlled trial, 29 youths (mean age = 13.9 years) lost 1.8 ± 2.0 kg (i.e., –2.7% body weight), which was significantly different from the average gain of 0.9 ± 1.4 kg on placebo (i.e., +1.4% body weight; DelBello et al., 2005). In an earlier 28-week chart review study, nine youths (mean age = 14.0 years) lost, on average, 5.0 ± 7.0 kg, which was significant compared with baseline weight. This suggests that weight loss on topiramate seems to continue beyond the acute treatment phase (DelBello, Kowatch, et al., 2002).

Divalproex plus Lithium

In each of the two trials that evaluated weight gain associated with the combined treatment of divalproex and lithium, weight gain was significant compared with baseline. In 38 children and adolescents (mean age = 10.5 years) treated with this combination for 8 weeks, weight increased by 1.2 kg (Findling et al., 2006). In the 20-week trial assessing the same treatment regimen in 90 youths (mean age = 10.9 years), a mean of 11 weeks of divalproex plus lithium was associated with 3.1 kg weight gain (Findling et al., 2003). The authors noted that the weight gain was greater in the first 8 weeks (average of 0.3 ± 0.4 kg per week) than in the second 8 weeks (i.e., 0.2 ± 0.5 kg per week), suggesting that weight gain began to level off slightly in the group as a whole.

Second-Generation Antipsychotics

All SGAs share a tendency to promote weight gain, especially in drug-naïve patients (Correll, 2005), but some of these agents appear to be more likely to do so than others. Preliminary data suggest that cotreatment with psychostimulants have only little, if any, relevant effect on SGA-related weight gain (Aman, Binder, & Turgay, 2004). Although larger, long-term studies are clearly needed to better define the relative risks of weight gain in children and adolescents, data from adults (American Diabetes Association et al., 2004; Allison et al., 1999; Casey et al., 2004) and from an ongoing large-scale naturalistic study in children and adolescents (Correll, 2005) suggest the following rank order in terms of the ability to promote weight gain and development of the metabolic syndrome (Correll & Carlson, 2006):

Clozapine = Olanzapine >> Risperidone >/= Quetiapine > Ziprasidone >/= Aripiprazole

To date, 10 published studies have reported on weight gain associated with SGAs (Table 18.5; Correll, 2007).

Aripiprazole

In one chart review, 14 children and adolescents (mean age = 13.0 years) with available weight data experienced a mean weight loss of 3.0 ± 6.0 kg during a mean treatment of 18 weeks of aripiprazole. It was not reported in this trial whether or not this change was significant compared with the baseline body weight in these patients (Barzman et al., 2004).

Clozapine

In another chart review, 10 children and adolescents (mean age = 14.8 years) experienced a mean weight gain of 7.0 ± 3.1 kg during a 28-week period. It was not reported whether or not this change was significant compared with the baseline, taking normal development during this medium-term follow-up period into account (Masi, Mucci, & Millepiedi, 2002).

Olanzapine

In a chart review of 23 children and adolescents (mean age = 10.3 years), 8 weeks of olanzapine treatment was associated with a significant weight gain of 5.0 ± 2.3 kg, translating into a BMI increase of 2.4 ± 1.3 kg/m^2 (Frazier et al., 2001). In a more recent open-label study of 15 preschoolers (mean age = 5.0 years), 8 weeks of olanzapine treatment was associated with a weight increase of 3.2 ± 0.7 kg or 12.9 ± 7.1% baseline body weight. It was not reported whether or not this change was significant (Biederman, Mick, Hammerness, 2005).

Quetiapine

In a randomized 4-week trial, quetiapine treatment in 25 adolescents (mean age = 15.0 years) was associated with 4.4 ± 5.0 kg weight gain (DelBello et al., 2006). Although it was not reported whether or not this change was significant compared with baseline, the weight gain was not significantly

TABLE 18.5. Studies Reporting on Atypical-Antipsychotic-Induced Weight Gain in Pediatric Patients with Bipolar Disorder

Atypical antipsychotic (N = 10, n = 225)	First author(s) (year)	Design	N^a	Age in years (range)	Duration in weeks[b] (mean)	Dropout (%)	Dose (mg/day)	Weight gain (kg)	Comparator	p
Antipsychotic monotherapy (N = 7, n = 152)										
Aripiprazole (n = 14)	Barzman (2004)	CR	14	13.0 (5–19)	17.6 (17.6)	N/A	10.0 ± 3.0	-3.0 ± 6.0	Baseline	NR
Clozapine (n = 10)	Masi (2002)	CR	10	14.8 (12–17)	24 (24)	N/A	142.5	7.0 ± 3.1 [10.7%]	Baseline	NR
Olanzapine (n = 38)	Frazier (2001)	OL	23	10.3 (5–14)	8 (7.9[c])	4.3	9.6 ± 4.3	5.0 ± 2.3 (BMI: 2.4 ± 1.3 kg/m^2)	Baseline	.001
	Biederman, Mick, Hammerness (2005)	OL	15	5.0 (4–6)	8 (NR)	40.0	6.3 ± 2.3	3.2 ± 0.7 (12.9 ± 7.1%)	Baseline	NR
Quetiapine (n = 44)	DelBello (2006)	DBRC	25	15.0 (12–18)	4 (3.4[c])	24.0	412 ± 83	4.4 ± 5.0	VPA: 3.6 ± 6.0 kg	.2
	Marchand (2004)	CR	19	10.8 (4–17)	24.4 (24.4)	N/A	397 ± 221	(BMI: 0.8 kg/m^2)	Baseline	NS
Risperidone (n = 46)	Biederman, Mick, Hammerness (2005)	OL	16	5.3 (4–6)	8 (NR)	6.2	1.4 ± 0.5	2.2 ± 0.4 (10.1 ± 6.1%)	Baseline	NR

(cont.)

TABLE 18.5. (continued)

Atypical antipsychotic (N = 10, n = 22.5)	First author(s) (year)	Design	N[a]	Age in years (range)	Duration in weeks[b] (mean)	Dropout (%)	Dose (mg/day)	Weight gain (kg)	Comparator	p
	Biederman, Mick, Wozniak (2005)	OL	30	10.6 (6–17)	8 (NR)	26.7	1.2 ± 1.5	2.1 ± 2.0	Baseline	.001
Antipsychotic–mood-stabilizer combination therapy (N = 3, n = 73)										
Quetiapine + divalproex (n = 15)	DelBello, Schwiers (2002)	DBRC	15	14.3 (12–18)	6 (4.7[c])	46.7	432 (DVPX: 104 µg/mL)	4.2 ± 3.2	VPA: 2.5 ± 2.1 kg	NS
Risperidone + divalproex (n = 20)	Pavuluri (2004)	OLR	20	12.1 (5–18)	24 (> 20)	0.0	0.7 ± 0.7	6.0 ± 3.8	Baseline	NR
Risperidone + lithium (n = 38)	Pavuluri (2004)	OLR	17	12.1 (5–18)	24 (12.2[c])	58.8	0.7 ± 0.7	6.8 ± 4.2	Baseline	NR
	Pavuluri (2006)	OL	21	10.5 (4–17)	44 (19.1[d])	NR	1.0 ± 0.5 (Li: 775 ± 400; 0.87 mEq/L)	3.7[d]	CDC growth curve Li: 3.3 kg	NS 0.34

Note. Adapted from Correll (2007). Copyright 2007 by the American Academy of Child and Adolescent Psychiatry. Adapted by permission. CR, chart review; DBRC, double-blind randomized controlled; N/A, not applicable; NR, not reported; NS, not significant; OL, open label; OLR, open label randomized; VPA, valproate; DVPX, divalproex; Li, lithium; CDC, Centers for Disease Control.

[a]Patient n may be larger in a given study, but only patients on index medication with data on weight gain are included.

[b]In ascending order of trial duration.

[c]Calculated.

[d]Individual data for lithium + risperidone group provided by the author (Pavuluri, personal communication, July 11, 2006).

374

different from divalproex treatment alone (3.6 ± 6.0). In a chart review study of 19 children and adolescents (mean age = 10.8 years), 24 weeks of quetiapine treatment were associated with a mean increase in BMI of 0.8 kg/m², which was not significant compared with baseline (DelBello, Schwiers, et al., 2002).

Risperidone

In an 8-week open-label trial of 16 preschoolers (mean age = 5.3 years), risperidone treatment was associated with a weight gain of 2.2 ± 0.4 kg or 10.1 ± 6.1% baseline body weight (Biederman, Mick, Hammerness, et al., 2005). It was not reported whether or not this change was significant compared with baseline. In a second open-label study of 30 children and adolescents (mean age = 10.6 years), weight increased significantly during 8 weeks of risperidone treatment by 2.1 ± 2.0 kg (Biederman, Mick, Wozniak, et al., 2005).

MOOD STABILIZER PLUS ANTIPSYCHOTIC COMBINATION

Three trials reported on weight gain in pediatric patients with bipolar disorder who were receiving combined mood stabilizer–antipsychotic treatment. In a 6-week, double-blind, randomized trial, quetiapine augmentation of divalproex was associated with a mean weight gain of 4.2 ± 3.2 kg in 15 adolescents (mean age = 14.3 years; DelBello, Schwiers, et al., 2002). Although the statistical significance of this weight increase compared with baseline was not reported, the weight gain was not statistically different from the randomized control treatment with quetiapine monotherapy (2.5 ± 2.1 kg). In an open-label study, 37 children and adolescents (mean age = 12.1 years) were sequentially assigned to 24 weeks of combined treatment with either lithium plus divalproex (n = 20) or lithium plus risperidone (n = 17), which were associated with weight gain of 6.0 ± 3.8 kg and 6.8 ± 4.2 kg, respectively (Pavuluri et al., 2004). The significance of this weight change compared with normal development over a 6-month period was not reported. Finally, the same group reported on combined lithium plus risperidone treatment for up to 11 months in 21 children and adolescents (mean age = 10.5 years; Pavuluri et al., 2006). The mean weight gain was 3.7 kg, which was not significant after adjustment for age-appropriate weight gain secondary to growth and similar to the 3.3 kg weight gain over up to 1 year of treatment in the group of 17 youngsters who did not get randomized to risperidone augmentation (Pavuluri et al., 2006; Pavuluri, personal communication, July 12, 2006).

COMPARISON OF WEIGHT GAIN ASSOCIATED WITH CONVENTIONAL MOOD STABILIZER AND SECOND-GENERATION ANTIPSYCHOTIC TREATMENT, ALONE OR IN COMBINATION

Pooling data from short-term trials, the weight gain between each medication class or their combinations was recently compared (Correll, 2007; Figure 18.1). In these analyses, the combined treatment of SGA + mood stabilizer ($N = 2$, $n = 32$, 5.5 ± 1.8) was associated with significantly greater weight gain compared with therapy with one mood stabilizer ($N = 6$, $n = 171$, 1.2 ± 1.9; Student's t test: $p < .05$, Cohen's effect size $d = 2.32$) and compared with therapy with two mood stabilizers ($N = 2$, $n = 128$, 2.1 ± 1.3 kg; Student's t test: $p < .05$, Cohen's effect size $d = 2.17$; Correll, 2007). Even after removal of the study with topiramate monotherapy ($n = 29$) from the mood-stabilizer monotherapy group, SGA + mood stabilizer was still associated with significantly greater weight gain than mood stabilizer treatment alone ($N = 5$, $n = 142$, 1.8 ± 1.3 kg; Student's t test: $p < .05$, Cohen's effect size $d = 2.36$). Short-term treatment with antipsychotic monotherapy ($N = 5$, $n = 109$) was associated with a mean weight gain of 3.4 ± 1.3 kg, which in pairwise comparisons was not significantly greater compared with treatment with SGA + mood stabilizer. Despite the lack of

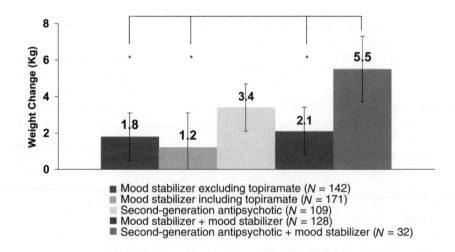

FIGURE 18.1. Comparison of weight gain in patients treated with mood stabilizers, second-generation antipsychotics, combined second-generation antipsychotics + mood stabilizers, and combined mood stabilizers for up to 12 weeks. *$p < .05$ for overall comparison and for combined second-generation antipsychotic + mood stabilizer treatment versus treatment with one mood stabilizer (including or excluding topiramate) and versus treatment with two mood stabilizers. Adapted from Correll (2007). Copyright 2007 by the American Academy of Child and Adolescent Psychiatry. Adapted by permission.

statistical significance for pairwise comparisons, effect sizes of weight gain with SGA therapy versus mood-stabilizer monotherapy or mood-stabilizer combination treatment ranged between 1.0 and 1.35, and combined mood-stabilizer treatment was associated with effect sizes of 0.23–0.55 compared with weight gain with one mood stabilizer alone (Correll, 2007). Unfortunately, in the currently available database, the total number of patients in each medication group during medium-term and long-term treatment is still too small for meaningful comparisons regarding weight effects.

CHANGES IN GLUCOSE METABOLISM ASSOCIATED WITH CONVENTIONAL MOOD STABILIZERS AND SECOND-GENERATION ANTIPSYCHOTICS

Blood glucose and lipid abnormalities, such as elevated triglyceride, total cholesterol, and low-density lipoprotein (LDL) cholesterol levels and/or decreased high-density lipoprotein (HDL) cholesterol levels, are potential consequences of significant weight gain and obesity, as well as of antipsychotic treatment (Henderson et al., 2005; Koro et al., 2002; Lindenmayer et al., 2003; Meyer & Koro, 2004; Newcomer, 2005; Wirshing et al., 2002). Consistent with the weight-related negative effect on glucose and lipid levels in adult populations, in adults olanzapine and clozapine have been associated with hyperglycemia and dyslipidemia (Lindenmayer et al., 2003; Newcomer, 2005).

However, because the mechanisms of antipsychotic-induced weight gain and glucose abnormalities are still unknown, it is also still a matter of debate how much antipsychotic treatment contributes independently to the increased baseline risk of obesity and diabetes/lipid abnormalities found in psychiatric patients. In nonpsychiatric pediatric populations, as in adults, being overweight is clearly linked to a higher incidence of glucose abnormalities and metabolic syndrome (Sinha et al., 2002; Weiss et al., 2004). It remains to be seen, however, whether antipsychotics affect insulin resistance and lipid dysregulation solely via weight gain and increased visceral adiposity or whether at least some antipsychotics can have a direct adverse effect on insulin secretion or glucose transport (Ader et al., 2005; Bergman & Ader, 2005; Henderson et al., 2005). Furthermore, cotreatment of antipsychotics with divalproex may increase the risk for development of diabetes and insulin resistance (Luef et al., 2002; Pylvanen et al., 2003; Roste et al., 2005; Saito & Kafantaris, 2002).

In pediatric populations, data on the adverse effect of SGAs on glucose metabolism (Bloch et al., 2003; Courvoisie, Cooke, & Riddle, 2004; Domon & Cargile, 2002; Domon & Webber, 2001; Koller, Weber, Doraiswamy, & Schneider, 2004; Selva & Scott, 2001) and lipid metabolism (Domon & Cargile, 2002; Domon & Webber, 2001; Martin & L'Ecuyer, 2002; Nguyen & Murphy, 2001) are limited to case reports and one larger retrospective chart review (Martin & L'Ecuyer, 2002). To date, only one published prospective study has reported on glucose and lipid changes in children and adolescents (Biederman, Mick, Hammerness, et al., 2005). In this 8-week, open-label study of preschoolers (mean age = 5.1 years, range 3–6 years) with bipolar disorder, the authors found no significant changes from baseline to end point during treatment with olanzapine ($n = 15$, 6.3 ± 2.3 mg/day) or risperidone ($n = 16$, 1.4 ± 0.5 mg/day). The lack of adverse changes in glucose and lipid levels is surprising, given the effect described in adults, and given the significant increase in weight with risperidone (2.2 ± 0.4 kg, 10.1 ± 6.1%) and olanzapine (3.2 ± 0.7 kg, 12.9 ± 7.1%) in that trial. These findings are also in contrast to significant adverse changes in lipid levels in youths treated with SGAs for a variety of psychiatric disorders (Correll, Parikh, Mughal, Kane, & Malhotra, 2005). However, this discrepancy could be explained by the fact that in this unpublished study laboratory assessments were strictly with fasting, whereas in the study by Biederman, Mick, Hammerness, et al. (2005), the testing appears to have been done without fasting. In addition, the stable glucose finding is also not entirely surprising, as in youngsters with intact pancreatic beta cell reserve, one would not expect to find an initial rise in glucose levels, as this is prevented by compensatory increases in insulin secretion, which is a state of insulin resistance. Presented subanalyses from an ongoing prospective, naturalistic study of antipsychotic-naive children and adolescents ages 5–19 years treated with olanzapine, risperidone, or quetiapine for a variety of psychiatric indications support the notion that SGA treatment in youths can lead to insulin resistance after as little as 3 months of treatment (Correll, Parikh, Mughal, Olshanisky, et al., 2005). Clearly, these findings need to be confirmed and extended in larger samples that include treatments with all available SGAs.

Finally, the metabolic syndrome, described in more detail earlier as a constellation of abdominal obesity, hyperglycemia, hypertension, and lipid abnormalities (Table 18.3), has been found to be more prevalent in adults treated with SGAs than the general public (Almeras et al., 2004; Basu et al., 2004; Cohn, Prud'homme, Streiner, Kameh, & Remington, 2004; Correll, Frederickson, Kane, & Manu, 2006; Heiskanen, Niskanen, Lyytikainen, Saarinen, & Hintikka, 2003; Straker et al., 2005). However, the relationship between atypical antipsychotics and metabolic syndrome has also been disputed, as illness, genetic, and unhealthy lifestyle factors may also be responsible (Mackin, Watkinson, & Young, 2005; Toalson, Ahmed, Hardy, & Kabinoff, 2004). Although, to date, data regarding the prevalence and incidence of metabolic syndrome are entirely lacking in children and adolescents with bipolar disorder or any other psychiatric condition, this risk clearly needs to be considered in youngsters receiving psychotropic medications that can increase weight, as inappropriate weight gain is the major pathway to the metabolic syndrome.

MONITORING STRATEGIES

Table 18.6 summarizes recently proposed monitoring practices for children and adolescents treated with SGAs and/or conventional mood stabilizers (Correll & Carlson, 2006). Monitoring of patients on atypical antipsychotic agents for diabetes should include a baseline fasting blood glucose measurement before the drug is instituted, if possible, and follow-up blood glucose determinations should be performed every 6 months. High-risk patients, that is, patients who are obese or non-Caucasian, who have family histories of diabetes, or who have gained a substantial amount of weight (see Table 18.6) should have fasting blood glucose measurements performed monthly or quarterly. Patients should be asked at each visit about weight loss, polyuria, and polydipsia, which, if present, could indicate the onset of hyperglycemia. A fasting serum lipid panel should be obtained at baseline before drug therapy is begun, at 3 months after starting the drug, and every 6 months thereafter if results are within normal limits and BMI percentile values are stable. Body height and weight should be measured at each visit and BMI calculated. The regular measurement of body composition is relevant, as several studies have found that early weight gain is predictive of later weight gain (Kinon, Kaiser, Ahmed, Rotelli, & Kollack-Walker, 2005). Thus patients with early significant weight increases should undergo intensive healthy-lifestyle counseling, and a change of treatments to agents with a lower propensity to cause weight gain and metabolic abnormalities should be considered.

Despite the importance of abnormal weight gain and obesity in childhood and adolescence (Dietz & Robinson, 2005), a generally accepted definition of clinically significant weight gain during development does not currently exist. Because it is of importance to determine when the weight gain that can occur with psychotropic medications becomes a health problem, the following set of criteria for clinically significant, abnormal weight gain in children and adolescents who are treated with psychotropic medications has recently been proposed (Correll & Carlson, 2006; Table 18.7).

The relative weight gain of 5% compared with baseline weight during the first 3 months of treatment was chosen because during this relatively short period normal growth does not contribute to weight change in a relevant way and also because this threshold is consistent with recent recommendations in adults (American Diabetes Association et al., 2004). For longer observation periods, however, the weight change needs to be adjusted for sex and age norms. An increase in BMI z score of 0.5 was proposed because Weiss et al. (2004) found that this degree of growth-adjusted weight gain increased the risk for metabolic syndrome by 55%. Finally, youngsters in the "at risk" weight category (i.e., > 85–94.9th BMI percentile) who already have at least one negative weight-related clinical outcome and youths with BMI or waist circumference percentiles in the overweight/obese category are at very high risk for adverse health outcomes and require close

TABLE 18.6. Endocrine and Metabolic Monitoring in Children and Adolescents Treated with Second-Generation Antipsychotics and Mood Stabilizers

Assessments prior to choosing SGA or mood stabilizer	Assessments prior to starting SGA or mood stabilizer	Follow-up assessments	Frequency of follow-up assessments[f]
Personal and family medical history	Height and weight	Height and weight	At each visit
Dietary habits	Blood pressure and pulse	Blood pressure and pulse	Every 3 months
Exercise habits	Fasting blood work[b]	Dietary habits	Monthly for 3 months, then every 3 months
Daytime sedation	Prolactin[c]	Exercise habits	Monthly for 3 months, then every 3 months
Appetite level		Daytime sedation	Monthly for 3 months, then every 3 months
Sexual symptoms/signs		Appetite level	Monthly for 3 months, then 3 months
Height, weight[a]		Sexual symptoms/ signs	Monthly for 3 months, then every 3 months
Blood pressure and pulse[a]		Fasting blood work[b]	At 3 months, then every 6 months
Fasting blood work[a,b]		Prolactin[c]	Only when symptomatic
Prolactin[a,c]		Thyroid-stimulating hormone[d,e]	At 1 month[d], 3 months[e], 6 months[d], and annually
Thyroid-stimulating hormone[a,d,e]		Serum calcium[d]	At 1 month, 6 months, and annually[d]
Serum calcium[a,d]			

Note. From Correll and Carlson (2006). Copyright 2006 by the American Academy of Child and Adolescent Psychiatry. Reprinted by permission.

[a]Optional assessments to inform choice of an SGA; will depend on patient condition and appropriateness of waiting for test results.

[b]Full blood count with differential, serum electrolytes, liver and kidney function, thyroid-stimulating hormone, glucose and lipid profile.

[c]In case of abnormal sexual symptoms or signs; draw fasting in the morning and approximately 12 hours after the last antipsychotic dose.

[d]If started on lithium.

[e]If started on valproic acid or quetiapine.

[f]Earlier and/or more frequent assessments are indicated if patients develop significant weight gain or metabolic abnormalities.

TABLE 18.7. Proposed Criteria for the Definition of Significant Weight Gain/Changes in Body Composition in Children and Adolescents

Duration of treatment	Threshold for significant change in body composition
First 3 months	> 5% of weight increase compared with baseline
Any duration	≥ 0.5 increase in BMI z score
Any duration	Crossing into the "at risk" weight category (i.e., $\geq$ 85–94.9 BMI percentile) *plus* presence of one other obesity-related complication, such as hypertension (i.e., $\geq$ 90th percentile), dyslipidemia (i.e., fasting cholesterol $\geq$ 200 mg/dL, LDL cholesterol $\geq$ 130 mg/dL, HDL cholesterol < 40 mg/dL, or triglycerides $\geq$ 150 mg/dL), hyperglycemia (i.e., fasting glucose $\geq$ 100 mg/dL), insulin resistance (i.e., fasting insulin > 20 µmol/L), orthopedic disorders, sleep disorders, or gall bladder disease
Any duration	Crossing into obesity (i.e., $\geq$ 95th BMI percentile) or abdominal obesity (i.e., $\geq$ 90th waist circumference percentile)

Note. From Correll and Carlson (2006). Copyright 2006 by the American Academy of Child and Adolescent Psychiatry. Reprinted by permission.

monitoring or interventions to reduce the risk, independently of where they started when psychotropic drug treatment began.

MANAGEMENT STRATEGIES

General strategies and principles of weight control described for youths include controlling the environment, monitoring behavior, setting goals, rewarding successful behaviors, identifying and solving problems, and adapting parental skills (Dietz & Robinson, 2005). Specific preventive and interventional strategies aimed at minimizing weight gain and related health problems associated with psychotropic medications are summarized in Table 18.8 (Correll & Carlson, 2006). These strategies include: (1) educating patients about, monitoring, and reinforcing healthy lifestyle behaviors; (2) choosing an agent with a lower likelihood of adverse effects on body composition and metabolic status, ideally at the beginning of treatment or when marked initial weight gain becomes apparent; and (3) initiating a formalized, nonpharmacological weight loss treatment (e.g., special diet, Weight Watchers, behavioral weight management program, etc.) or pharmacological intervention, in case the first and second steps insufficiently addressed weight gain and metabolic complications. Therapies that have had some success in producing weight loss in pediatric patients receiving antipsychotics include metformin (Morrison, Cottingham, & Barton, 2002; Klein, Cottingham, Sorter, Barton & Morrison, 2006), topiramate (DelBello et al., 2005), amantadine (Gracious, Krysiak, & Youngstrom, 2002), and orlistat (Chanoine,

TABLE 18.8. Strategies for the Prevention and Management of Weight Gain
and the Metabolic Abnormalities in Patients Receiving Psychotropic Medications

I. Healthy lifestyle behaviors
   1. Replace all drinks containing sugar (soda, punch, juice), "diet" drinks, and whole
      milk with at least 2 L of water and moderate amounts of unsweetened tea or low-
      fat milk.
   2. Eat every 3–4 hours, with no more than 2 meals in the evening or at night.
   3. Eat small portions at each meal.
   4. Eat breakfast every morning.
   5. Eat slowly, drink an ample amount of water between bites, and take second helpings
      only after a delay.
   6. Eat no more than one fast-food meal per week.
   7. Replace refined white flour and processed sugar products with whole-grain and
      other food items that have a low glycemic index (i.e., of 55 or less;
      http://www.glycemicindex.com)
   8. Do not snack when full and replace high-fat, high-calorie snacks with ample
      amounts of fruits or vegetables.
   9. Limit saturated fat intake, but avoid extensive consumption of processed
      fat-free food items.
   10. Eat at least 25–30 grams of soluble fiber from fruits, vegetables, and/or whole grains
      per day.
   11. Limit watching TV or playing computer/video games to less than 2 hours per day.
   12. Perform moderate to vigorous physical activity for at least 30–60 minutes/day.

II. Medication choice
   1. Avoid starting treatment with medications that are associated with marked or
      extreme weight gain.
   2. Consider switching to an agent that is associated with less weight gain potential.

III. Additional weight-loss treatment (if weight gain/obesity remain problematic despite the
   first and second strategies)
   1. Initiate/refer to formalized, nonpharmacological weight-loss program.
   2. Initiate adjunctive pharmacological weight-loss treatment.

Note. From Correll and Carlson (2006). Copyright 2006 by the American Academy of Child and Adolescent Psychiatry. Reprinted by permission.

Hampl, Jensen, Boldrin, & Hauptman, 2005). Dyslipidemia should be treated
initially with dietary measures. If this is not sufficient, a referral to a specialist
may become necessary, and drug therapy may include a fibric acid derivative
(gemfibrozil or fenofibrate), a statin, fish oil, or niacin. Once diabetes devel-
ops, patients should be comanaged with a pediatric specialist and may be
treated with diet, oral hypoglycemic agents, or insulin, as needed. However, it
should also be remembered that diabetes induced by antipsychotics may
sometimes disappear when the drug is stopped or changed (Cheng-Shannon,
McGough, Pataki, & McCraken, 2004; Domon & Webber, 2001).

For the prevention of weight gain and related metabolic complications,
the initial choice of a psychotropic agent with the least negative impact, as
well as healthy-lifestyle counseling and promoting healthy diet and regular

exercise, should be an integral part of any treatment with a mood stabilizer or antipsychotic medication. Therapeutic lifestyle changes have shown modest efficacy in reducing weight gain that has already occurred in adults (Ball et al., 2003; Menza et al., 2004; Vreeland et al., 2003), and these measures may be even more effective in the prevention or attenuation of weight gain due to psychotropic medications, particularly in normal-weight individuals who have not yet failed multiple attempts at implementing therapeutic lifestyle changes. However, data on the effectiveness of healthy lifestyle intervention in youths treated with weight-inducing psychotropic medications are lacking.

For these strategies to be successful, interventions have to be simple, realistic, and measurable. Moreover, the entire family system should be involved (Hopper, Munoz, Gruber, & Nguyen, 2005). Not unsurprisingly, studies have shown strong associations between parental BMI, food intake, and attitudes toward activity and those observed in their children (Davison & Birch, 2001; Francis, Lee, & Birch, 2003). Furthermore, the entire spectrum of unhealthy lifestyle behaviors should be targeted in youngsters and their parents, as focusing on the remediation of just one aspect of weight-gain-promoting behavior, such as a high-fat diet, for example, is easily counterbalanced by other behaviors, such as deriving up to one-third of daily calories from fast food, snacks, and desserts (Van Horn, Obarzanek, Friedman, Gernhofer, & Barton, 2005). In general, to limit weight gain associated with psychotropic medications, parents and children should pay attention to the amount, frequency, and type of foods and drinks consumed. At the same time, families should decrease the amount of sedentary behaviors and increase exercise.

CONCLUSIONS

Conventional mood stabilizers and SGAs that are central to the treatment of bipolar disorder are frequently associated with significant weight gain. In addition, vulnerable patient groups are also at risk for the development of abnormalities in blood sugar and blood lipids. Adults with bipolar disorder and, most likely even more so, pediatric patients are prone to these adverse events. Importantly, in youths such medication effects occur in the context of physiological changes in hormonal and endocrine levels and body composition. Practically, this means that normal adult values have to be adjusted to account for age- and sex-appropriate developmental changes. These include use of the BMI percentiles or z scores instead of weight or BMI to assess the youngster's body composition. In addition, lipid thresholds need to be adjusted and percentile cutoffs are to be used for waist circumference and blood pressure. In view of the long-term consequences of age-inappropriate weight gain and metabolic abnormalities, pediatric patients require a careful selection of lower-risk treatments, regular monitoring, and early interventions to mitigate anthropometric and metabolic adverse events that can have detrimental effects on long-term health and survival. Management of these vulnerable youngsters needs to be individualized by weighing risks and benefits of specific medications against the often devastating effects of untreated or suboptimally treated bipolar disorder.

ACKNOWLEDGMENTS

This work was supported by the Zucker Hillside Hospital National Institute of Mental Health Advanced Center for Intervention and Services Research for the Study of Schizophrenia (Grant No. MH 074543-01) and the NSLIJ Research Institute National Institutes of Health General Clinical Research Center (Grant No. MO1RR018535). I would like to thank Hanna M. Kester for her assistance with the manuscript.

REFERENCES

Ader, M., Kim, S. P., Catalano, K. J., Ionut, V., Hucking, K., Richey, J. M., et al. (2005). Metabolic dysregulation with atypical antipsychotics occurs in the absence of underlying disease: A placebo-controlled study of olanzapine and risperidone in dogs. *Diabetes, 54*, 862–871.

Allison, D. B., & Casey, D. E. (2001). Antipsychotic-induced weight gain: A review of the literature. *Journal of Clinical Psychiatry, 62*(Suppl. 7), 22–31.

Allison, D. B., Mentore, J. L., Heo, M., Chandler, L. P., Cappelleri, J. C., Infante, M. C., et al. (1999). Antipsychotic-induced weight gain: A comprehensive research synthesis. *American Journal of Psychiatry, 156*, 1686–1696.

Almeras, N., Despres, J. P., Villeneuve, J., Demers, M. F., Roy, M. A., Cadrin, C., et al. (2004). Development of an atherogenic metabolic risk factor profile associated with the use of atypical antipsychotics. *Journal of Clinical Psychiatry, 65*, 557–564.

Aman, M. G., Binder, C., & Turgay, A. (2004). Risperidone effects in the presence/absence of psychostimulant medicine in children with ADHD, other disruptive behavior disorders, and subaverage IQ. *Journal of Child and Adolescent Psychopharmacology, 14*, 243–254.

American Diabetes Association. (2006). Position statement on the diagnosis and classification of diabetes mellitus. *Diabetes Care, 29*, S43–S48.

American Diabetes Association; American Psychiatric Association; American Association of Clinical Endocrinologists; North American Association for the Study of Obesity. (2004). Consensus Development Conference on Antipsychotic Drugs and Obesity and Diabetes. (2004). *Journal of Clinical Psychiatry, 65*, 267–272.

Ascher-Svanum, H., Stensland, M., Zhao, Z., & Kinon, B. J. (2005). Acute weight gain, gender, and therapeutic response to antipsychotics in the treatment of patients with schizophrenia. *BMC Psychiatry, 5*, 3.

Ball, S. D., Keller, K. R., Moyer-Mileur, L. J., Ding, Y. W., Donaldson, D., & Jackson, W. D. (2003). Prolongation of satiety after low versus moderately high glycemic index meals in obese adolescents. *Pediatrics, 111*, 488–494.

Bao, W., Srinivasan, S. R., Wattigney, W. A., & Berenson, G. S. (1994). Persistence of multiple cardiovascular risk clustering related to syndrome X from childhood to young adulthood: The Bogalusa Heart Study. *Archives of Internal Medicine, 154*, 1842–1847.

Barzman, D. H., DelBello, M. P., Kowatch, R. A., Gernert, B., Fleck, D. E., Pathak, S., et al. (2004). The effectiveness and tolerability of aripiprazole for pediatric bipolar disorders: A retrospective chart review. *Journal of Child and Adolescent Psychopharmacology, 14,* 593–600.

Basu, R., Brar, J. S., Chengappa, K. N., John, V., Parepally, H., Gershon, S., et al. (2004). The prevalence of the metabolic syndrome in patients with schizoaffective disorder—bipolar subtype. *Bipolar Disorders, 6,* 314–318.

Berenson, G. S., Srinivasan, S. R., Bao, W., Newman, W. P., III, Tracy, R. E., & Wattigney, W. A. (1998). Association between multiple cardiovascular risk factors and atherosclerosis in children and young adults: The Bogalusa Heart Study. *New England Journal of Medicine, 338,* 1650–1656.

Bergman, R. N., & Ader, M. (2005). Atypical antipsychotics and glucose homeostasis. *Journal of Clinical Psychiatry, 66,* 504–514.

Biederman, J., Faraone, S. V., Wozniak, J., Mick, E., Kwon, A., & Aleardi, M. (2004). Further evidence of unique developmental phenotypic correlates of pediatric bipolar disorder: Findings from a large sample of clinically referred preadolescent children assessed over the last 7 years. *Journal of Affective Disorders, 82*(Suppl. 1), S45–S58.

Biederman, J., Mick, E., Hammerness, P., Harpold, T., Aleardi, M., Dougherty, M., et al. (2005). Open-label, 8-week trial of olanzapine and risperidone for the treatment of bipolar disorder in preschool-age children. Biological Psychiatry, *58,* 589–594.

Biederman, J., Mick, E., Wozniak, J., Aleardi, M., Spencer, T., Faraone, S. V. (2005), An open-label trial of risperidone in children and adolescents with bipolar disorder. *Journal of Child and Adolescent Psychopharmacology, 15,* 311–317.

Bloch, Y., Vardi, O., Mendlovic, S., Levkovitz, Y., Gothelf, D., & Ratzoni, G. (2003). Hyperglycemia from olanzapine treatment in adolescents. *Journal of Child and Adolescent Psychopharmacology, 13,* 97–102.

Bray, G. A. (2004). Medical consequences of obesity. *Journal of Clinical Endocrinology and Metabolism, 89,* 2583–2589.

Brown, S., Inskip, H., & Barraclough, B. (2000). Causes of the excess mortality of schizophrenia. *British Journal of Psychiatry, 177,* 212–217.

Calabrese, J. R., Hirschfeld, R. M., Reed, M., Davies, M. A., Frye, M. A., Keck, P. E., et al. (2003). Impact of bipolar disorder on a U.S. community sample. *Journal of Clinical Psychiatry, 64,* 425–432.

Carlson, G. A., & Meyer, S. E. (2000). Bipolar disorder in youth. *Current Psychiatry Reports, 2,* 90–94.

Casey, D. E., Haupt, D. W., Newcomer, J. W., Henderson, D. C., Sernyak, M. J., Davidson, M., et al. (2004). Antipsychotic-induced weight gain and metabolic abnormalities: Implications for increased mortality in patients with schizophrenia. *Journal of Clinical Psychiatry, 65*(Suppl. 7), 4–20.

Chang, K., Saxena, K., & Howe, M. (2006). An open-label study of lamotrigine adjunct or monotherapy for the treatment of adolescents with bipolar depression. *Journal of the American Academy of Child and Adolescent Psychiatry, 45,* 298–304.

Chanoine, J. P., Hampl, S., Jensen, C., Boldrin, M., & Hauptman, J. (2005). Effect of orlistat on weight and body composition in obese adolescents: A randomized controlled trial. *Journal of the American Medical Association, 293,* 2873–2883.

Cheng-Shannon, J., McGough, J. J., Pataki, C., & McCracken, J. T. (2004). Second-generation antipsychotic medications in children and adolescents. *Journal of Child and Adolescent Psychopharmacology, 14,* 372–394.

Cohn, T., Prud'homme, D., Streiner, D., Kameh, H., & Remington, G. (2004). Characterizing coronary heart disease risk in chronic schizophrenia: High prevalence of the metabolic syndrome. *Canadian Journal of Psychiatry, 49,* 753–760.

Cook, S., Weitzman, M., Auinger, P., Nguyen, M., & Dietz, W. H. (2003). Prevalence of a metabolic syndrome phenotype in adolescents: Findings from the third National Health and

Nutrition Examination Survey, 1988–1994. *Archives of Pediatric and Adolescent Medicine, 157,* 821–827.

Cooper, W. O., Arbogast, P. G., Ding, H., Hickson, G. B., Fuchs, D. C., & Ray, W. A. (2006). Trends in prescribing of antipsychotic medications for U.S. children. *Ambulatory Pediatrics, 6,* 79–83.

Cooper, W. O., Hickson, G. B., Fuchs, C., Arbogast, P. G., & Ray, W. A. (2004). New users of antipsychotic medications among children enrolled in TennCare. *Archives of Pediatric and Adolescent Medicine, 158,* 753–759.

Correll, C. U. (2005). Metabolic side effects of second-generation antipsychotics in children and adolescents: A different story? *Journal of Clinical Psychiatry, 66,* 1331–1332.

Correll, C. U. (2007). Weight gain and metabolic effects of mood stabilizers and antipsychotics in pediatric bipolar disorder: A systematic review and pooled analysis of short-term trials. *Journal of the American Academy of Child and Adolescent Psychiatry, 46*(6), 687–700.

Correll, C. U., & Carlson, H. E. (2006). Endocrine and metabolic adverse effects of psychotropic medications in children and adolescents. *Journal of the American Academy of Child and Adolescent Psychiatry, 45,* 771–791.

Correll, C. U., Frederickson, A. M., Kane, J. M., & Manu, P. (2006). Metabolic syndrome and the risk of coronary heart disease in 367 patients treated with second-generation antipsychotic drugs. *Journal of Clinical Psychiatry, 67,* 575–583.

Correll, C. U., Leucht, S., & Kane, J. M. (2004). Lower risk for tardive dyskinesia associated with second-generation antipsychotics: A systematic review of 1-year studies. *American Journal of Psychiatry, 161,* 414–425.

Correll, C. U., Parikh, U. H., Mughal, T., Kane, J. M., & Malhotra, A. K. (2005). New onset dyslipidemia in antipsychotic-naive youngsters treated with atypical antipsychotics. *Biological Psychiatry, 57,* 36.

Correll, C. U., Parikh, U. H., Mughal, T., Olshanisky, V., Moroff, M., Pleak, R. R., et al. (2005). Development of insulin resistance in antipsychotic-naive youngsters treated with novel antipsychotics. *Biological Psychiatry, 57,* 35–36.

Courvoisie, H. E., Cooke, D. W., & Riddle, M. A. (2004). Olanzapine-induced diabetes in a seven-year-old boy. *Journal of Child and Adolescent Psychopharmacology, 14,* 612–616.

Czobor, P., Volavka, J., Sheitman, B., Lindenmayer, J. P., Citrome, L., McEvoy, J., et al. (2002). Antipsychotic-induced weight gain and therapeutic response: A differential association. *Journal of Clinical Psychopharmacology, 22,* 244–251.

Davison, K. K., & Birch, L. L. (2001). Weight status, parent reaction, and self-concept in five-year-old girls. *Pediatrics, 107,* 46–53.

de Ferranti, S. D., Gauvreau, K., Ludwig, D. S., Neufeld, E. J., Newburger, J. W., & Rifai, N. (2004). Prevalence of the metabolic syndrome in American adolescents: Findings from the third National Health and Nutrition Examination Survey. *Circulation, 110,* 2494–2497.

DelBello, M. P., Findling, R. L., Kushner, S., Wang, D., Olson, W. H., Capece, J. A., et al. (2005). A pilot controlled trial of topiramate for mania in children and adolescents with bipolar disorder. *Journal of the American Academy of Child and Adolescent Psychiatry, 44,* 539–547.

DelBello, M. P., Kowatch, R. A., Adler, C. M., Stanford, K. E., Welge, J. A., Barzman, D. H., et al. (2006). A double-blind randomized pilot study comparing quetiapine and divalproex for adolescent mania. *Journal of the American Academy of Child and Adolescent Psychiatry, 45,* 305–313.

DelBello, M. P., Kowatch, R. A., Warner, J., Schwiers, M. L., Rappaport, K. B., Daniels, J. P., et al. (2002). Adjunctive topiramate treatment for pediatric bipolar disorder: A retrospective chart review. *Journal of Child and Adolescent Psychopharmacology, 12,* 323–330.

DelBello, M. P., Schwiers, M. L., Rosenberg, H. L., & Strakowski, S. M. (2002). A double-blind, randomized, placebo-controlled study of quetiapine as adjunctive treatment for adolescent mania. *Journal of the American Academy of Child and Adolescent Psychiatry, 41,* 1216–1223.

Dietz, W. H., & Robinson, T. N. (2005). Clinical practice: Overweight children and adolescents. *New England Journal of Medicine, 352,* 2100–2109.

Domon, S. E., & Cargile, C. S. (2002). Quetiapine-associated hyperglycemia and hypertriglyceridemia. *Journal of the American Academy of Child and Adolescent Psychiatry, 41,* 495–496.

Domon, S. E., & Webber, J. C. (2001). Hyperglycemia and hypertriglyceridemia secondary to olanzapine. *Journal of Child and Adolescent Psychopharmacology, 11,* 285–288.

Duncan, G. E., Li, S. M., & Zhou, X. H. (2004). Prevalence and trends of a metabolic syndrome phenotype among U.S. adolescents, 1999–2000. *Diabetes Care, 27,* 2438–2443.

Ebbeling, C. B., Pawlak, D. B., & Ludwig, D. S. (2002). Childhood obesity: Public-health crisis, common sense cure. *Lancet, 360,* 473–482.

Executive summary of the third report of the National Cholesterol Education Program (NCEP) Expert Panel on Detection, Evaluation, and Treatment of High Blood Cholesterol in Adults (Adult Treatment Panel III). (2001). *Journal of the American Medical Association, 285,* 2486–2497.

Fedorowicz, V. J., & Fombonne, E. (2005). Metabolic side effects of atypical antipsychotics in children: A literature review. *Journal of Psychopharmacology, 19,* 533–550.

Fernandez, J. R., Redden, D. T., Pietrobelli, A., & Allison, D. B. (2004). Waist circumference percentiles in nationally representative samples of African-American, European-American, and Mexican-American children and adolescents. *Journal of Pediatrics, 145,* 439–444.

Findling, R. L. (2005). Update on the treatment of bipolar disorder in children and adolescents. *Euopean Psychiatry, 20,* 87–91.

Findling, R. L., & Calabrese, J. R. (2000). Rapid-cycling bipolar disorder in children. *American Journal of Psychiatry, 157,* 1526–1527.

Findling, R. L., Gracious, B. L., McNamara, N. K., Youngstrom, E. A., Demeter, C. A., Branicky, L. A., et al. (2001). Rapid, continuous cycling and psychiatric co-morbidity in pediatric bipolar I disorder. *Bipolar Disorders, 3,* 202–210.

Findling, R. L., McNamara, N. K., Gracious, B. L., Youngstrom, E. A., Stansbrey, R. J., Reed, M.D., et al. (2003). Combination lithium and divalproex sodium in pediatric bipolarity. *Journal of the American Academy of Child and Adolescent Psychiatry, 42,* 895–901.

Findling, R. L., McNamara, N. K., Stansbrey, R., Gracious, B. L., Whipkey, R. E., Demeter, C. A., et al. (2006). Combination lithium and divalproex sodium in pediatric bipolar symptom re-stabilization. *Journal of the American Academy of Child and Adolescent Psychiatry, 45,* 142–148.

Findling, R. L., Steiner, H., & Weller, E. B. (2005). Use of antipsychotics in children and adolescents. *Journal of Clinical Psychiatry, 66*(Suppl. 7), 29–40.

Fontaine, K. R., Redden, D. T., Wang, C., Westfall, A. O., & Allison, D. B. (2003). Years of life lost due to obesity. *Journal of the American Medical Association, 289,* 187–193.

Fourth report on the diagnosis, evaluation, and treatment of high blood pressure in children and adolescents. (2004). *Pediatrics, 114,* 555–576.

Francis, L. A., Lee, Y., & Birch, L. L. (2003). Parental weight status and girls' television viewing, snacking, and body mass indexes. *Obesity Research, 11,* 143–151.

Frazier, J. A., Biederman, J., Tohen, M., Feldman, P. D., Jacobs, T. G., Toma, V., et al. (2001). A prospective open-label treatment trial of olanzapine monotherapy in children and adolescents with bipolar disorder. *Journal of Child and Adolescent Psychopharmacology, 11,* 239–250.

Freedman, D. S., Khan, L. K., Serdula, M. K., Dietz, W. H., Srinivasan, S. R., & Berenson, G. S. (2005). The relation of childhood BMI to adult adiposity: The Bogalusa Heart Study. *Pediatrics, 115,* 22–27.

Geller, B., Craney, J. L., Bolhofner, K., Nickelsburg, M. J., Williams, M., & Zimerman, B. (2002). Two-year prospective follow-up of children with a prepubertal and early adolescent bipolar disorder phenotype. *American Journal of Psychiatry, 159,* 927–933.

Goldberg, J. F., & Ernst, C. L. (2002). Features associated with the delayed initiation of mood stabilizers at illness onset in bipolar disorder. *Journal of Clinical Psychiatry, 63,* 985–991.

Goldberg, J. F., & Harrow, M. (2004). Consistency of remission and outcome in bipolar and unipolar mood disorders: A 10-year prospective follow-up. *Journal of Affective Disorders*, *81*, 123–131.

Gracious, B. L., Krysiak, T. E., & Youngstrom, E. A. (2002). Amantadine treatment of psychotropic-induced weight gain in children and adolescents: Case series. *Journal of Child and Adolescent Psychopharmacology*, *12*, 249–257.

Grundy, S. M. (2004). What is the contribution of obesity to the metabolic syndrome? *Endocrinology and Metabolism Clinics of North America*, *33*, 267–282.

Grundy, S. M., Cleeman, J. I., Daniels, S. R., Donato, K. A., Eckel, R. H., Franklin, B. A., et al. (2005). Diagnosis and management of the metabolic syndrome: An American Heart Association/National Heart, Lung, and Blood Institute scientific statement. *Circulation*, *112*, 2735–2752.

Guo, S. S., Roche, A. F., Chumlea, W. C., Gardner, J. D., & Siervogel, R. M. (1994). The predictive value of childhood body mass index values for overweight at age 35 y. *American Journal of Clinical Nutrition*, *59*, 810–819.

Guo, S. S., Wu, W., Chumlea, W. C., & Roche, A. F. (2002). Predicting overweight and obesity in adulthood from body mass index values in childhood and adolescence. *American Journal of Clinical Nutrition*, *76*, 653–658.

Heiskanen, T., Niskanen, L., Lyytikainen, R., Saarinen, P. I., & Hintikka, J. (2003). Metabolic syndrome in patients with schizophrenia. *Journal of Clinical Psychiatry*, *64*, 575–579.

Henderson, D. C., Cagliero, E., Copeland, P. M., Borba, C. P., Evins, E., Hayden, D., et al. (2005). Glucose metabolism in patients with schizophrenia treated with atypical antipsychotic agents: A frequently sampled intravenous glucose tolerance test and minimal model analysis. *Archives of General Psychiatry*, *62*, 19–28.

Hennen, J., Perlis, R. H., Sachs, G., Tohen, M., & Baldessarini, R. J. (2004). Weight gain during treatment of bipolar I patients with olanzapine. *Journal of Clinical Psychiatry*, *65*, 1679–1687.

Hopper, C. A., Munoz, K. D., Gruber, M. B., & Nguyen, K. P. (2005). The effects of a family fitness program on the physical activity and nutrition behaviors of third-grade children. *Research Quarterly for Exercise and Sport*, *76*, 130–139.

Kafantaris, V., Coletti, D. J., Dicker, R., Padula, G., & Kane, J. M. (2003). Lithium treatment of acute mania in adolescents: A large open trial. *Journal of the American Academy of Child and Adolescent Psychiatry*, *42*, 1038–1045.

Kane, J. M. (2001). Extrapyramidal side effects are unacceptable. *Euopean Neuropsychopharmacology*, *11*(Suppl. 4), S397–403.

Keck, P. E., & McElroy, S. L. (2003). Bipolar disorder, obesity, and pharmacotherapy-associated weight gain. *Journal of Clinical Psychiatry*, *64*, 1426–1435.

Kinon, B. J., Kaiser, C. J., Ahmed, S., Rotelli, M. D., & Kollack-Walker, S. (2005). Association between early and rapid weight gain and change in weight over one year of olanzapine therapy in patients with schizophrenia and related disorders. *Journal of Clinical Psychopharmacology*, *25*, 255–258.

Klein, D. J., Cottingham, E. M., Sorter, M., Barton, B. A., & Morrison, J. A. (2006). A randomized, double-blind, placebo-controlled trial of metformin treatment of weight gain associated with initiation of atypical antipsychotic therapy in children and adolescents. *American Journal of Psychiatry*, *163*, 2072–2079.

Koller, E. A., Weber, J., Doraiswamy, P. M., & Schneider, B. S. (2004). A survey of reports of quetiapine-associated hyperglycemia and diabetes mellitus. *Journal of Clinical Psychiatry*, *65*, 857–863.

Koro, C. E., Fedder, D. O., L'Italien, G. J., Weiss, S., Magder, L. S., Kreyenbuhl, J., et al. (2002). An assessment of the independent effects of olanzapine and risperidone exposure on the risk of hyperlipidemia in schizophrenic patients. *Archives of General Psychiatry*, *59*, 1021–1026.

Krebs, N. F., & Jacobson, M. S. (2003). Prevention of pediatric overweight and obesity. *Pediatrics*, *112*, 424–430.

Leibenluft, E., Charney, D. S., & Pine, D. S. (2003). Researching the pathophysiology of pediatric bipolar disorder. *Biological Psychiatry*, *53*, 1009–1020.

Li, S., Chen, W., Srinivasan, S. R., Bond, M. G., Tang, R., Urbina, E. M., et al. (2003). Childhood cardiovascular risk factors and carotid vascular changes in adulthood: The Bogalusa Heart Study. *Journal of the American Medical Association, 290*, 2271–2276.

Lindenmayer, J. P., Czobor, P., Volavka, J., Citrome, L., Sheitman, B., McEvoy, J. P., et al. (2003). Changes in glucose and cholesterol levels in patients with schizophrenia treated with typical or atypical antipsychotics. *American Journal of Psychiatry, 160*, 290–296.

Lish, J. D., Dime-Meenan, S., Whybrow, P. C., Price, R. A., & Hirschfeld, R. M. (1994). The National Depressive and Manic-Depressive Association (DMDA) survey of bipolar members. *Journal of Affective Disorders, 31*, 281–294.

Luef, G., Abraham, I., Hoppichler, F., Trinka, E., Unterberger, I., Bauer, G., et al. (2002). Increase in postprandial serum insulin levels in epileptic patients with valproic acid therapy. *Metabolism, 51*, 1274–1278.

Mackin, P., Watkinson, H. M., & Young, A. H. (2005). Prevalence of obesity, glucose homeostasis disorders and metabolic syndrome in psychiatric patients taking typical or atypical antipsychotic drugs: A cross-sectional study. *Diabetologia, 48*, 215–221.

Marchand, W. R., Wirth, L., & Simon, C. (2004). Quetiapine adjunctive and monotherapy for pediatric bipolar disorder: A retrospective chart review. *Journal of Child and Adolescent Psychopharmacology, 14*(3), 405–411.

Martin, A., & L'Ecuyer, S. (2002). Triglyceride, cholesterol and weight changes among risperidone-treated youths: A retrospective study. *Euopean Child and Adolescent Psychiatry, 11*, 129–133.

Masi, G., Cosenza, A., Mucci, M., & Brovedani, P. (2003). A 3-year naturalistic study of 53 preschool children with pervasive developmental disorders treated with risperidone. *Journal of Clinical Psychiatry, 64*, 1039–1047.

Masi, G., Mucci, M., & Millepiedi, S. (2002). Clozapine in adolescent inpatients with acute mania. *Journal of Child and Adolescent Psychopharmacology, 12*, 93–99.

McIntyre, R. S., Konarski, J. Z., Misener, V. L., & Kennedy, S. H. (2005). Bipolar disorder and diabetes mellitus: Epidemiology, etiology, and treatment implications. *Annals of Clinical Psychiatry, 17*, 83–93.

Menza, M., Vreeland, B., Minsky, S., Gara, M., Radler, D. R., & Sakowitz, M. (2004). Managing atypical antipsychotic-associated weight gain: 12-month data on a multimodal weight control program. *Journal of Clinical Psychiatry, 65*, 471–477.

Meyer, J. M., & Koro, C. E. (2004). The effects of antipsychotic therapy on serum lipids: A comprehensive review. *Schizophrenia Research, 70*, 1–17.

Morrison, J. A., Cottingham, E. M., & Barton, B. A. (2002). Metformin for weight loss in pediatric patients taking psychotropic drugs. *American Journal of Psychiatry, 159*, 655–657.

Morriss, R., & Mohammed, F. A. (2005). Metabolism, lifestyle and bipolar affective disorder. *Journal of Psychopharmacology, 19*, 94–101.

Must, A., Jacques, P. F., Dallal, G. E., Bajema, C. J., & Dietz, W. H. (1992). Long-term morbidity and mortality of overweight adolescents: A follow-up of the Harvard Growth Study of 1922 to 1935. *New England Journal of Medicine, 327*, 1350–1355.

Must, A., & Strauss, R. S. (1999). Risks and consequences of childhood and adolescent obesity. *International Journal of Obesity and Related Metabolic Disorders, 23*(Suppl. 2), S2–S11.

Newcomer, J. W. (2005). Second-generation (atypical) antipsychotics and metabolic effects: A comprehensive literature review. *CNS Drugs, 19*(Suppl. 1), 1–93.

Nguyen, M., & Murphy, T. (2001). Olanzapine and hypertriglyceridemia. *Journal of the American Academy of Child and Adolescent Psychiatry, 40*, 133.

Olfson, M., Blanco, C., Liu, L., Moreno, C., & Laje, G. (2006). National trends in the outpatient treatment of children and adolescents with antipsychotic drugs. *Archives of General Psychiatry, 63*, 679–685.

Osby, U., Correia, N., Brandt, L., Ekbom, A., & Sparen, P. (2000). Mortality and causes of death in schizophrenia in Stockholm county, Sweden. *Schizophrenia Research, 45*, 21–28.

Patel, N. C., Hariparsad, M., Matias-Akthar, M., Sorter, M. T., Barzman, D. H., Morrison, J. A., et al. (2007). Body mass indexes and lipid profiles in hospitalized children and adolescents exposed to atypical antipsychotics. *Journal of Child and Adolescent Psychopharmacology, 17*, 303–311.

Pavuluri, M. N., Henry, D. B., Carbray, J. A., Naylor, M. W., & Janicak, P. G. (2005). Divalproex sodium for pediatric mixed mania: A 6-month prospective trial. *Bipolar Disorders, 7*, 266–273.

Pavuluri, M. N., Henry, D. B., Carbray, J. A., Sampson, G., Naylor, M. W., & Janicak, P. G. (2004). Open-label prospective trial of risperidone in combination with lithium or divalproex sodium in pediatric mania. *Journal of Affective Disorders, 82*(Suppl. 1), S103–S111.

Pavuluri, M. N., Henry, D. B., Carbray, J. A., Sampson, G. A., Naylor, M. W., & Janicak, P. G. (2006). A one-year open-label trial of risperidone augmentation in lithium nonresponder youth with preschool-onset bipolar disorder. *Journal of Child and Adolescent Psychopharmacology, 16*, 336–350.

Perlis, R. H., Miyahara, S., Marangell, L. B., Wisniewski, S. R., Ostacher, M., DelBello, M. P., et al. (2004). Long-term implications of early onset in bipolar disorder: Data from the first 1,000 participants in the systematic treatment enhancement program for bipolar disorder (STEP-BD). *Biological Psychiatry, 55*, 875–881.

Post, R. M., Denicoff, K. D., Leverich, G, S,, Altshuler, L. L., Frye, M. A., Suppes, T. M., et al. (2003). Morbidity in 258 bipolar outpatients followed for 1 year with daily prospective ratings on the NIMH life chart method. *Journal of Clinical Psychiatry, 64*, 680–690, 738–739.

Pylvanen, V., Knip, M., Pakarinen, A. J., Turkka, J., Kotila, M., Rattya, J., et al. (2003). Fasting serum insulin and lipid levels in men with epilepsy. *Neurology, 60*, 571–574.

Raitakari, O. T., Juonala, M., Kahonen, M., Taittonen, L., Laitinen, T., Maki-Torkko, N., et al. (2003). Cardiovascular risk factors in childhood and carotid artery intima-media thickness in adulthood: The Cardiovascular Risk in Young Finns Study. *Journal of the American Medical Association, 290*, 2277–2283.

Ratzoni, G., Gothelf, D., Brand-Gothelf, A., Reidman, J., Kikinzon, L., Gal, G., et al. (2002). Weight gain associated with olanzapine and risperidone in adolescent patients: A comparative prospective study. *Journal of the American Academy of Child and Adolescent Psychiatry, 41*, 337–343.

Robinson, T. N., Chang, J. Y., Haydel, K. F., & Killen, J. D. (2001). Overweight concerns and body dissatisfaction among third-grade children: The impacts of ethnicity and socioeconomic status. *Journal of Pediatrics, 138*, 181–187.

Roste, L. S., Tauboll, E., Morkrid, L., Bjornenak, T., Saetre, E. R., Morland, T., et al. (2005). Antiepileptic drugs alter reproductive endocrine hormones in men with epilepsy. *European Journal of Neurology, 12*, 118–224.

Safer, D. J. (2004). A comparison of risperidone-induced weight gain across the age span. *Journal of Clinical Psychopharmacology, 24*, 429–436.

Saito, E., & Kafantaris, V. (2002). Can diabetes mellitus be induced by medication? *Journal of Child and Adolescent Psychopharmacology, 12*, 231–236.

Selva, K. A., & Scott, S. M. (2001). Diabetic ketoacidosis associated with olanzapine in an adolescent patient. *Journal of Pediatrics, 138*, 936–938.

Sikich, L., Hamer, R. M., Bashford, R. A., Sheitman, B. B., & Lieberman, J. A. (2004). A pilot study of risperidone, olanzapine, and haloperidol in psychotic youth: A double-blind, randomized, 8-week trial. *Neuropsychopharmacology, 29*, 133–145.

Simon, G .E., Von Korff, M., Saunders, K., Miglioretti, D. L., Crane, P. K., van Belle, G., et al. (2006). Association between obesity and psychiatric disorders in the U.S. adult population. *Archives of General Psychiatry, 63*, 824–830.

Sinaiko, A. R., Donahue, R. P., Jacobs, D. R., Jr., & Prineas, R. J. (1999). Relation of weight and rate of increase in weight during childhood and adolescence to body size, blood pressure, fasting insulin, and lipids in young adults: The Minneapolis Children's Blood Pressure Study. *Circulation, 99*, 1471–1476.

Sinha, R., Fisch, G., Teague, B., Tamborlane, W. V., Banyas, B., Allen, K., et al. (2002). Prevalence of impaired glucose tolerance among children and adolescents with marked obesity. *New England Journal of Medicine, 346*, 802–810.

Sporn, A. L., Bobb, A. J., Gogtay, N., Stevens, H., Greenstein, D. K., Clasen, L. S., et al. (2005). Hormonal correlates of clozapine-induced weight gain in psychotic children: An exploratory study. *Journal of the American Academy of Child and Adolescent Psychiatry, 44,* 925–933.

Srinivasan, S. R., Myers, L., & Berenson, G. S. (2002). Predictability of childhood adiposity and insulin for developing insulin resistance syndrome (syndrome X) in young adulthood: The Bogalusa Heart Study. *Diabetes, 51,* 204–209.

Straker, D., Correll, C. U., Kramer-Ginsberg, E., Abdulhamid, N., Koshy, F., Rubens, E., et al. (2005). Cost-effective screening for the metabolic syndrome in patients treated with second-generation antipsychotic medications. *American Journal of Psychiatry, 162,* 1217–1221.

Strassnig, M., Brar, J. S., & Ganguli, R. (2003). Body mass index and quality of life in community-dwelling patients with schizophrenia. *Schizophrenia Research, 62,* 73–76.

Toalson, P., Ahmed, S., Hardy, T., & Kabinoff, G. (2004). The metabolic syndrome in patients with severe mental illnesses. *Primary Care Companion to the Journal of Clinical Psychiatry, 6,* 152–158.

Vanhala, M. J., Vanhala, P. T., Keinanen-Kiukaanniemi, S. M., Kumpusalo, E. A., & Takala, J. K. (1999). Relative weight gain and obesity as a child predict metabolic syndrome as an adult. *International Journal of Obesity and Related Metabolic Disorders, 23,* 656–659.

Van Horn, L., Obarzanek, E., Friedman, L. A., Gernhofer, N., & Barton, B. (2005). Children's adaptations to a fat-reduced diet: The Dietary Intervention Study in Children (DISC). *Pediatrics, 115,* 1723–1733.

Vreeland, B., Minsky, S., Menza, M., Rigassio Radler, D., Roemheld-Hamm, B., & Stern, R. (2003). A program for managing weight gain associated with atypical antipsychotics. *Psychiatric Services, 54,* 1155–1157.

Wagner, K. D., Kowatch, R. A., Emslie, G. J., Findling, R. L., Wilens, T. E., McCague, K., et al. (2006). A double-blind, randomized, placebo-controlled trial of oxcarbazepine in the treatment of bipolar disorder in children and adolescents. *American Journal of Psychiatry, 163,* 1179–1186.

Weiden, P. J., Daniel, D. G., Simpson, G., & Romano, S. J. (2003). Improvement in indices of health status in outpatients with schizophrenia switched to ziprasidone. *Journal of Clinical Psychopharmacology, 23,* 595–600.

Weiss, R., Dziura, J., Burgert, T. S., Tamborlane, W. V., Taksali, S. E., Yeckel, C. W., et al. (2004). Obesity and the metabolic syndrome in children and adolescents. *New England Journal of Medicine, 350,* 2362–2374.

Williams, C. L., Hayman, L. L., Daniels, S. R., Robinson, T. N., Steinberger, J., Paridon, S., et al. (2002). Cardiovascular health in childhood: A statement for health professionals from the Committee on Antherosclerosis, Hypertension, and Obesity in the Young (Attoy) of the Council on Cardiovascular Disease in the Young, American Heart Association. *Circulation, 106,* 143–160.

Wirshing, D. A., Boyd, J. A., Meng, L. R., Ballon, J. S., Marder, S. R., & Wirshing, W. C. (2002), The effects of novel antipsychotics on glucose and lipid levels. *Journal of Clinical Psychiatry, 63,* 856–865.

Wozniak, J. (2005). Recognizing and managing bipolar disorder in children. *Journal of Clinical Psychiatry, 66*(Suppl. 1), 18–23.

Zipursky, R. B., Gu, H., Green, A. I., Perkins, D. O., Tohen, M. F., McEvoy, J. P., et al. (2005). Course and predictors of weight gain in people with first-episode psychosis treated with olanzapine or haloperidol. *British Journal of Psychiatry, 187,* 537–543.

Zito, J. M., Safer, D. J., DosReis, S., Gardner, J. F., Magder, L., Soeken, K., et al. (2003). Psychotropic practice patterns for youth: A 10-year perspective. *Archives of Pediatric and Adolescent Medicine, 157,* 17–25.

CHAPTER 19

Ethical and Regulatory Aspects in the Treatment of Children and Adolescents with Bipolar Disorder

Benedetto Vitiello

Treatment of children (i.e., persons under age 19 years) with bipolar disorder, either in usual practice or for research purposes, presents a number of ethical and regulatory concerns. Some of these concerns are common to pediatric treatment in general or to the use of psychotropic medications in children. This chapter addresses ethical and regulatory issues that are especially relevant to the treatment of childhood bipolar disorder within the broader context of pediatric psychopharmacology.

THE CHILD AS A PATIENT AND THE ROLE OF THE PARENT

Children do not usually seek treatment themselves; rather, they are brought to medical attention by adults responsible for their care. From an ethical and legal perspective, the relationship between clinician and child is mediated by the parent (or other guardian). In addition, as with for many other psychiatric conditions, the formulation of a diagnosis of bipolar disorder relies on the parents as key informants. In the current absence of diagnostic biological markers of bipolar disorder, the diagnosis rests on careful clinical evaluation. As the symptoms of the illness typically wax and wane, it is not always possible for the clinician to directly witness the child displaying the cardinal signs of the disorder, and younger children especially may lack the insight or the cognitive skills to report symptoms. Thus parental report typically plays a critical role in the diagnostic process.

Decisions about treatment are also made by the parent. Not uncommonly, the child with bipolar disorder sees no problems with her or his mood or behavior and therefore no need for treatment. Although attempts to explain the nature of the disorder and the purpose of treatment to the child should always be made as allowed by her or his developmental stage, cognitive capacities, and clinical status, the ultimate decision to start treatment rests with the parent.

Clinical guidelines for the treatment of children with bipolar disorder have been recently published (Kowatch et al., 2005). These guidelines, however, are primarily informed by expert opinion and only in part by evidence from well-controlled studies, which are still too few in childhood bipolar disorder. Rather than an absolute standard of care, these parameters represent a general guide to clinicians with the understanding that there may be wide variability in the way individual patients are treated. It is also understood that these guidelines may be subject to change and updates based on emerging new information from research in progress. Parents should be informed of the current state-of-the-science of treatment for bipolar disorder and made aware that, though there is expert consensus that children with bipolar disorder should receive pharmacological treatment to stabilize mood, the effectiveness of treatment in preventing recurrence and improving ultimate prognosis remains to be documented. Because response to treatment is highly variable across individuals, finding an effective treatment regimen for a patient is still very much a process of trial and error. It is important that patients and their parents be aware of these limitations.

Besides contributing essential information to the diagnostic process and making treatment decisions, parents are also responsible for implementing treatment as prescribed, monitoring for possible adverse effects of treatment, and reporting both benefits and potential toxicities to the attention of the clinician. These functions are especially important given that some of the medications used in the treatment of bipolar disorder have a narrow therapeutic index (e.g., lithium) or can induce infrequent but serious adverse effects (e.g., valproate). It is therefore critical that the treating clinician inform the parents not only about the potential benefits and harms of treatment and about possible alternatives but also about the monitoring procedures that need to be implemented during treatment in order to minimize risks. To this end, a substantial amount of time and effort needs to be devoted to parent education.

Particularly challenging are those situations in which the family context, due to environmental stressors or parental psychopathology, is not conducive to an orderly approach to treatment. Although it would not be appropriate to prescribe medications to children without evidence of responsible parental supervision, no general guidelines currently exist for these situations, and each case has to be considered based on individual needs and characteristics.

Adolescents are expected to become more actively involved in the treatment decision process and to gradually take more responsibility for their care. Parents remain legally responsible for treatment decisions, but adolescents should actively participate in the decision process and provide their "assent" to treatment. Bipolar disorder, however, often impairs insight and judgment.

Adolescents may refuse treatment or not adhere to it as prescribed. Adolescents with bipolar disorder are at increased risk for engaging in alcohol and substance abuse and a number of risky behaviors. Unprotected sexual activity is problematic not only because of the risks of infections and unwanted pregnancy, which apply to the general adolescent population, but also because a number of mood stabilizers are teratogenic, causing harm to a developing fetus. These factors can make the management of bipolar disorder in adolescence particularly challenging.

Involuntary treatment, although not a major issue for younger children, becomes more problematic for adolescents. As persons under the legal age of 18, adolescents do not have full right to self-determination, and parental permission for evaluation, treatment, or release of information is required unless waived by law or the court. Based on state law, a minor can be "emancipated." For instance, in many jurisdictions, teenagers older than 15 living independently from their parents and financially self-sufficient, or minors who are married or serving on active military duty, are considered "emancipated" and given complete right of self-determination. For most adolescents, however, parents remain legally responsible for treatment decisions. Conflict between the adolescent and her or his parents can be the source of considerable disruption and constitute a major threat to successful treatment implementation.

OFF-LABEL USE OF MEDICATIONS

By off-label use of a medication, we mean its use to treat conditions or groups of patients other than those included in the official drug label approved by the Food and Drug Administration (FDA). As the federal drug regulatory agency, the mission of the FDA is to ensure that drug products are accurately labeled. The information contained in the drug label is derived from various sources, including both research studies and clinical practice, and the evidence about its efficacy typically comes from controlled clinical trials. Pharmaceutical companies can market and advertise a drug only for the specific indications that have been approved by the FDA and listed in the official label. It happens, however, that drugs marketed for certain indications (e.g., seizure disorder) or only for a certain age group (e.g., adults) are prescribed also for other indications (e.g., bipolar disorder) or age groups (e.g., children) in the community.

In the case of bipolar disorder in children, lithium is currently FDA approved for the treatment of bipolar disorder in patients age 12 years and older (although this is based more on extrapolation of adult data to adolescents than on adolescent research data). Thus use of lithium in a child under age 12 constitutes off-label use. Other drugs often prescribed off-label to children with bipolar disorders are valproate, carbamazepine, oxcarbazepine, and lamotrigine, which are approved for the treatment of seizure disorders in children. Antipsychotic medications, such as risperidone, olanzapine, and quetiapine, are also used off-label to control symptoms of mania in children. Risperidone was approved for the treatment of mania in children age 10 and older in 2007.

It must be pointed out that the off-label use of medications is quite common in general pediatrics and in child psychiatry and is not *per se* an inappropriate practice on the part of the clinician, who is faced with the difficult task of treating severe conditions with only limited therapeutic options. Off-label use does, however, identify the need for systematic research in order to acquire the necessary evidence for efficacy and safety. Following the recognition of the widespread and increasing off-label use of medications in children, a number of initiatives have been recently launched to remedy the current situation.

The Food and Drug Administration Modernization Act (1997) first provided financial incentives (i.e., a 6-month extension in the drug's patent exclusivity) to pharmaceutical companies in return for conducting pediatric studies. The initiative was further expanded and extended until 2008 by the Best Pharmaceuticals for Children Act (2002). In addition, the Pediatric Research Equity Act (2003) requires the conduct of pediatric studies as part of new drug applications submitted to the FDA on or after April 1, 1999, unless this requirement is waived or deferred by the FDA.

A number of pediatric pharmacokinetics and clinical trials have been conducted under the additional exclusivity program. For instance, clinical trials to test the efficacy of citalopram, sertraline, venlafaxine, and nefazodone in pediatric depression have been conducted. Medications for child bipolar disorder, such as risperidone, olanzapine, quetiapine, and aripiprazole are receiving increasing attention. Research on older medications that are no longer covered by patent exclusivity, such as lithium, cannot benefit from the additional patent exclusivity program. For this reason, the Best Pharmaceuticals for Children Act mandated the establishment of a program by the National Institutes of Health (NIH) to conduct pediatric research on off-patent medications with public funding. Pursuant to this initiative, a contract was recently awarded by the NIH to study the pharmacokinetics, effectiveness, and tolerability of lithium carbonate in children (ages 7–17 years) with bipolar I disorder in a manic or mixed episode.

THE CHILD AS A RESEARCH PARTICIPANT

Research involving children with bipolar disorder is necessary in order to understand the benefits and risks of possible treatment interventions. Data collected in adults, though informative, are not sufficient for guiding treatment of children. Differences in pharmacokinetics, metabolism, pharmacodynamics, and psychopathological manifestations between adults and children and between younger children and adolescents can have clinical implications for the efficacy and safety of treatments. Thus it cannot be assumed that a medication is effective or safe in children based only on experience with adults. For example, tricyclic antidepressants have not been found to be effective in children in spite of their proven antidepressant activities in adults (Hazell, O'Connell, Heathcote, & Henry, 2002), and the risk of valproate-induced hepatoxicity is inversely related to age (Bryant & Dreifuss, 1996).

Whereas child research in general finds ethical justification in the need to acquire the necessary knowledge for a rational approach to treatment, the ethical acceptability of individual research projects must be carefully examined according to the existing norms. Research involving human participants that is conducted, supported, or regulated by the U.S. Department of Health and Human Services (DHHS) and many other federal departments or agencies must be conducted in accordance to the basic policy for the protection of research participants, which is often referred to as the "Common Rule" (U.S. Department of Health and Human Services, 1991). In addition, children's participation in research is subject to special protections (U.S. Department of Health and Human Services, 1983; Office for Human Research Protections, 2005). Studies conducted under FDA investigational new drug procedures are subject to similar regulations (U.S. Food and Drug Administration, 2000). These codes of federal regulations may also be used for reviewing the ethics of human research in nonfederally funded or regulated studies.

Individual research projects must be reviewed by an independent ethical committee, usually referred to as Institutional review board (IRB). IRBs have the challenging task of applying the code of ethical regulations to the specific study under review. Granted that only scientifically sound research investigations utilizing valid methodology and having the potential to acquire important new knowledge may be ethically acceptable, each project must be systematically examined to determine whether it meets all the ethical requirements (Vitiello, Jensen, & Hoagwood, 1999; Emmanuel, Wedler, & Grady, 2000; Vitiello, 2003).

Child research can be broadly classified into two categories according to whether it does or does not offer a "prospect of direct benefit" to study participants. *Direct benefit* refers to a concrete and personal health improvement. General acquisition of knowledge does not meet the requirement for "direct benefit." Research with the prospect of direct benefit must have a favorable balance between anticipated benefits and foreseeable harms. Clinical trials testing the therapeutic benefits of a treatment intervention typically have potential for direct benefit to research participants. In this case, the main criterion for determining whether the study is ethically acceptable is the *risk–benefit ratio*, which must be favorable.

In evaluating the risk–benefit ratio of a clinical trial in child bipolar disorder, one needs to consider both the potential for symptomatic and functional improvement, vis-à-vis the seriousness of the condition and its pervasive negative impact on the life of the child, and the potential for harm from the treatment in light of the possible alternatives. The presence of detailed protocol procedures for safety monitoring and early detection of adverse effects substantially contribute to making the risk–benefit ratio more favorable.

Inclusion of a placebo control arm in a clinical trial in bipolar disorder is a potentially contentious issue. On the one hand, bipolar disorder is a serious condition requiring treatment. On the other hand, there is no officially approved medication for bipolar disorder in children. Medications are used in the community based mainly on experience with adults but very limited empirical evidence from pediatric investigations. These medications are also known for their potential toxicity. In fact, the lack of adequate pediatric data on the efficacy and safety of mood stabilizers constitutes the rationale for conducting clinical trials in children with bipolar disorder, and the inclusion of a placebo control group may provide the most efficient and valid way of assessing drug effects. Moreover, placebo treatment does not usually equal absence of treatment, as children receive nonspecific clinical management with regular monitoring. Thus, although extended use of placebo in the absence of symptom improvement would seem unacceptable, brief exposure to placebo in a context of a carefully controlled and monitored trial can be considered acceptable. In fact, placebo-controlled trials of mood stabilizers in child bipolar disorder are in progress.

An important component of a clinical trial that substantially affects the risk–benefit ratio of the study is the presence of a Data and Safety Monitoring Board (DSMB). A DSMB is an independent committee of experts that, separately from the study investigators, have access to the cumulative data from the study and periodically review the safety and the risk–benefit ratio of the trial. The DSMB can be unblinded to treatment assignments, and it exercises the important function of ensuring the continuing scientific validity and ethics of the investigation for the duration of the study. DSMBs are in general required only for phase III clinical trials as defined by the NIH and are not mandatory for smaller, single-site studies, in which less formal data and safety monitoring procedures can be considered instead.

Discontinuation designs, in which children are first treated with active medication until improved and then randomly assigned to continuing active medication or a switch to a placebo, are an important way of assessing whether continuous treatment is effective in preventing relapse or recurrence of manic or depressive symptoms. These designs are particularly relevant to bipolar disorder because of the recurrent nature of this condition and the fact that long-term use of antimanic medications may have clinically important adverse effects, such as weight gain, hypothyroidism, renal dysfunction, or dyskinesias. Discontinuation designs, however, raise ethical concerns because a treatment that has been apparently effective is being discontinued, with consequent risk for relapse. Close monitoring of participants in discontinuation trials is critical for prompt identification of early signs of relapse. The role of the study DSMB in periodically reviewing the available study data for possible differences in relapse rates is especially critical in the case of discontinuation trials. Certain protocols for discontinuation studies that are submitted to the National Institute of Mental Health (NIMH) for possible funding go through a special ethical review process, in addition to the usual scientific and administrative program reviews.

The other broad category of child research is constituted by studies that do not offer a prospect of direct benefit to the participants. Pharmacokinetics and pharmacodynamics studies fall into this category. Other studies in this group include those in which participants are exposed to a chemical challenge or experience so that researchers can investigate basic physiological or psychopathological processes. The process of determining whether a study without prospect of direct benefit is ethically acceptable includes several sequential steps. First, it must be determined whether the study does or does not have the potential for generating essential knowledge *relevant to the disorder or condition* of the research participant.

A study aimed at acquiring information that is not directly relevant to the children participating in the research (e.g., a pharmacokinetics of a drug study in children not suffering from a condition for which the drug is indicated) can be approved only if it entails *no more than minimal risk.* Minimal risk is defined as "risk for harm not greater than ordinarily encountered in daily life, or during routine physical or psychological examinations or tests" (U.S. Department of Health and Human Services, 1983, Section 46.102(i)). The daily life, exams, and tests of a normal child are used as a reference, even though a precise quantification of risk in ordinary daily life is not easy and remains a matter of discussion (Wendler, Belsky, Thompson, & Emanuel, 2005).

A study aimed at acquiring information that is relevant to the participants' condition (e.g., the pharmacokinetics of a mood stabilizer in children with bipolar disorder) is approvable if the estimated research risk is not greater than *a minor increase over minimal risk*. A *minor increase over minimal risk* can be considered acceptable only if: (1) it presents "experiences to the subjects that are commensurate with those inherent in their actual or expected medical, dental, psychological, social, or educational situations," and (2) it has the potential to generate new knowledge considered of "vital importance" for understanding or treating the child's disorder or condition (U.S. Department of Health and Human Services, 1983, 46.405).

Research not otherwise approvable based on these criteria but that presents an opportunity to understand, prevent, or alleviate a serious problem affecting the health or welfare of children can be referred to the Secretary of Health and Human Services for further review under the DHHS regulations at 45 C.F.R. 46.407 (U.S. Department of Health and Human Services, 1983) and FDA regulations at 21 C.F.R. 50.56 (U.S. Food and Drug Administration, 2000). Studies in which psychotropic medications are given to normal children in order to better understand their mechanisms of action on the brain would fall into this category, as nontherapeutic administration of a psychotropic drug would generally be considered to pose more than minimal risk. For example, a protocol for a brain magnetic resonance imaging study of normal children age 9 and older receiving a single oral dose of dextroamphetamine was referred by the IRB of the NIMH under the 45 C.F.R. 46.407 regulation in 2004 (Couzin, 2004). Because, on the one hand, a single administration of dextroamphetamine 10 mg to a school-age child was considered to entail no more than a minor increase over minimal risk and because, on the other hand, the study had the potential to generate critically important information on the brain effects of a commonly used medication in children, the study was approved (U.S. Food and Drug Administration, 2004).

Parental permission is generally necessary for child participation in research. Parents and children (depending on age and level of cognitive development) must be informed of the aims, procedures, expected benefits, foreseeable risks, and discomforts of research participation, the presence of alternatives, the voluntary nature of research participation, and their rights as research participants. The rights include the right to withdraw from the research at any time and for any reason; the right to be kept informed of any new, relevant, and clinically important information that may become available after entering the study; and the right to have all personal data maintained confidential. When applicable, children's assent may be documented in writing with an appropriate "assent form" written in a developmentally appropriate language.

MONITORING FOR SAFETY

Central to the ethics of child psychopharmacology is the concern about exposing children to potentially toxic drugs. In fact, pharmacological treatment during a period of rapid development such as childhood can result in unwanted effects that are not predictable based on adult data. For example, prolonged administration of phenobarbital to young children to prevent recurrence of febrile seizures impairs their cognitive development (Farwell et al. 1990).

Safety, however, is a relative concept. The risk of treatment-induced harms must be weighed against its potential for benefit, the benefit–risk of alternative treatments, and the risk of leaving psychopathology untreated. Unfortunately, the current state-of-the-science of childhood bipolar disorder does not allow a complete analysis of risk and benefits of treatment to be conducted. In a way, the current status of relative ignorance contributes to the rationale for conducting research in childhood bipolar disorder. At a time when the full extent of the potential benefit of treatment remains unclear, safety monitoring appears especially important when prescribing medications to children in either research studies or usual practice.

It has become apparent that the methodology for eliciting, interpreting, classifying, recording, and analyzing clinical data relevant to safety has lagged behind that for assessing efficacy (Greenhill et al., 2003; Vitiello et al., 2003). This situation is not surprising given that the main purpose of clinical trials is usually to demonstrate efficacy, whereas safety evaluation has been considered a secondary aim. The recent experience with antidepressant-associated suicidality, however, has shown the importance of systematically assessing for possible adverse effects of treatments (Hammad, Laughren, & Racoosin, 2006). The reported association between pediatric antidepressant treatment and increased risk of "suicidality" (i.e., suicidal thinking and suicide attempts), as well as the consequent regulatory warnings, are relevant to childhood bipolar disorder (U.S. Food and Drug Administration, 2007). Children with bipolar disorder may receive antidepressant medication, together with a mood stabilizer, for the treatment of the depressive component of the disorder and are at increased risk for suicidal behavior.

Besides antidepressants, atypical antipsychotics, such as olanzapine, risperidone, and clozapine, have been the object of safety concerns because they often induce weight gain and can lead to a metabolic syndrome characterized by hyperlipidemia, decreased glucose tolerance, insulin resistance, and diabetes (Morrison et al., 2005). Antipsychotics have been increasingly prescribed to children also for the treatment of bipolar disorder. Thus special attention to weight gain and possible metabolic adverse effects is necessary when these medications are used.

The establishment of a safety monitoring plan before the treatment is initiated and its careful implementation during treatment can help alleviate ethical concerns about pharmacological treatment in children.

PROTECTION OF CONFIDENTIALITY

Personal medical information is confidential, and its release to third parties is regulated by both federal and local laws. In particular, the Health Insurance Portability and Accountability Act sets the procedures for protecting the confidentiality of health records when some of these data are transmitted electronically (U.S. Department of Health and Human Services, 2002). Although these regulations apply to all health-related information and are by no means specific to a particular condition, they have important implications for the management of childhood bipolar disorder.

A diagnosis of bipolar disorder can be considered especially sensitive information because of the potential practical implications that such diagnosis may have on the child and her or his future life. Bipolar disorder is a chronic condition whose symptoms are controllable with treatment but for which no cure is as yet available. Because judgment and functioning can be impaired, a diagnosis of bipolar disorder may put a person at a disadvantage in certain situations, for example, when pursuing certain occupations that involve high levels of responsibility, applying for life insurance, or arguing legal matters such as child custody. It is therefore particularly important to ensure the confidentiality of the clinical information obtained during the diagnostic assessment and the treatment of children with bipolar disorder. Medical records can be released only with the consent of the parents or of the patient (after he or she achieves the legal age) or upon a valid and binding court order.

When research data are published, no personally identifiable information can be released. Likewise, before research databases are put into the public domain, all personal identifiers, such as birthdate and geographical location, are removed. Confidentiality of research data can be further protected by study-specific "certificates of confidentiality" issued by a government agency under the authority vested in the Secretary of Health and Human Services by Section 301(d) of the Public Health Service Act (1988). These documents certify that the investigators involved in the specified research project cannot be compelled to release any personally identifiable information in federal, state, or local civil, criminal, administrative, legislative, or other legal proceedings.

Together with the duty to protect the confidentiality of personal information as privileged communication also comes the duty to report situations of child abuse, neglect or mistreatment and to take appropriate action to prevent suicidal and homicidal acts that the patient might have threatened to commit (i.e., the duty to protect third parties). Local statutes provide immunity regarding the consequences of reporting, as well as penalties for failure to report. Thus a clinician may be liable in case of harm to the patient or other person if the clinician was aware of the danger and could have been prevented the harm. In the landmark case of Tarasoff vs. Regents of the University of California (1976), the California supreme court ruled that, if a clinician determines that a patient represents a serious danger to another person, he or she has the duty to use reasonable care to protect the intended victim. This may include warning the intended victim, informing the police, and other reasonable preventive steps. This duty to warn applies to the protection of the identifiable persons against which a threat has been made and not to nonspecific, general threats.

CONCLUSION

Treating children with bipolar disorder, in clinical practice or for research purposes, requires attention to a number of ethical and regulatory issues, which, though not unique to this disorder, are extremely relevant to it. The limitations in the current knowledge about the efficacy and safety of the interventions for childhood bipolar disorder make the treatment of this condition particularly challenging and the need to conduct relevant research especially pressing. A number of controlled clinical trials in childhood bipolar disorder are under way and are expected to inform us on the therapeutic benefits of mood stabilizers in children with mania. As research on bipolar disorder in children is an area of rapid expansion, the interpretation and application of ethical and regulatory requirements will need to be constantly revisited in light of new findings.

DISCLAIMER

The opinions and assertions contained in this chapter are the private views of Benedetto Vitiello and are not to be construed as official or as reflecting the views of the National Institute of Mental Health, the National Institutes of Health, or the Department of Health and Human Services.

REFERENCES

Best Pharmaceuticals for Children Act, Pub. L. No. 107-109.

Bryant, A. E., & Dreifuss, F. E. (1996). Valproic acid hepatic fatalities: III. I.S. experience since 1986. *Neurology, 46,* 465–469.

Couzin, J. (2004). Pediatric study of ADHD drug draws high-level public review. *Science, 305,* 1088–1089.

Emmanuel, E. J., Wedler, D., & Grady, C. (2000). What makes clinical research ethical? *Journal of the American Medical Association, 283,* 2701–2711.

Farwell, J. R., Lee, Y. J., Hirtz, D. G., Sulzbacher, S. I., Ellenberg, J. H., & Nelson, K. B. (1990). Phenobarbital for febrile seizures—Effects on intelligence and on seizure recurrence. *New England Journal of Medicine, 322,* 364–369.

Food and Drug Administration Modernization Act, Pub. L. No. 105-115 (1997).

Greenhill, L. L., Vitiello, B., Riddle, M. A., Fisher, P., Shockey, E., March, J. S., et al. (2003). Review of safety assessment methods used in pediatric psychopharmacology. *Journal of the American Academy of Child and Adolescent Psychiatry, 42,* 627–633.

Hammad, T. A., Laughren, T., & Racoosin, J. (2006). Suicidality in pediatric patients treated with antidepressant drugs. *Archives of General Psychiatry, 63,* 332–339.

Hazell, P., O'Connell, D., Heathcote, D., & Henry, D. (2002). Tricyclic drugs for depression in children and adolescents. *Cochrane Database Systematic Review, 2* CD002317.

Kowatch, R. A., Fristad, M., Birmaher, B., Wagner, K. D., Findling, R. L., Hellander, M., et al. (2005). Treatment guidelines for children and adolescents with bipolar disorder. *Journal of the American Academy of Child and Adolescent Psychiatry, 44,* 213–235.

Morrison, J. A., Friedman, L. A., Harlan, W. R., Harlan, L. C., Barton, B. A., Schreiber, G. B., et al. (2005). Development of the metabolic syndrome in black and white adolescent girls: A longitudinal assessment. *Pediatrics, 116,* 1178–1182.

Pediatric Research Equity Act of 2003, Pub. L. No. 108-155.

Public Health Service Act 301(d), U.S.C. 241 (d), as amended by Pub. L. No. 100-607, §163, November 4, 1988.

Office for Human Research Protections. (2005). Special protections for children as research subjects. Retrieved November 2, 2007, from *www.hhs.gov/ohrp/children/guidance_407process.html.*

Tarasoff v. Regents of the University of California. 17 Cal. 3d 425; 551P. 2d 334, 131 Cal Rptr 14 (1976).

U.S. Department of Health and Human Services. (1983). Protection of Human Subjects. Code of Federal Regulations, Title 45, Public Welfare: Part 46, Subpart D, 88 FR, 9818, March 8, 1983; revised June 23, 2005. Retrieved November 2, 2007, from *www.dhhs.gov/ohrp/humansubjects/guidance/45cfr46.htm.*

U.S. Department of Health and Human Services. (1991). Protection of Human Subjects. Code of Federal Regulations, Title 45, Public Welfare: Part 46, Subpart A; revised June 23, 2005. Retrieved November 2, 2007, from *www.dhhs.gov/ohrp/humansubjects/guidance/45cfr46.htm.*

U.S. Department of Health and Human Services. (2002). Office of Civil Rights: Standards for privacy of individually identifiable health information: Final rules. *Fed. Reg., 67*(157), 53182–53272.

U.S. Food and Drug Administration. (2000). Additional safeguards for children in clinical investigations of FDA-regulated products,21 C.F.R. Parts 51 and 56. Retrieved November 2, 2007, from *www.fda.gov/OHRMS/DOCKETS/98fr/042401a.pdf.*

U.S. Food and Drug Administration. (2004). Summary Minutes of the Pediatric Ethics Subcommittee of the Pediatric Advisory Committee, September 10th, 2004. Retrieved January 31, 2008, from *www.fda.gov/ohrms/dockets/ac/04/minutes/2004-@reftext = 4066m1_summary %20Minutes.doc.*

U.S. Food and Drug Administration. (2007). Medication guide–antidepressants medicines, depression and other serious mental illnesses, and suicidal thoughts or actions. Retrieved November 2, 2007, from *www.fda.gov/cder/drug/antidepressants_MG_2007.pdf*.

Vitiello, B. (2003). Ethical considerations in psychopharmacological research involving children and adolescents. *Psychopharmacology, 171*, 86–91.

Vitiello, B., Jensen, P. S., & Hoagwood, K (1999). Integrating science and ethics in child and adolescent psychiatry research. *Biological Psychiatry, 46*, 1044–1049.

Vitiello, B., Riddle, M. A., Greenhill, L. L., March, J. S., Levine, J., Schachar, R., et al. (2003). How can we improve the assessment of safety in child and adolescent psychopharmacology? *Journal of the American Academy of Child and Adolescent Psychiatry, 42*, 634–641.

Wendler, D., Belsky, L., Thompson, K. M., & Emanuel, E. J. (2005). Quantifying the federal minimal risk standard: Implications for pediatric research without a prospect of direct benefit. *Journal of the American Medical Association, 294*, 826–832.

Index

405